Contents

Preface to the Third Edition

It is now 10 years since the first edition of *Data Interpretation for Medical Students* hit the shelves, and it was a great honour to be asked to update the book for 2017.

The pace of change in medicine is, in many ways, awe-inspiring. The sheer volume of new information published in journals each month is staggering, and it is a continual struggle to keep up to date with even the most important changes in a single specialty. It is in this environment that modern medical students must learn their trade. Arguably now, more than ever before, it is critical that students must be able to 'sort the wheat from the chaff', and pick out the key information to process and digest.

The accurate interpretation of key laboratory, imaging and other data is an essential skill for a newly qualified doctor. The number of potential tests that medics now have at their disposal is phenomenal, and it would be very easy to get bogged down in minutiae. We hope that readers continue to find this book a useful guide in learning how to interpret the data that are requested most frequently in modern medicine.

Paul Hamilton
Ian Bickle

DATA INTER[illegible]ATION FOR MEDICAL STUDENTS

Third Edition

Paul K Hamilton

BSc(Hons), MB BCh BAO(Hons)
PGDip Toxicol, MD,
FRCP (Edin), FRCPath

Ian C Bickle

MB BCh BAO(Hons), FRCR

Egerton Court
Parkgate Estate
Knutsford
Cheshire
WA16 8DX

Telephone: 01565 752000

First published 2006, reprinted 2007, second edition 2012, reprinted 2013, 2015, third edition 2017

ISBN 9781784140007

eISBN: 9781784140014 ePUB

9781784140021 MobiPocket

A catalogue record for this book is available from the British Library.

Illustrations by Ben Stockham and Ivan Frontani
Text prepared by Carnegie Book Production, Lancaster, UK

Printed and bound in the UK by Bell & Bain Limited, Glasgow

Acknowledgements

Many thanks to Cathy Dickens and Lily Atkins at Pastest who commissioned this third edition, and whose patience and dedication at all stages were much appreciated. Cathy, we will miss you dearly, and wish you a long and happy retirement. Many thanks also to Michael Upchurch who has been very helpful and patient during the preparation of the latest edition of this book. We also extend thanks to Dr Barry Kelly who assisted with the preparation of the radiology material in earlier editions of the book, and whose influence persists in this latest edition.

Reference ranges for adults

Reference ranges for tests vary from laboratory to laboratory. You should always refer to the ranges from your laboratory when interpreting results for real patients.

Biochemistry

Arterial blood gas analysis

Anion gap	12–16 mmol/l
Arterial partial pressure of oxygen breathing room air (PaO_2)	11–13 kPa
Arterial partial pressure of carbon dioxide ($PaCO_2$)	4.7–6.0 kPa
Base excess (BE)	-2 to +2 mmol/l
pH	7.35–7.45

Bone profile

Adjusted calcium (Ca^{2+})	2.10–2.65 mmol/l
Albumin	35–50 g/l
Alkaline phosphatase (ALP)	30–150 U/l
Phosphate (PO_4^{3-})	0.8–1.45 mmol/l

Cerebrospinal fluid

Glucose	Approximately 40–60% of plasma value
Red cell count (RCC)	0/mm^3
Total protein	0.15–0.45 g/l
White cell count (WCC)	<5/mm^3

Haematinics

Folate	>2 µg/l
Iron studies	
Iron	11–32 µmol/l
Total iron-binding capacity (TIBC)	42–80 µmol/l
Ferritin (age- and gender-specific reference range often quoted)	12–200 µg/l
Transferrin saturation	20–50%
Vitamin B_{12}	191–663 ng/l

Immunoglobulins

IgA	0.8–4.0 g/l
IgG	7.0–14.5 g/l
IgM	0.45–2.0 g/l

Free light chains

κ	3.3–19.4 mg/l
λ	5.7–26.3 mg/l
$\kappa:\lambda$ ratio	0.26–1.65

Lipids

HDL-cholesterol	>1.0 mmol/l
LDL-cholesterol	<3.0 mmol/l
Total cholesterol	<5.0 mmol/l
Triglyceride	<2.2 mmol/l

Liver function tests

Albumin	35–50 g/l
Alkaline phosphatase (ALP)	30–150 U/l
Aspartate aminotransferase (AST)	5–35 U/l
Alanine aminotransferase (ALT)	5–35 U/l
γ-Glutamyl transpeptidase (GGT)	
Males	11–58 U/l
Females	7–33 U/l
Total bilirubin	3–17 μmol/l

Other

Amylase	25–125 U/l
C-reactive protein (CRP)	<10 mg/l
Creatine kinase (CK)	
Male	25–195 U/l
Female	25–170 U/l
CK-MB	<25 U/l
Glucose (random)	4.0–8.0 mmol/l
High sensitivity troponin T	<14 ng/l
Lactate dehydrogenase (LDH)	70–250 U/l
Lactate	0.5–2.0 mmol/l
N-terminal pro-brain natriuretic peptide (NT-proBNP)	<125 ng/l
Osmolality (serum)	280–300 mosmol/kg
Total protein	60–80 g/l
Urate	0.15–0.50 mmol/l

Tumour markers

α-Fetoprotein (AFP)	
<50 years	<10 kU/l
50–70 years	<15 kU/l
70–90 years	<20 kU/l
β Human chorionic gonadotrophin (β-hCG)	<5 U/l
CA-125	<35 U/ml
CA-19-9	<37 U/ml
Carcinoembryonic antigen (CEA)	<10 ng/ml
Prostate-specific antigen (PSA; males)	
40–49 years	<2.5 ng/ml
50–59 years	<3.5 ng/ml
60–69 years	<4.5 ng/ml
70–79 years	<6.5 ng/ml

Urea and electrolytes (U+E)

Bicarbonate (HCO_3^-)	24–30 mmol/l
Chloride (Cl^-)	95–105 mmol/l
Creatinine	79–118 μmol/l (dependent on muscle mass)
Magnesium (Mg^{2+})	0.7–1.0 mmol/l
Potassium (K^+)	3.5–5.0 mmol/l
Sodium (Na^+)	135–145 mmol/l
Urea	2.5–6.7 mmol/l

Urine

Creatinine clearance	
Males	85–125 ml/min
Females	75–115 ml/min

Haematology

Full blood picture

Erythrocyte sedimentation rate (ESR) (age-related range often quoted)	
Males	0–15 mm/h
Females	0–22 mm/h
Haemoglobin (Hb)	
Males	130–180 g/l
Non-pregnant females	120–160 g/l
HbA1c (glycated haemoglobin)	23.5–43.2 mmol/mol
Mean cell volume (MCV)	76–96 fl
Packed cell volume (PCV)	
Males	0.4–0.54
Females	0.37–0.47
Platelets	150–400 × 10^9/l
Red cell distribution width (RDW)	12–15%
Reticulocytes	0.5–2.5% of red blood cells
White cell count (WCC)	4.0–11.0 × 10^9/l
Basophils	0.0–0.1 × 10^9/l
Eosinophils	0.04–0.4 × 10^9/l
Lymphocytes	1.5–4.0 × 10^9/l
Monocytes	0.2–0.8 × 10^9/l
Neutrophils	2.0–7.5 × 10^9/l

Tests of clotting

Activated partial thromboplastin time (APTT)	24–38 s
Bleeding time	3–9 min
D-dimer	<0.5 mg/l
Fibrinogen	2–4 g/l
Prothrombin time (PT)	12–16 s

Endocrinology

Adrenal hormones

Aldosterone	<46 ng/l
Cortisol	
9am	200–700 nmol/l
10pm	50–250 nmol/l
Renin	3.2–32.6 pg/ml

Sex hormones

Young adult males

Follicle stimulating hormone (FSH)	1.5–12.4 U/l
Luteinising hormone (LH)	1.7–8.6 U/l
Prolactin	86–324 mU/l
Testosterone	11.4–27.9 nmol/l

Females

Follicle stimulating hormone (FSH)	Depends on menstrual status
Luteinising hormone (LH)	Depends on menstrual status
Mono-prolactin	102–496 mU/l
Oestradiol	Depends on menstrual status
Progesterone	Depends on menstrual status
Prolactin	102–496 mU/l
Testosterone	0.28–1.7 nmol/l

Thyroid hormones

Free thyroxine (T_4)	7.6–19.7 pmol/l
Thyroid-stimulating hormone (TSH)	0.4–4.5 mU/l
Total thyroxine (T_4)	70–140 nmol/l

Toxicology/therapeutic drug levels

Alcohol	Nil
Carboxyhaemoglobin	0.5–1.5% of total haemoglobin in non-smokers
Digoxin (6 hours post-dose)	0.8–2.0 μg/l
Lithium	0.5–1.5 mmol/l
Paracetamol	Nil
Salicylates	Nil

INTERPRETING LABORATORY RESULTS

1

1

BIOCHEMISTRY

Urea and electrolyte profile

A urea and electrolyte profile (U+E) is the most commonly requested panel of biochemical tests, and generally comprises measures of sodium, potassium, chloride, total carbon dioxide (which is predominantly a measure of bicarbonate), urea and creatinine. It is now common for laboratories to additionally report an estimated glomerular filtration rate (eGFR). We first consider disorders of sodium and potassium, before detailing the assessment of renal function (incorporating the interpretation of urea, creatinine and eGFR results). Measures of chloride and total bicarbonate are helpful in interpreting results in conditions involving disturbances of acid-base balance (see page 23).

Sodium

When the sodium concentration falls below the reference interval, hyponatraemia is present. Hypernatraemia is the term used to describe an elevated sodium concentration.

Hyponatraemia

Hyponatraemia is common and potentially life threatening because, when it develops rapidly, water can shift into the brain causing cerebral oedema. Hyponatraemia is the end-result of a great many conditions and differentiating between them is crucially important to enable the correct treatment to be given to a patient. The steps that should be taken when faced with hyponatraemia are as follows:

1. Measure and interpret the serum osmolality (see page 11 for more details). In this situation, the osmolality of the serum should be measured in the laboratory, not calculated from results. If the osmolality is low, you can assume that the patient is truly hyponatraemic. If the osmolality is not low, the apparently low sodium level may well be a 'falsely' low result. This situation is called pseudohyponatraemia, and is most commonly seen when the triglyceride level or protein level in the blood is extremely high (eg with genetic disorders of lipid metabolism or multiple myeloma). In such conditions, laboratory analysers measure sodium concentrations as artificially low.

   High glucose levels are also associated with hyponatraemia, and the sodium concentration tends to normalise when the glucose disturbance is brought under control.

2. Assess the patient's fluid status to decide if he or she is dehydrated (hypovolaemic), fluid overloaded (hypervolaemic) or normally hydrated (isovolaemic). The likely cause of the hyponatraemia varies depending into which group the patient falls. The diagnosis and common causes of hyponatraemia are illustrated in the flow diagram in Fig 1.1.

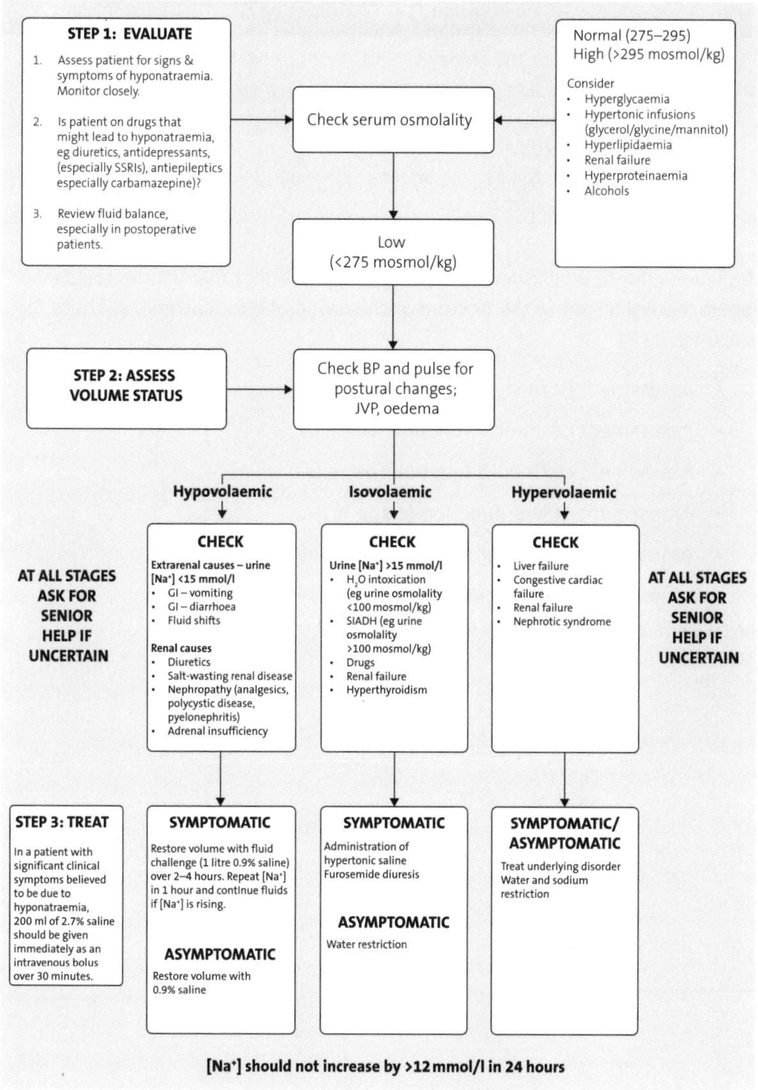

Fig 1.1: The assessment of hyponatraemia in adult patients.
From GAIN. *Hyponatraemia in Adults (on or after 16th birthday)*. GAIN, 2010. Available at: http://www.gain-ni.org/Library/Guidelines/Hyponatraemia_guideline.pdf.

Sometimes it can be difficult to classify a patient's volume status with certainty. In this instance, measurement of the urinary sodium concentration can be helpful.

USING URINARY SODIUM CONCENTRATION TO HELP CLASSIFY VOLUME STATUS

In hypovolaemic states, the kidney will attempt to hold on to sodium and water. The urinary sodium will be low (eg <15 mmol/l). Beware the following caveats:

- If a patient has taken a diuretic, the urinary sodium may be high due to the effects of the medication.
- In heart and liver failure, low effective circulating volume can also cause low urinary sodium.

Following the flow diagram in Fig 1.1, you can see that many more tests may be necessary to get to the bottom of the cause of hyponatraemia. These include:

- Assessment of renal function (page 8)
- Assessment of adrenal function (page 62)
- Assessment of thyroid function (page 60)
- Assessment of liver function (page 16)
- Assessment of cardiac function (page 36)
- Urine osmolality (pages 11 and 39).

THE SYNDROME OF INAPPROPRIATE ANTIDIURETIC HORMONE SECRETION (SIADH)

SIADH is all too often diagnosed incorrectly. It is a diagnosis of exclusion. It can be thought of as the opposite of diabetes insipidus (see page 59), with excessive ADH action causing the body to retain water, thus diluting the serum and causing hyponatraemia.

In order to diagnose SIADH, the following criteria should be met:

1. Clinically isovolaemic
2. Normal renal function
3. Normal adrenal function
4. Normal thyroid function
5. Normal pituitary function
6. Absence of diuretic therapy
7. Low serum osmolality (<275 mosmol/kg)
8. Inappropriately concentrated urine (>100 mosmol/kg)

COMMON CAUSES OF SIADH	
Intrathoracic causes: • Infection • Tumour Intracranial causes: • Infection • Tumour • Head injury	Medications: • Carbamazepine • Antipsychotics

It would seem intuitive that ADH levels should be measured in these patients, but this is not common practice due to the difficulties in measuring the hormone.

DON'T FORGET

Hyponatraemia does not mean SIADH!

Hypernatraemia

Hypernatraemia is a very strong stimulus for thirst, so in normal circumstances (ie a healthy person with access to adequate fluid), it should not develop. If you think about a glass containing water and a certain amount of salt, the salt concentration will rise if more salt is put in the glass or if water is removed from the glass. This can help when thinking about causes of hypernatraemia.

CAUSES OF HYPERNATRAEMIA
Poor water intake (eg an elderly person with dementia who cannot pour a glass of water or tell anyone that he or she is thirsty)
Diabetes insipidus - causing excessive water loss in the urine
Excessive salt administration (eg in intravenous fluids, or orally)

Diabetes insipidus is dealt with on page 59.

Potassium

Hypokalaemia and hyperkalaemia are the terms used to describe the situation when the potassium is below or above the reference interval, respectively. Maintaining a normal potassium concentration is critical for normal functioning of the heart, so potassium disorders can cause characteristic changes on ECG (see page 333). It is convenient to think about causes of potassium disorders under the headings ‘intake’, ‘shifts’ and ‘losses’, as illustrated in Figs 1.2 and 1.3.

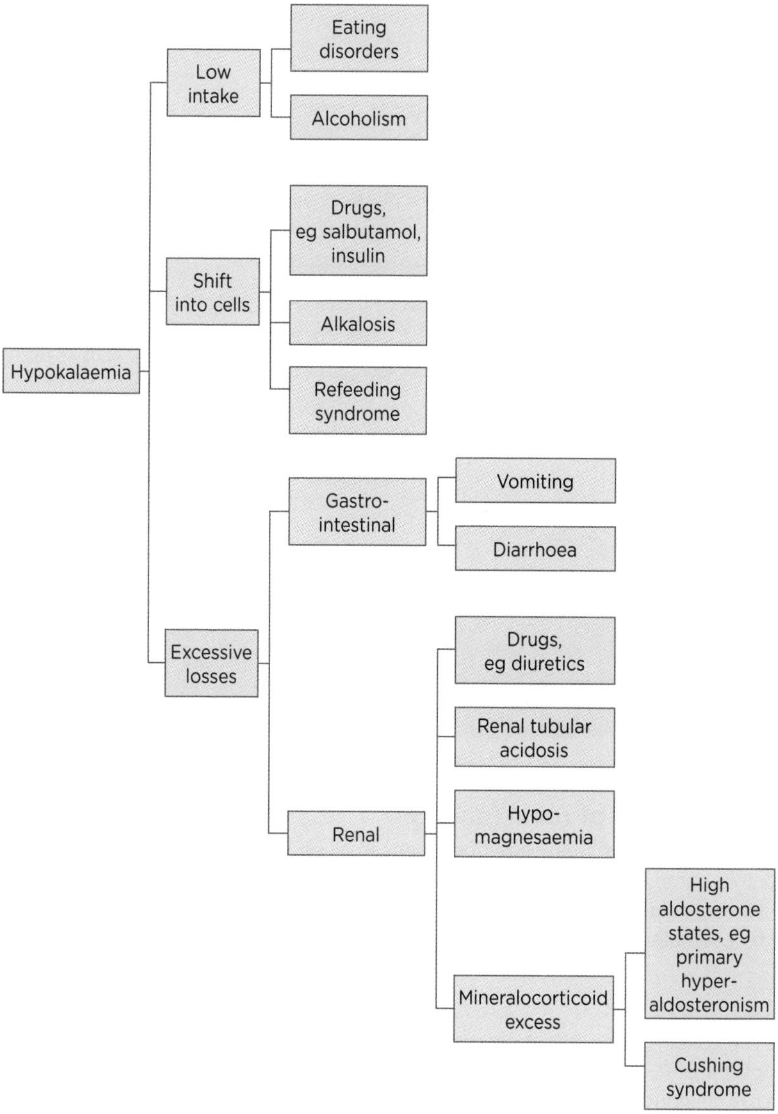

Fig 1.2: Common causes of hypokalaemia.

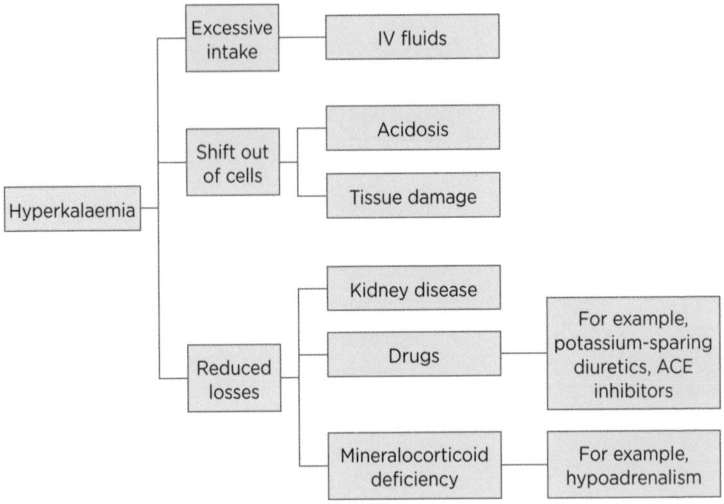

Fig 1.3: Common causes of hyperkalaemia.

DON'T FORGET

Hyperkalaemia is a medical emergency with levels of potassium of more than 6.5 mmol/l requiring immediate attention and lesser levels requiring immediate attention if the ECG is abnormal.

Assessment of renal function

The kidneys have many functions that can all be investigated in detail. The most commonly assessed aspect of kidney function is the GFR, which is used to stage chronic kidney disease. There are many ways in which the GFR can be estimated or measured, as detailed below.

Creatinine

The concentration of creatinine in serum is often used as a crude indicator of the GFR. Creatinine is produced by muscles and eliminated from the body by the kidneys. If a person's muscle mass and GFR remain constant, his or her creatinine level will be stable. If a patient develops acute kidney injury causing a reduction in GFR, his or her creatinine level will increase. However, there are several problems when using creatinine as a marker of GFR. First, one must pay attention to the age, sex and muscle bulk of a patient when interpreting the result. A small, frail, elderly woman with a creatinine level of 120 μmol/l will probably have a markedly reduced GFR, whereas a 25-year-old male body-builder with the same result could well have healthy kidneys. Furthermore, consuming meat and undertaking exercise can both raise creatinine levels in the presence of a stable GFR.

Urea

Urea is made in the liver as a product of protein metabolism. It tends to increase when the GFR falls, but urea is a poor indicator of GFR because its concentration can vary in various situations, as detailed in the table below, and also because it can be reabsorbed by renal tubules after it has been filtered at glomerular level.

CAUSES OF AN ABNORMAL UREA CONCENTRATION	
LOW	HIGH
Malnutrition Liver disease	Renal failure Dehydration High protein intake Gastrointestinal tract bleeding Catabolic states, eg severe burns

Estimated GFR

Research has shown that a person's GFR can be estimated reasonably accurately if their age, sex, serum creatinine concentration and ethnicity are known. These parameters can be combined using a formula, which is rather laborious to use without the aid of a computer. It would be unlikely that you would be asked to calculate the eGFR.

CALCULATING eGFR
eGFR (ml/min per 1.73 m^2) = 186 x (serum creatinine in μmol/l × 0.011312)$^{-1.154}$ x (age in years)$^{-0.203}$ × 0.742 (if female) × 1.21 (if African-Caribbean)
Levey AS et al. A more accurate method to estimate glomerular filtration rate from serum creatinine: a new prediction equation. Modification of diet in Renal Disease Study Group. *Ann Intern Med* 1999;**130**:461–70.

Example eGFR calculation
For an 80-year-old African-Caribbean woman with a serum creatinine of 180 μmol/l: eGFR = 186 × (180 × 0.011312)$^{-1.154}$ × 80$^{-0.203}$ × 0.742 × 1.21 = 30 ml/min per 1.73 m^2

The eGFR is commonly used to define the stage of chronic kidney disease (CKD), as follows:

eGFR (ml/min per 1.73 m^2)	STAGE OF CKD
>90	1 (if other signs of kidney damage present)
60–89	2
45–59	3a
30–44	3b
15–29	4
<15	5

The formulae listed here are known as the 'Modification of Diet in Renal Disease' (MDRD) formulae. An alternative formula, known as the CKD-EPI formula, is gaining popularity (Levey AS et al. A new equation to estimate glomerular filtration rate. *Ann Intern Med* 2009;150:604–12).

Creatinine clearance

Creatinine clearance can be used as another estimate of GFR. It can be measured directly using urine and blood results, or estimated using serum creatinine, age and weight.

CALCULATING CREATININE CLEARANCE USING A TIMED URINE COLLECTION

$$\text{Creatinine clearance (ml/min)} = \frac{U \times V}{P}$$

where U is urinary creatinine (mmol/l), V is urine flow rate (ml/min) and P is serum creatinine (mmol/l).

Difficulties with this method of calculation arise for two reasons:

1. The plasma creatinine is usually measured in μmol/l, not mmol/l, as required by the formula.
2. The urine flow rate is usually measured in litres per day.

A correction factor can be used to adjust for these factors, making the formula:

$$\text{Creatinine clearance (ml/min)} = \frac{U \times V \times 0.694}{P}$$

Where P is now serum creatinine (μmol/l).

The most problematic issue with using a timed urine collection is inaccuracies in collection. Patients may not collect all their urine, or may collect for more or less than what they report. Timing is critical if an accurate result is to be returned.

CALCULATING CREATININE CLEARANCE USING THE 'COCKCROFT AND GAULT FORMULA'

$$\text{Creatinine clearance (ml/min)} = \frac{(140 - \text{age in years}) \times \text{weight (kg)} \times 0.85 \text{ (if female)}}{0.81 \times \text{serum creatinine } (\mu\text{mol/l})}$$

Other methods

Cystatin C is a substance that can be measured in blood. Its level reflects GFR and, unlike creatinine, it is not affected by muscle bulk. It is becoming increasingly popular, but is not yet in widespread use.

It is possible to inject certain substances (eg inulin or radiolabelled EDTA) into a patient and measure his or her levels in the urine. Such techniques are expensive and labour intensive, and used rarely in clinical practice.

Osmolality

Osmolality is a measure of the number of osmotically active particles in a solution. The measurement gives an idea of how many particles are in a solution, but it does not tell you the nature of these particles. Thus, a sample of serum with a high glucose level and normal other constituents might have the same osmolality as a different sample with a high concentration of sodium.

> There is a technical difference between the terms osmolality (measured in mosmol/kg) and osmolarity (measured in mosmol/l), but for practical purposes the two terms are almost equivalent and can be considered synonymous.

The following formulae can be useful when dealing with osmolality.

OSMOLALITY FORMULAE

An estimate of serum osmolality can be made using the following:
Serum osmolality = 2 × (sodium + potassium) + urea + glucose (all in mmol/l)

The osmolar gap is defined as:
Osmolar gap = osmolality measured in lab – osmolality calculated as above

Measures of osmolality are useful in the following scenarios:

- Hyponatraemia - see page 2
- Diagnosing hyperosmolar hyperglycaemic state
- Toxic alcohol poisoning - see page 55.

The 'bone profile' and magnesium

Calcium, phosphate and alkaline phosphatase (ALP) concentrations are often reported together in what is commonly called a 'bone profile'. Looking at these three results in combination points to a diagnosis in patients with metabolic bone disease, if the common patterns of abnormalities are known. Please note that ALP is not specific to bone, meaning that an elevated ALP level can be seen in a patient with no bone disease whatsoever. The other common cause of the finding of raised ALP is disease of the liver or biliary tree. If a patient has a high ALP but a normal γ-glutamyl transpeptidase (GGT) concentration (measured as part of 'liver function tests', see page 16), it is likely that the ALP is of bony origin. Similarly if both the ALP and the GGT are high, the ALP is likely to have arisen from the liver.

BONE DISEASES	ADJUSTED CALCIUM	PHOSPHATE	ALP
Osteoporosis	N	N	N
Osteomalacia	N/↓	↓	↑
Paget's disease of bone	N	N	↑
Bony metastases	↑/N	N/↑	↑
Primary hyperparathyroidism	↑	↓	↑
Secondary hyperparathyroidism	N	↑	↑
Tertiary hyperparathyroidism	↑	↓	↑

DON'T FORGET

The bone profile is normal in osteoporosis.

Calcium

Adjusting calcium for abnormal albumin states

Around one-third of calcium in the blood is bound to albumin, but it is free calcium ions that are physiologically active. It is therefore conventional to 'adjust' calcium when the albumin concentration falls outside the reference interval. This can be done simply, using the formula in the box.

ADJUSTING CALCIUM FOR ABNORMAL ALBUMIN CONCENTRATIONS
If albumin <40 g/l: adjusted calcium (mmol/l) = calcium in mmol/l + 0.02 × (40 − albumin in g/l)
If albumin >45 g/l: adjusted calcium (mmol/l) = calcium in mmol/l − 0.02 × (albumin in g/l − 45)

Abnormal calcium concentration

'Hypocalcaemia' and 'hypercalcaemia' are terms used to describe the situation when the calcium is below or above the reference interval, respectively. Common causes for these calcium disorders are detailed in the boxes below.

COMMON CAUSES OF HYPOCALCAEMIA
Vitamin D deficiency
Renal failure
Hypomagnesaemia
Hypoparathyroidism

COMMON CAUSES OF HYPERCALCAEMIA
Cancer (especially with bone metastases, and in multiple myeloma)
Hyperparathyroidism (primary or tertiary)
Thiazide diuretics
Sarcoidosis
Familial hypercalciuric hypercalcaemia

Useful tests in a patient with hypocalcaemia are therefore: vitamin D, U+E, magnesium and PTH.

Parathyroid hormone

The most useful first-line investigation in a patient found to have hypercalcaemia is measurement of the parathyroid hormone (PTH) level. If the PTH level is normal or elevated, the patient probably has hyperparathyroidism. In hypercalcaemia caused by other diseases, the parathyroid glands should shut off production of PTH, and the measured concentration should be low. Other useful investigations include imaging for cancer, angiotensin-converting enzyme (ACE) levels (often raised in sarcoidosis) and urinary calcium:creatinine ratio.

DON'T FORGET

A normal or high PTH level in the setting of hypercalcaemia is abnormal, and usually indicates hyperparathyroidism.

Phosphate

Hypophosphataemia and hyperphosphataemia are the terms used to describe the situation when the phosphate level is below or above the reference interval, respectively. Common causes are detailed in the boxes below.

COMMON CAUSES OF HYPOPHOSPHATAEMIA
Refeeding syndrome
Respiratory alkalosis of any cause
Glucose infusion
Alcoholism
Renal tubular leak

COMMON CAUSES OF HYPERPHOSPHATAEMIA
Renal failure
Tissue damage, eg tumour lysis syndrome, rhabdomyolysis
(Excessive use of phosphate-containing medication and vitamin D)

Magnesium

Hypermagnesaemia (a high serum magnesium concentration) is generally seen only after a patient receives a magnesium infusion. Hypomagnesaemia (low magnesium) occurs much more frequently, and common causes are shown in Fig 1.4.

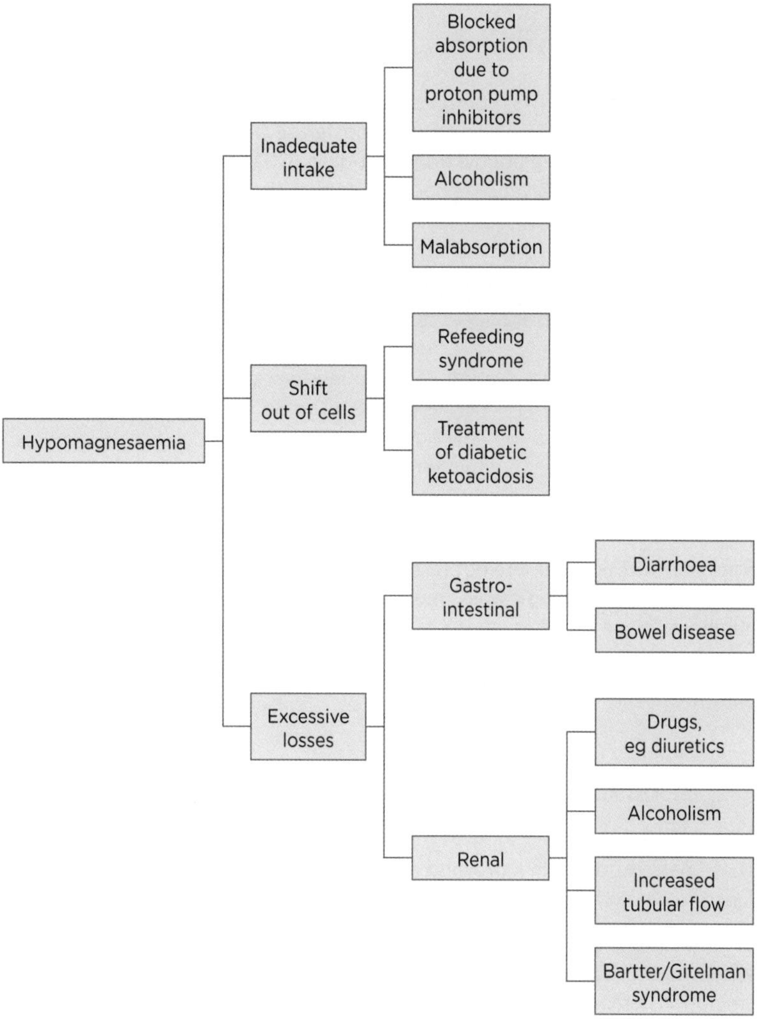

Fig 1.4: Common causes of hypomagnesaemia.

Liver function tests

Liver function tests (LFTs) comprise six measurements: bilirubin, aspartate aminotransferase (AST), alanine aminotransferase (ALT), alkaline phosphatase (ALP), γ-glutamyl transpeptidase (GGT) and albumin. Prothrombin time (PT) which is part of a coagulation screen is an important addition (see page 84).

COMPONENTS OF LIVER FUNCTION TESTS
Bilirubin
Aspartate aminotransferase
Alanine aminotransferase
Alkaline phosphatase
γ-Glutamyl transpeptidase
Albumin

Note that AST and ALP are not tests specific to the liver. AST is also released when muscle (including cardiac muscle) is damaged. ALP is raised in a number of bone diseases, hence its presence in a bone profile (see page 12).

Broadly speaking, disturbances of liver function may be classified into 3 patterns:

1. Hepatitic (parenchymal)
2. Cholestatic
3. Mixed.

These patterns assist in narrowing the differential diagnosis of altered liver function. An understanding of the different causes allows an appropriate sequence of investigation.

When hepatocellular damage occurs, hepatocytes 'spill out' aminotransferases (AST and ALT). A rise in these indices alone may be termed a 'transaminitis'.

When there is obstruction to the outflow of bile from the liver, a cholestatic pattern (elevated ALP and GGT) will be seen. The bilirubin level would also be expected to be high.

Bilirubin is conjugated in the liver with the attachment of a glucuronide group. Measured bilirubin may be conjugated (direct bilirubin) or unconjugated (indirect bilirubin). Total bilirubin is the sum of both types.

Confusion sometimes arises in cholestatic liver disease when the AST and ALT are also elevated. This occurs because of back pressure on the liver. In such instances the elevation of ALP and GGT will be out of proportion to that of the aminotransferases.

In cholestatic jaundice, conjugated bilirubin can be detected in the urine using urinalysis.

CAUSES OF HEPATITIC LFTs
• Viral hepatitis • Autoimmune hepatitis • Drugs and toxins • Alcohol • Metabolic disorders (eg Wilson's disease) • Fatty liver • Malignancy (both primary and metastatic) • Congestive cardiac failure

CAUSES OF CHOLESTATIC LFTs
Obstruction in the bile duct lumen • Bile duct gallstone **An abnormal bile duct wall** • Bile duct stricture • Cholangiocarcinoma **Compression of the bile duct by an extrinsic lesion** • Pancreatic carcinoma • Nodes at the porta hepatis • Ampullary carcinoma

One of the functions of the liver is protein synthesis. In a failing liver, synthetic function is often affected. This will manifest as low albumin levels and a raised prothrombin time (since the liver manufactures clotting factors).

COMMON CAUSES OF JAUNDICE	
Pre-hepatic • Haemolysis **Hepatic** • Gilbert's syndrome • Hepatitis (which itself has many causes) • Cirrhosis • Drugs • Liver cancer	**Post-hepatic** • Gallstones • Pancreatic cancer • Cholangiocarcinoma • Bile duct stricture

As such a large number of conditions can cause liver disease, it is common practice to order a panel of investigative tests if the cause of the liver disease is not apparent. These include those in the table below.

TEST	DISEASE	EXPECTED RESULT
Autoantibody test	Autoimmune hepatitis	Anti-nuclear Anti-smooth muscle Anti-liver/kidney microsomal-I
	Primary biliary cirrhosis	Anti-mitochondrial
	Coeliac disease	Anti-transglutaminase
Iron profile	Haemochromatosis	High iron, ferritin and transferrin saturation Low TIBC
Copper studies	Wilson's disease	Low ceruloplasmin and elevated 24-hour urine copper concentration is suggestive
Viral hepatitis 'screen': hepatitis B virus, hepatitis C virus, Epstein–Barr virus, cytomegalovirus	Viral hepatitis	Positive viral tests
α_1-Antitrypsin	α_1-Antitrypsin deficiency	Low level
α-Fetoprotein	Hepatocellular carcinoma	High level
Immunoglobulins	Several liver diseases	Specific pattern of immunoglobulin rise can give a clue to underlying disease but will not be diagnostic

Arterial blood gas analysis

Arterial blood gas (ABG) analysis provides a wealth of information about a patient's state of health. The test is most commonly used in acute illness but may also be used in the assessment of patients with chronic respiratory disease. In acute situations, multiple analyses are often made to assess response to treatment. Trends are usually more helpful than one-off readings. Never forget to consult old medical records if possible, since the patient's baseline may be well outside 'normal' limits.

Interpretation of four key indices - pH, partial pressure of oxygen (PaO_2), partial pressure of carbon dioxide ($PaCO_2$) and bicarbonate (HCO_3^-) - will provide most of the information needed in clinical practice. Other measures such as 'standard bicarbonate' and 'base excess' are calculated by many analysers, and are known as derived indices. They are not considered here.

Sophisticated blood gas analysers will provide other useful information such as blood levels of lactate and methaemoglobin.

NORMAL RANGES (BREATHING ROOM AIR AT SEA LEVEL)	
pH	7.35-7.45
PaO_2	11-13 kPa
$PaCO_2$	4.7-6.0 kPa
HCO_3^-	24-30 mmol/l
Base excess	-2 to +2 mmol/l
Anion gap	12-16 mmol/l

Of all the normal reference ranges for values listed in this book, it is recommended that all students learn the reference ranges in an ABG sample. This is for two reasons:

1. ABGs are commonly tested, so knowing the reference ranges for adults will help you as an undergraduate.
2. More importantly, in real medical practice, ABGs are often encountered in stressful situations involving critically unwell patients. Knowing reference ranges can speed up analysis and reduce stress.

Oxygen levels in the air fall with increasing altitude. Bear this in mind if you are interpreting ABGs taken at any significant height above sea level. For the purposes of simplicity, for the remainder of this chapter, it will be assumed that samples have been taken at sea level.

Systematic interpretation of an ABG

The two main steps involved are to assess oxygenation, then acid-base status.

Step 1: assessing oxygenation

You will note that the normal range for PaO_2 given in the box above was 11–13 kPa. This value holds true for a patient breathing air that contains 21% oxygen. It is crucial to appreciate that a patient with normal lungs will have a much higher PaO_2 if their inspired oxygen concentration (FiO_2) is increased. The physiology behind this is summarised in the alveolar gas equation, which will be dealt with shortly.

Unless you are someone who particularly enjoys equations, a useful rule of thumb is that, for a healthy person at sea level, the expected PaO_2 (kPa) is roughly 10 less than the FiO_2 (%). This will not compute exactly, but will highlight patients with serious problems. Exact expected values are shown in the table below. Thus, a patient who is receiving 85% oxygen and has a PaO_2 of 11 kPa has a serious problem.

INSPIRED OXYGEN CONCENTRATION (%)	RULE OF THUMB METHOD FOR ESTIMATING PaO_2	EXPECTED PaO_2 WITH HEALTHY LUNGS (kPa)
28	18	21
35	25	27
40	30	32
60	50	51
85	75	75
100	90	89

MEMORY AID

As a rule of thumb,
the expected PaO_2 (kPa) is roughly 10 less than the FiO_2 (%).

It is therefore impossible to interpret the PaO_2 without knowing the FiO_2. If the PaO_2 is lower than expected, this implies that a disease process in the lungs is interfering with gas exchange. This can occur with a variety of conditions, from pulmonary fibrosis to pulmonary embolism, and pneumonia to pulmonary oedema, to name but a few.

DON'T FORGET

Always interpret the PaO_2 with the FiO_2 in mind.

The first step in interpreting an ABG sample is to assess oxygenation. So, with the above in mind, decide whether oxygenation is normal or abnormal.

The label of 'respiratory failure' is used when the PaO_2 is less than 8 kPa. It is divided into two types depending on the $PaCO_2$, as follows:

RESPIRATORY FAILURE TYPE	PaO_2 (kPa)	$PaCO_2$ (kPa)
Type 1	<8	<6.5
Type 2	<8	>6.5

MEMORY AID

In type **ONE** respiratory failure, **ONE** gas is abnormal (ie low O_2, without high CO_2).

In type **TWO** respiratory failure, **TWO** gases are abnormal (low O_2 and high CO_2).

COMMON CAUSES OF RESPIRATORY FAILURE	
TYPE 1	**TYPE 2**
Pulmonary oedema Pneumonia Pulmonary embolism Pulmonary fibrosis	Chronic obstructive pulmonary disease Respiratory centre depression Respiratory muscle weakness Abnormal chest wall architecture

THE ALVEOLAR GAS EQUATION AND THE ALVEOLAR-ARTERIAL GRADIENT

The assessment of oxygenation described above will suffice in most situations. It is possible to be more precise, however, so, if you are particularly interested in this subject, there are two further equations that are of interest.

The alveolar gas equation

This equation allows the calculation of the expected oxygen level in the alveoli of an individual ($P\text{A}O_2$). It is rarely used in clinical practice:

$$P\text{A}O_2 = FiO_2\,(P_{atm} - P_{H_2O}) - \frac{PaCO_2\,(1 - FiO_2) \times (1 - \text{RQ})}{\text{RQ}}$$

where P_{atm} = atmospheric pressure, P_{H_2O} = saturated vapour pressure of water at that particular temperature and pressure, and RQ = respiratory quotient (a ratio of CO_2 eliminated to O_2 consumed).

So, for example, for someone breathing 21% oxygen at sea level with $PaCO_2$ of 5 kPa:

$$P\text{A}O_2 = 0.21 \times (101\text{ kPa} - 6.25\text{ kPa}) - \frac{5\text{ kPa}\,(1 - 0.21) \times (1 - 0.8)}{0.8}$$

$$P\text{A}O_2 = 0.21 \times 94.75\text{ kPa} - 5.99$$

$$P\text{A}O_2 = 13.91\text{ kPa}$$

The alveolar-arterial gradient

This equation allows the calculation of the difference in oxygen concentration between alveoli and the arterial system:

$$\text{A-a gradient} = \left[FiO_2 \times (P_{atm} - P_{H_2O}) - \left(\frac{PaO_2}{0.8}\right)\right] - PaO_2$$

So, for example, for someone breathing 40% oxygen at sea level with PaO_2 of 12 kPa and $PaCO_2$ of 5 kPa:

$$\text{A-a gradient} = \left[0.4 \times (101\text{ kPa} - 6.25\text{ kPa}) - \left(\frac{5\text{ kPa}}{0.8}\right)\right] - 12$$

$$\text{A-a gradient} = (0.4 \times 94.75\text{ kPa} - 6.25\text{ kPa}) - 12$$

$$\text{A-a gradient} = 19.65\text{ kPa}$$

There is no established normal range for the A-a gradient. It has been variably defined in the following ways:

- No more than 2.66 kPa. This is a simplistic approach, however, as the A-a gradient normally increases with age.
- No more than $\left(\frac{\text{Age in years}}{4} + 4\right) \times 0.13$ kPa.
- Or compare the value with 'normal' age-based values in the literature.

Stein PD et al. Alveolar-arterial oxygen gradient in the assessment of acute pulmonary embolism. *Chest* 1995;**107**:139–43.

Step 2: assess acid-base status

The human body works best when its acid-base status is kept tightly controlled - the pH of the blood is normally held between 7.35 and 7.45. A pH lower than this is termed 'acidosis' (or 'acidaemia'), and a high pH is termed an 'alkalosis' ('alkalaemia'). A clear understanding of the bicarbonate buffering system makes understanding of acid-base problems much easier. This system comprises carbonic acid (H_2CO_3) in equilibrium with bicarbonate ions (HCO_3^-):

$$H^+ + HCO_3^- \rightleftharpoons H_2CO_3 \rightleftharpoons H_2O + CO_2$$

The pH is directly dependent on the concentration of hydrogen ions (H^+) in a solution. If there were no buffer present in the blood and the H^+ concentration were to rise, the pH would fall proportionately and the solution would become more acidic. If the H^+ concentration were to fall, pH would rise and a more alkaline state would result. With an adequately functioning bicarbonate buffer system, any modest rise or fall in H^+ concentration will be resisted. Should the H^+ concentration increase, excess H^+ will combine with bicarbonate ions and effectively be removed from the system (the equation above is driven to the right). Should the concentration decrease, the equation is driven to the left, and extra H^+ will be generated.

You might find it helpful to remember the following formula:

$$H^+ \text{ is proportional to } \frac{PaCO_2}{HCO_3^-}$$

This makes it easy to see that the concentration of hydrogen ions increases (and therefore an acidosis will result) in two settings: an increase in carbon dioxide, CO_2, or a reduction in bicarbonate.

When assessing acid-base status, it is recommended that a logical system be used, as detailed below.

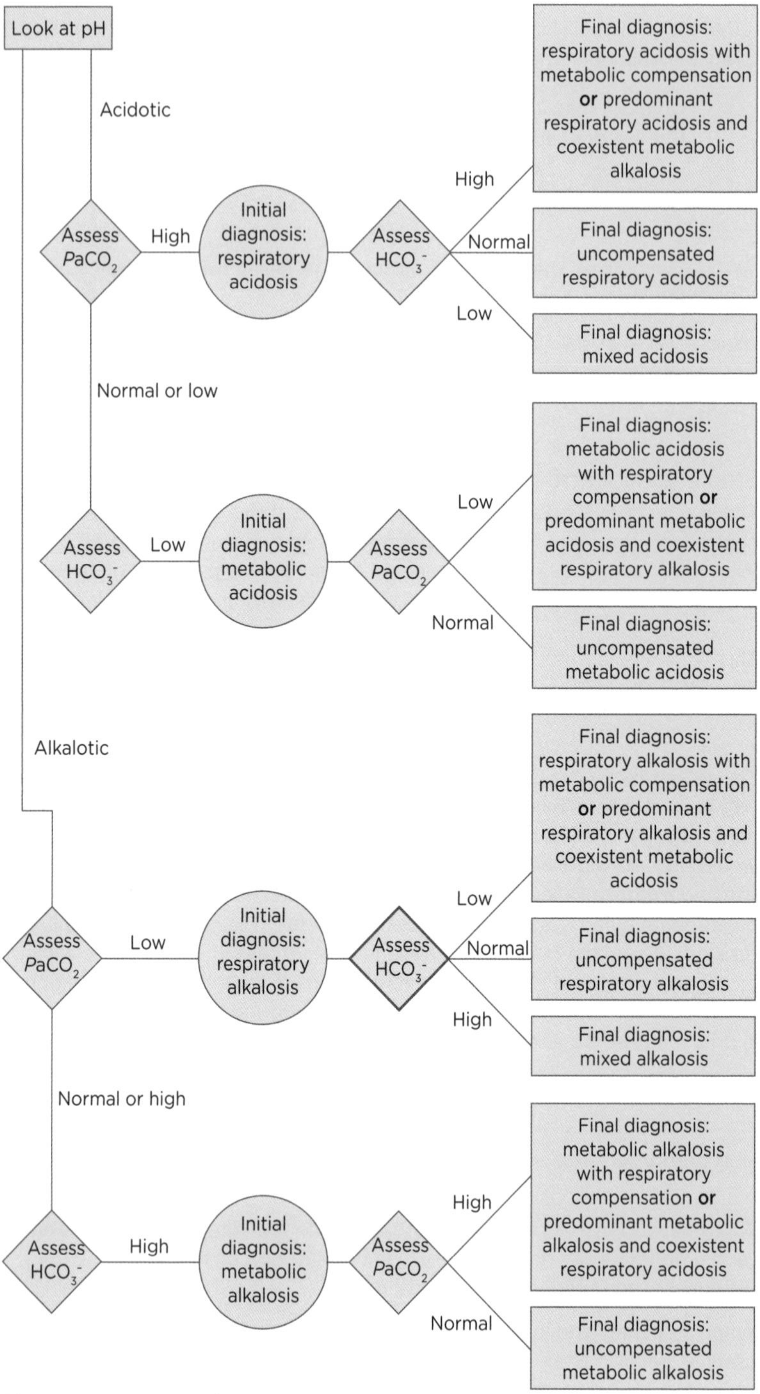

Fig 1.5: Interpretation of common arterial blood gas abnormalities.

a. Look at the pH

Is it:

- normal (7.35–7.45)?
- low (<7.35) indicating acidosis?
- high (>7.45) indicating alkalosis?

Acid-base disorders are classified into problems involving metabolic processes and problems of respiration. Proceed to the next steps to work out what type of disturbance is present.

b. Look at the $PaCO_2$

Is it normal, low or high? You should recall from the earlier description that, when the $PaCO_2$ rises, the H^+ concentration rises, ie acidosis ensues.

If you find this difficult to recall, remember that carbon dioxide is an 'acidic gas' (carbon dioxide plus water → carbonic acid), so:

- If the pH is acid and the CO_2 is high, the problem is a respiratory acidosis.
- If the pH is alkaline and the CO_2 is low, the problem is a respiratory alkalosis.

c. Look at the HCO_3^-

Is it normal, low or high? Recall from earlier that, when HCO_3^- falls the H^+ concentration rises. A low HCO_3^- will occur if it is buffering ('mopping up') acids, if it is not being made correctly or if it is being lost in excessive quantities. If you find this difficult to recall, remember that, bicarbonate is an alkaline substance (some people take sodium bicarbonate to combat stomach acid), so an excess of it is seen in alkalosis and a shortage in acidosis. Therefore:

- If the pH is acid and the bicarbonate is low, the problem is a metabolic acidosis (lack of alkaline bicarbonate).
- If the pH is alkaline and the bicarbonate is high, the problem is a metabolic alkalosis (excess alkaline bicarbonate).

DON'T FORGET

In some circumstances, patients can have more than one abnormality, eg a combined respiratory and metabolic acidosis.

d. Look for compensation

The body adapts (compensates) in situations of acid-base disturbance. If the problem is metabolic, the compensatory mechanism is respiratory. The respiratory rate is altered over the course of a few minutes to attempt to keep the hydrogen ion concentration normal. If the primary problem is respiratory, the kidneys adapt to counteract the change by altering their handling of hydrogen ions. This process takes place over several days. **The body will never overcompensate.** The following patterns are commonly seen:

- In an acute metabolic acidosis, the body responds by getting rid of extra CO_2, thus losing acid and shifting the pH towards normality.
- In a chronic respiratory acidosis, the body responds by holding on to extra bicarbonate.

e. Try to determine the cause

Respiratory acidosis

Respiratory acidosis can be due to any of the causes of respiratory failure.

Respiratory alkalosis

Respiratory alkalosis is always due to hyperventilation. Be wary of attributing hyperventilation exclusively to anxiety, however, since it may occur secondary to an underlying severe disease process, such as sepsis or stroke.

Metabolic acidosis

There is a wide range of causes for a metabolic acidosis. To narrow down this list, and help you come to a diagnosis, it is helpful to calculate the anion gap. If this is high (>16 mmol/l), the acidosis is usually due to the presence of excess acids in the body that are not routinely analysed in the laboratory. The anion gap is calculated as follows:

$$\text{Anion gap} = (Na^+ + K^+) - (Cl^- + HCO_3^-)$$

A patient with the following biochemical findings - Na^+ 136 mmol/l, K^+ 3.5 mmol/l, Cl^- 100 mmol/l, HCO_3^- 24 mmol/l - would therefore have an anion gap of 15.5 mmol/l.

Some experts in this area omit the potassium component of the equation which then becomes:

$$\text{Anion gap} = Na^+ - (Cl^- + HCO_3^-)$$

Either form of the equation is acceptable, but the normal value will differ slightly.

DON'T FORGET

Always calculate the anion gap in a patient with a metabolic acidosis.

COMMON CAUSES OF A METABOLIC ACIDOSIS	
NORMAL ANION GAP	**RAISED ANION GAP**
HCO_3^- loss from gut, eg diarrhoea	Ketoacidosis
Renal tubular acidosis	Renal failure
	Lactic acidosis
	Salicylate toxicity
	Methanol ingestion
	Ethylene glycol (antifreeze) ingestion

Metabolic alkalosis

There are several causes of metabolic alkalosis (see box below). Most commonly, it is seen in patients with excessive vomiting.

COMMON CAUSES OF A METABOLIC ALKALOSIS
Losses from the gut, particularly vomiting (classically pyloric stenosis)
Primary or secondary hyperaldosteronism
Hypercalcaemia
Use of diuretics
Bicarbonate ingestion

Markers of nutrition

It is possible to measure a wide range of substances (vitamins, trace metals, etc) in the blood in an attempt to quantify a patient's nutritional status. Although the interpretation of many of these test results might appear simplistic (the results are low, normal or high), bear in mind that blood levels of many substances are poor indicators of total body stores. It is a common misconception that albumin is a good marker of nutrition. It is not: a patient can be profoundly malnourished but have a normal serum albumin level.

Assessment of the status of the three key nutrients (haematinics) necessary for red blood cell formation - iron, folic acid and vitamin B_{12} - is particularly important.

Finding a haematinic deficiency is only the first part of establishing the cause of anaemia. Where possible, the cause of the nutrient deficiency should also be sought. For example, iron deficiency is often due to blood loss from the gastrointestinal tract, and endoscopy is often used to search for this.

Knowledge of exactly where haematinics are absorbed from the gastrointestinal tract can sometimes help localise the pathology underlying anaemia. These sites are shown in the box below.

HAEMATINIC	ABSORBED FROM
Iron	Duodenum and jejunum
Vitamin B_{12}	Terminal ileum
Folate	Small bowel

Iron studies

A good understanding of how the body handles iron is required before iron studies can be interpreted.

Iron is best absorbed from the upper small bowel in the ferrous (Fe^{2+}) state. Iron is transported across the intestinal cell and into the plasma. Iron in the plasma is carried to developing red cells in the bone marrow by a protein called transferrin. Iron is stored in the body as ferritin and haemosiderin. Red cells have transferrin receptors (soluble transferrin receptors, sTfRs) which can be measured in plasma.

COMPONENTS OF AN IRON PROFILE
Serum iron
Serum total iron-binding capacity (serum TIBC)
Serum ferritin
Transferrin saturation
Serum soluble transferrin receptors

In iron deficiency states, iron studies are as follows:

IRON PARAMETER	RESULT
Serum iron	Reduced
Serum total iron-binding capacity	Increased - the body tries hard to bind any iron around the system
Serum ferritin	Reduced - since iron stores are low
Transferrin saturation	Reduced
Serum sTfRs	Increased - since red cells attempt to absorb any iron in the system

The serum ferritin level is the single best test for iron deficiency. To make matters a little more confusing, ferritin behaves as an acute phase reactant - its level increases with active inflammation, in the same way as the erythrocyte sedimentation rate (ESR) and C-reactive protein (CRP) (see pages 81 and 34). This means that, in states of iron deficiency associated with an ongoing inflammatory process (eg an active infection), the serum ferritin level may be high. However, the sTfR will reveal the true state of affairs.

Unfortunately the sTfR assay is not routinely available, and often clinical judgement is required in such situations. Sometimes, it can be difficult to be sure that a patient is iron deficient, and in such circumstances a trial of iron treatment may be necessary. Once the diagnosis has been established, it is imperative that a reason for the iron deficiency be sought.

In cases of diagnostic uncertainty, a bone marrow biopsy can be obtained and stained for the presence of iron. In iron deficiency states, little or no iron will be seen in the marrow.

Iron studies are also abnormal in states of iron overload. This is commonly seen in haemochromatosis and in haematological conditions that require frequent blood transfusions. In such cases, serum iron, ferritin and transferrin saturation are raised. The total iron-binding capacity (TIBC) is usually low.

In anaemia of chronic disease, iron studies are commonly as follows:

IRON PARAMETER	RESULT
Serum iron	Normal or slightly reduced
Serum total iron-binding capacity	Reduced
Serum ferritin	May be raised as acute phase reactant
Transferrin saturation	Reduced
Serum sTfRs	Normal - reflecting the true state of body iron levels

Goddard AG, James MW, McIntyre AS, et al. Guidelines for the management of iron deficiency anaemia. *Gut* 2011;**60**;1309-16

Vitamin B_{12}

Vitamin B_{12} deficiency may result from inadequate intake, but the most common reason for deficiency relates to poor absorption.

In health, vitamin B_{12} is bound to a protein called intrinsic factor secreted by gastric parietal cells. The vitamin is then absorbed from the ileum. Poor absorption generally results from the absence of intrinsic factor or disease of the ileum.

The most common disease causing vitamin B_{12} deficiency is pernicious anaemia, in which there is defective intrinsic factor production. The disease is associated with autoantibodies against gastric parietal cells and intrinsic factor (see Chapter 6).

It used to be standard practice to investigate low vitamin B_{12} levels with a Schilling test (see box), but this is rarely performed in modern medicine. Details of the Schilling test are included here for interest only.

Schilling test

The Schilling test may be used to distinguish between the various causes of vitamin B_{12} deficiency. In this test, patients are given two doses of vitamin B_{12}. One dose is radioactively labelled and given orally. The other dose is given intramuscularly with the aim of flushing absorbed radiolabelled vitamin B_{12} into the urine. The urine is collected over a period of 24 hours. Normally, a proportion of the oral vitamin B_{12} dose will be absorbed and excreted, so that more than 10% of the oral dose will be excreted in the urine. With vitamin B_{12} malabsorption, this amount will be reduced.

The test is repeated with an oral preparation of intrinsic factor being given at the same time as the oral dose of vitamin B_{12}. If the test results are now normal, one can assume that the patient's problem lies with inadequate intrinsic factor. If the test is still abnormal, the problem most likely lies in the ileum.

One possible cause of ileal disease is bacterial overgrowth. In order to test for this possibility, the patient can be given a course of antibiotics. If the Schilling test returns to normal after this, the diagnosis of bacterial overgrowth can be made. Alternatively, bacterial overgrowth can be diagnosed using a breath test. The most commonly used test is the hydrogen breath test. A carbohydrate load is given orally. Bacteria in the small bowel metabolise the carbohydrate, liberating hydrogen which is absorbed and detected in exhaled air.

Folate

Folate analysis is simple. Serum folate levels are measured with a deficiency identified if levels are low.

Refeeding syndrome

If a malnourished patient is suddenly given food to eat, he or she may be at risk of refeeding syndrome. This is manifest by a rapid fall in several biochemical markers, most noticeably phosphate, potassium and magnesium. This condition should be anticipated and careful monitoring undertaken of at-risk patients, to minimise the chance of harm.

Enzymes

It is common to measure the concentration or activity of several enzymes in the body. The most common tests requested are listed below.

Amylase and lipase

There are two main sources of amylase in the body: the pancreas and the salivary glands. Amylase is generally measured in patients suspected of having acute pancreatitis, with markedly raised levels being typical of this disorder. The finding of a high blood amylase level is not, however, specific to pancreatitis, and other causes should be considered, particularly if the clinical picture is not typical.

CAUSES OF ELEVATED AMYLASE
Pancreatic disease, eg acute pancreatitis, pancreatic cancer
Salivary gland disease, eg mumps, salivary gland tumours, stones
Other abdominal disease, eg acute cholecystitis, perforated peptic ulcer, bowel obstruction, ruptured ectopic pregnancy
Kidney disease
Diabetic ketoacidosis (DKA)
Other cancers, eg lung cancer
Drugs, eg morphine

Lipase is also secreted by the pancreas. The finding of an elevated lipase level in the blood is a more specific indicator that the diagnosis is acute pancreatitis, but this test is not offered by many laboratories.

Creatine kinase

Creatine kinase (CK) is released from damaged skeletal muscle, and will be detected in elevated quantities in a range of conditions as shown in the box. CK is also found in cardiac muscle, and it may therefore also rise after a myocardial infarction (see page 37). Subtypes of CK can be measured.

CAUSES OF ELEVATED CK
Muscle disease, eg rhabdomyolysis, muscular dystrophy, polymyositis
Vigorous exercise
Drugs, eg statins, fibrates, antipsychotics
Hypothyroidism

Lactate dehydrogenase

Lactate dehydrogenase (LDH) is most commonly measured when looking for evidence of haemolysis, since red blood cells normally contain a high concentration of this enzyme. See page 75 for more details. It is also commonly measured in patients with haematological malignancies, where an elevated level can indicate a poor prognosis.

Plasma proteins and enzymes

Albumin

Albumin is normally the protein that is present in the highest concentration in the plasma. Abnormally high levels are usually due to dehydration. Low levels can result from a variety of causes as shown in the box.

COMMON CAUSES OF LOW ALBUMIN
Malabsorption
Liver failure
Sepsis
Nephrotic syndrome
Protein-losing enteropathy
Burns
Chronic malnutrition

M-protein

M-protein, or paraprotein, is the hallmark feature of multiple myeloma and related disorders (see pages 87–88 for more information). The term refers to an abnormal protein secreted by cancerous plasma cells. Interpreting the results of tests for M-protein can be difficult if you are unaware of the terminology.

Serum protein electrophoresis

This is a specialist test run in the laboratory that results in the generation of a tracing that is interpreted manually. The initial output resembles a series of stripes, one on top of the other. Software is used to convert the stripes into a trace comprising several peaks that correspond to proteins in the serum. Abnormal peaks may be due to the presence of M-protein. The language used in reporting these samples can be confusing. Terms incorporating the Greek letters α, β or γ simply indicate where on the tracing the abnormal peaks occur. 'Fast' and 'slow' are sometimes used to refine the description of the location of the abnormal peak. The peak itself is referred to as a 'band', and can be further defined as 'light' or 'heavy' depending on the size of the peak. Usually, the report will quantify the amount of M-protein present, so that severity can be gauged and progress with time monitored. Further testing of samples can then be performed in the laboratory to investigate the subtype of immunoglobulin (Ig) being produced (ie IgG, IgM, IgA, IgE or IgD).

Serum-free light chains

Immunoglobulins are made up of heavy and light chains. Occasionally the malignant plasma cells secrete light chains only, and these can be tested for. There are two types of light chains - κ and λ - and, in myeloma and related disorders, either κ or λ chains will be secreted excessively. In this situation, the $\kappa:\lambda$ ratio will be raised.

Urinary Bence Jones protein

Bence Jones protein is the name given to light chains that are detected in the urine.

Immunoglobulins

The subtypes of Ig molecules (IgG, IgA, IgM, IgD and IgE) can be quantified. This can be helpful in diagnosing immunodeficiency states (where one or more subtypes may be low), liver disease (see page 18) and investigating IgE-mediated diseases, such as hypersensitivity disorders.

Other proteins

Many other proteins can be measured. Some of the most important of these are detailed in the box below.

PROTEIN	NOTES
α_1-Antitrypsin	An antiprotease protein; high in inflammatory states; low in α_1-antitrypsin deficiency, a cause of emphysema and liver cirrhosis
Haptoglobin	Involved in mopping up free haemoglobin from damaged red blood cells; high in inflammatory states; low in haemolysis
Ceruloplasmin	Copper-carrying protein; high in inflammatory states; low in Wilson's disease (see page 18)
Transferrin	Part of an iron profile; see page 29

C-reactive protein

C-reactive protein (CRP) is a protein produced in the liver. It is an acute phase reactant, being raised in inflammation and infection. It is often thought of in a similar manner to the erythrocyte sedimentation rate (ESR) (see page 81). The CRP and ESR are together termed inflammatory markers. There are a few recognised conditions in which the ESR is raised, but the CRP is normal.

CAUSES OF A RAISED ESR WITH A NORMAL CRP
Systemic lupus erythematosus
Multiple myeloma

The level of the CRP does not necessarily reflect the severity of a disease process.

Lipids

The human body has an extremely intricate system for processing lipids, which are vital for many essential physiological processes, eg cell membrane formation and steroid hormone synthesis. Lipid profiles are, however, normally requested in the setting of preventing or treating cardiovascular disease due to atherosclerosis. The main components measured on a standard 'lipid profile' are as follows:

- Total cholesterol
- High-density lipoprotein (HDL)-cholesterol
- Triglyceride.

In addition to these, low-density lipoprotein (LDL)-cholesterol and non-HDL-cholesterol are often reported. The LDL is usually calculated using a formula that incorporates total cholesterol, HDL and triglyceride. The formula does not apply when triglycerides exceed 4.5 mmol/l, hence the LDL will not be reported in patients with severe hypertriglyceridaemia. Non-HDL-cholesterol is a relatively recently introduced concept. It is calculated simply as total cholesterol minus HDL-cholesterol. Recent clinical guidelines stipulate targets for reductions in non-HDL-cholesterol for patients receiving lipid-lowering therapy. Another easily calculated index is the total cholesterol:HDL ratio, but this is slowly going out of favour.

There are very many individual disorders of lipid metabolism, some common and some rare. It is very important to investigate patients with dyslipidaemia for a secondary cause. Common causes include:

- Alcohol excess
- Diabetes mellitus
- Drugs, eg thiazide diuretics
- Hypothyroidism
- Kidney disease
- Liver disease
- Obesity.

The following are some of the more common primary causes of dyslipidaemia:

- Familial hypercholesterolaemia (FH): this is an umbrella term for a variety of genetic abnormalities that predispose the affected individual to a very high LDL-cholesterol level, and hence a markedly raised cardiovascular risk. The condition is inherited in an autosomal dominant manner, and genetic testing for common mutations is undertaken as part of the routine care of these patients. This disease should be particularly considered if there is a strong family history of premature ischaemic heart disease.
- Polygenic hypercholesterolaemia: affected individuals tend to have high LDL-cholesterol levels, but this condition is not due to a simple genetic mutation, and the family history is usually not as dramatic as in FH.
- Familial hypertriglyceridaemia: in this disorder, the primary problem is hypertriglyceridaemia.
- Familial dysbetalipoproteinaemia: the characteristic lipid profile pattern in this condition is high LDL-cholesterol and high triglyceride concentrations, which are approximately equal numerically when measured in the same units. Affected individuals are at very high risk of cardiovascular disease. The disease can be confirmed by genetic testing.
- Familial combined hyperlipidaemia: again, both LDL-cholesterol and triglyceride concentrations tend to be raised, but there is no easily defined genetic basis for this.

Cardiac biomarkers

Testing for the presence of the cardiac contractile protein troponin (type I or T) is currently the test most commonly performed to assess for myocardial cell damage. Troponin is normally involved in cardiac muscle cell contraction, and is released systemically when cardiac muscle cells are damaged. Troponin may be elevated after 2 hours, and can stay elevated for up to 7 days. Levels are generally measured 12 hours after the onset of symptoms. 'High-sensitivity' troponin is now being measured commonly. This can allow myocardial infarction to be diagnosed very early. Unfortunately, elevated troponin levels are not specific to myocardial infarction, and may be found in conditions such as those listed in the box:

CAUSES OF RAISED TROPONIN	
• Myocardial infarction • Heart failure • Myocarditis • Pulmonary embolism	• Renal failure • Severe sepsis • Supraventricular tachycardia

A variety of enzymes rise after a myocardial infarction and were, in the past, used to diagnose this condition. The enzymes differ in terms of time taken to peak and how long they stayed elevated in the circulation, but are now rarely measured in this setting due to the widespread measurement of troponin.

TEST	TIME TO PEAK (h)	DURATION OF ELEVATED BLOOD LEVEL AFTER CARDIAC EVENT
Creatine kinase (CK)	24	48
AST	30	60
Lactate dehydrogenase (LDH)	72	240

Creatine kinase is also released from damaged skeletal muscle (see page 32). The subtype (isoenzyme) released mainly from cardiac muscle is called CK-MB, and a high level of this enzyme should raise suspicions of cardiac damage.

B-type natriuretic peptide (BNP)

In heart failure, heart chambers are stretched more than normal. In such circumstances, substances are released that cause increased sodium excretion (natriuresis) in an attempt to improve the situation for the failing heart. One such substance is BNP. BNP, and its inactive cleavage fragment (N-terminal pro-BNP), tend to be elevated in patients with heart failure to such an extent that, if the level of these hormones is normal, then heart failure is an unlikely diagnosis. The extremely low likelihood of heart failure in a patient who has the combination of a normal ECG and a normal BNP or N-terminal pro-BNP level makes this approach a very effective screening test for this condition.

Tumour markers

Tumour markers are substances that can be associated with cancer. Some markers are used for making a diagnosis, whereas others are useful in predicting prognosis, charting response to treatment or monitoring for recurrence of disease. Panels of tumour markers are sometimes requested in an attempt to find a primary cancer. This approach is not to be encouraged, however, because tumour markers are not perfect tests and the finding of an elevated marker does not mean that a patient has a disease.

TUMOUR MARKER	ASSOCIATED TUMOURS
CA-125	Ovarian
CA-19-9	Pancreatic
Calcitonin	Medullary thyroid
Carcinoembryonic antigen (CEA)	Colorectal
Catecholamines	Phaeochromocytoma
α-Fetoprotein (FP)	Hepatocellular carcinoma; testicular teratoma
Human chorionic gonadotrophin (β-hCG)	Testicular teratoma and seminoma Choriocarcinoma
5-Hydroxyindoleacetic acid (5-HIAA)	Carcinoid syndrome
M-protein (paraprotein)	Multiple myeloma
Prostate-specific antigen (PSA)	Prostate

Examination of urine

Examination of a patient's urine can provide a wealth of information. For bedside tests involving urine, see pages 342–344. Microbiological examination is commonly performed on urine, and this is considered on page 95.

Protein quantification

The protein content of urine is often measured as a test of glomerular integrity. A 24-hour collection of urine can be analysed and results given in terms of grams of protein excreted in 24 h. It is often more convenient, however, to collect a 5-ml urine sample from a patient and measure either total protein or albumin, together with creatinine. In this way a protein:creatinine ratio (PCR) or albumin:creatinine ratio (ACR) can be determined. Exact reference ranges differ from lab to lab and between sexes, but, as a rule of thumb, an ACR <3 mg/mmol is normal, between 3 and 30 mg/mmol equates to microalbuminuria and >30 mg/mmol to proteinuria. In nephrotic syndrome, patients excrete >3 g protein every 24 h.

Urinary biochemistry in acute kidney injury

Acute kidney injury is a common problem in clinical practice. A common cause of this is renal hypoperfusion. Urine is often analysed for electrolyte content in such patients to enable the differentiation of prerenal uraemia from acute tubular necrosis. Patients with prerenal uraemia would be expected to recover faster than those with acute tubular necrosis when appropriate therapy is initiated.

The key to correct interpretation of urinary electrolytes is understanding that, in prerenal uraemia, normal renal regulatory mechanisms remain intact and attempt to maintain homeostasis. The juxtaglomerular apparatus senses the reduction in renal blood flow and activates the renin-angiotensin-aldosterone system. The end-product, aldosterone, acts to promote sodium reabsorption in the distal convoluted tubule. This results in an increase in the circulating volume. Therefore, in prerenal uraemia, the urinary sodium is low.

In acute tubular necrosis, the normal physiological mechanisms break down. Urinary sodium is therefore high.

It is difficult to interpret urinary sodium levels when a patient is taking a diuretic.

The fractional sodium excretion (FE_{Na}) is sometimes measured in addition. This is simply a measure of the proportion of sodium that is filtered at the glomerulus that ends up in the urine. The FE_{Na} will therefore be low in prerenal uraemia and high in acute tubular necrosis.

The following table summarises the differences.

	PRERENAL URAEMIA	ACUTE TUBULAR NECROSIS
Urinary sodium (mmol/l)	<20	>40
FE_{Na} (%)	<1	>1
Urine concentration	Concentrated	Relatively dilute

The measurement of urinary sodium can also be helpful in patients with hyponatraemia, and in those in whom assessment of volume status is necessary (see page 3).

Osmolality

Urinary osmolality can be measured in the same way as serum osmolality. Very dilute urine has an osmolality <100 mosmol/kg. Urinary osmolality can be helpful in assessing patients with disturbances of serum sodium.

Analysis of pleural fluid

In health, only a small volume of fluid surrounds the pleural lining of the lung. In various pathological states, excess fluid can accumulate forming a pleural effusion. When a significant volume has collected it may be detected on clinical examination or seen on a chest radiograph. Approximately 300 ml of fluid must be present before a pleural effusion is apparent on a chest radiograph. Pleural fluid is not the only fluid that can collect within the pleural cavity. Blood in the pleural space is termed a haemothorax, lymph a chylothorax, and pus an empyema.

Analysis of this fluid may help determine the cause of the effusion, knowledge of which is vital in planning treatment. If significant volumes of fluid are removed there can also be symptomatic benefit to the patient. Fluid is collected by performing pleural aspiration ('a pleural tap') which should be performed under imaging guidance.

A number of key parameters are analysed routinely, with many additional tests being possible on request. The first fundamental point to establish is whether the effusion is unilateral or bilateral. Unilateral effusions are more likely to be 'exudates' and bilateral effusions are more likely to be 'transudates', but this is not always the case. The protein concentration of the pleural fluid is a good starting point for fluid analysis.

DON'T FORGET

Unilateral pleural effusions are more likely to be exudates.

For pleural effusions

Exudate ≥30 g/l of protein
Transudate <30 g/l of protein

Reliance on the fluid protein concentration is most useful when there is a clear clinical suspicion of either exudate or transudate, and when the protein concentration of the fluid is either much higher or much lower than 30 g/l. Occasionally, reliance on the protein concentration can result in misclassifying an exudate as a transudate, or vice versa. For this reason, 'Light's criteria' can be used to make the distinction with greater certainty. This requires knowledge of pleural fluid and serum protein levels, as well as lactate dehydrogenase (LDH) levels.

'LIGHT'S CRITERIA'
A pleural effusion is likely to be an exudate if one or more of the following conditions are met: • Pleural fluid:serum protein ratio >0.5 • Pleural fluid LDH >200 U/l (commonly taken as more than two-thirds of the upper limit of normal for blood) • Pleural fluid:serum LDH ratio >0.6 Light RW, MacGregor MI, Luchsinger PC, et al. Pleural effusions: the diagnostic separation of transudates and exudates. *Ann Intern Med* 1972;**77**:507–13.

COMMON BIOCHEMICAL PARAMETERS ANALYSED IN PLEURAL FLUID	REASON FOR ANALYSIS
Total protein	Differentiate exudate and transudate
Lactate dehydrogenase (LDH)	Differentiate exudate and transudate
pH	Low in empyema. If pH <7.2, chest drain insertion should be strongly considered

ADDITIONAL PARAMETERS ANALYSED IN PLEURAL FLUID	INTERPRETATION
Glucose	Low in rheumatoid disease
Rheumatoid factor	High in rheumatoid disease
Amylase	High in pancreatitis
Haematocrit	High in haemothorax
Lipids	High triglyceride with low cholesterol in chylothorax

COMMON CAUSES OF A TRANSUDATE PLEURAL EFFUSION
Cardiac failure Liver failure Nephrotic syndrome (think 'renal failure' for ease of memory) Hypoalbuminaemia ('nutritional failure') Hypothyroidism ('thyroid failure')

Hooper C, Lee YC, Maskell N. Investigation of a unilateral pleural effusion in adults: British Thoracic Society pleural disease guideline 2010. *Thorax* 2010;**65**(suppl 2):ii4–17.

DON'T FORGET

Transudates are usually associated with FAILURE.

COMMON CAUSES OF AN EXUDATE PLEURAL EFFUSION
Cancer
Pneumonia (parapneumonic effusion)
Pulmonary embolus/infarction
Tuberculosis
Connective tissue disease (eg rheumatoid disease)
Acute pancreatitis

DON'T FORGET

An exudate exudes (pumps out) protein so the protein content is normally high.

The colour of the fluid aspirated from a pleural effusion also gives useful information as to the potential cause.

COLOUR OF FLUID	DIAGNOSIS
Straw	Normal
Yellow	Infected
Blood stained	Traumatic, malignancy
Frank blood	Mesothelioma, trauma, other malignancy
Pus	Empyema
Food debris	Oesophageal rupture

Pleural fluid is commonly sent to culture when infection is suspected.

Analysis of peritoneal fluid

In health, peritoneal fluid is present only in small volumes. In illness it may collect in vast quantities, in which case it should be detected on clinical examination. Smaller volumes may be detected on imaging. An abnormal collection of peritoneal fluid is termed 'ascites'.

Paracentesis (often termed 'peritoneal tap') may be undertaken for diagnostic purposes. Alternatively, large volumes of fluid can be removed to provide symptomatic benefit to the patient.

Analysis of peritoneal fluid has two main purposes:

- To characterise the disease causing ascites
- To detect infection.

Characterising the disease causing ascites

The most common cause of ascites by far is portal hypertension secondary to liver cirrhosis. However, there are a great many other causes. It is important to be able to distinguish between these. In a method analogous to pleural fluid analysis, the causes of ascites can be divided into whether they cause an exudate or a transudate. The total protein content is used to differentiate between the two, with a cut-off level of 25 g/l.

FOR ASCITES
Exudate ≥25 g/l of protein
Transudate <25 g/l of protein

CAUSES OF TRANSUDATE ASCITES
Cirrhosis
Cardiac failure
Hypoalbuminaemia
Nephrotic syndrome

CAUSES OF EXUDATE ASCITES
Intraperitoneal malignancy (primary or secondary)
Intraperitoneal infection including tuberculosis
Pancreatitis
Hypothyroidism
Chylous ascites

Characterising ascites is, however, notoriously unreliable. Accuracy can be improved by comparing the albumin content of the ascitic fluid with its level in the serum. This yields a serum-ascites albumin gradient (SAAG) as shown in the box.

Serum-ascites albumin gradient

SAAG (g/l) = Serum albumin (g/l) - Ascites albumin (g/l)

If the SAAG is ≥11 g/l, one can say that the patient is very likely to have portal hypertension. Bear in mind, however, that a patient may have portal hypertension alongside another cause of ascites. Other causes listed in the 'Transudate' box are possibilities. If the SAAG is <11 g/l, the causes listed in the 'Exudate' box are more likely.

The detection of infection in ascitic fluid is extremely important. The white cell count (WCC) of the ascites is increased in peritonitis. In most patients with ascites associated with cirrhosis, peritonitis is a primary problem, and is termed 'spontaneous bacterial peritonitis' (SBP). Occasionally another cause of peritonitis, such as a subphrenic abscess or perforated bowel, can be mistaken for SBP.

The diagnosis of SBP can be made when bacteria are identified after culturing ascitic fluid. However, this process takes some time, so the ascites WCC is usually used to guide treatment. This result should be available within a matter of hours. An ascites neutrophil count ≥250 cells/mm^3 (0.25 x 10^9/l) is in keeping with SBP. If the clinical setting fits with this diagnosis, treatment with an appropriate antibiotic should be commenced.

DON'T FORGET

Ascites neutrophil count of ≥250 cells/mm^3 is in keeping with SBP.

An alternative cause for peritonitis (eg perforated bowel) should be suspected when multiple organisms are seen on Gram staining.

Other biochemical tests commonly performed on peritoneal fluid are shown in the table below.

PARAMETER	PURPOSE
Total protein content and albumin	To distinguish exudates and transudates To calculate the serum-ascites albumin gradient
Culture	To identify bacteria
Glucose	Low in malignant ascites
Amylase	Raised in ascites associated with pancreatitis

Analysis of cerebrospinal fluid

Biochemical investigations are commonly performed on cerebrospinal fluid (CSF). Please refer to page 347 for consideration of this topic.

Analysis of synovial fluid

Patients with acute monoarthritis often have synovial fluid aspirated for diagnostic purposes. It is important to be able to differentiate between the common causes of the acutely red, hot and swollen joint on the basis of fluid analysis.

DIAGNOSIS	APPEARANCE	LEUKOCYTE COUNT (/mm^3)	APPEARANCE ON PLANE POLARISED LIGHT MICROSCOPY
Septic arthritis	Purulent	>750 000	
Haemarthrosis	Heavily blood stained		
Gout	Cloudy	3000–40 000	Negatively birefringent needle-shaped crystals
Pseudogout	Cloudy	3000–40 000	Weakly positively birefringent rhomboidal crystals

MEMORY AID

Gout – remember the letter 'N' – **N**egatively birefringent, **N**eedle-shaped crystals of sodium urate

Pseudogout – remember the letter 'P' – weakly **P**ositively birefringent rhomboidal crystals of sodium **P**yrophosphate

Other common tests

Urate (uric acid)

Urate is produced during the metabolism of purines, and is excreted by the kidneys. High levels in the blood (hyperuricaemia) can occur through two mechanisms:

- Increased purine consumption or uric acid production
- Impaired excretion of uric acid.

A modest amount of the body's purines is ingested in food and drink. A patient with a raised urate level may be asymptomatic or may be troubled with gout. It is common practice to measure serum urate levels in any patient with an acute monoarthritis. High levels of urate support a diagnosis of gout. However, urate levels can be normal during an acute attack of gout.

DON'T FORGET

Urate levels may be normal during an acute attack of gout.

Faecal elastase

The measurement of the elastase content of faeces is an excellent test for detecting pancreatic insufficiency. Low faecal elastase suggests exocrine pancreatic insufficiency, such as is seen in some patients with chronic pancreatitis. Patients with this problem may need to take enzymes with their meals to help with digestion.

Sweat testing

Cystic fibrosis results from a mutation in the gene that encodes the cystic fibrosis transmembrane conductance regulator (CFTR). CFTR is responsible for chloride ion transport across epithelial cells, and abnormalities in its structure result in viscous secretions, particularly in the lung and pancreas.

Abnormal sweat gland function leads to high concentrations of sodium and chloride in the sweat. Indeed, excessively salty tasting sweat was noted to be a clinical feature of cystic fibrosis long before the genetics were fully understood. This feature underlies the diagnostic test for cystic fibrosis – the sweat test.

In this test, sweating is stimulated, and sweat collected for analysis. Sufficient sweat (100 mg) must be collected for the test to be reliable. The test is positive if more than 60 mmol/l of chloride is present, and the test should always be repeated before a conclusion is reached. Measurements of sweat sodium concentration are less reliable, but a concentration of greater than 90 mmol/l is in keeping with cystic fibrosis.

There are instances when a false-positive sweat test can occur. The most common of these are listed below.

COMMON CAUSES OF A FALSE-POSITIVE SWEAT TEST
Adrenal insufficiency
Anorexia nervosa
Coeliac disease
Hypothyroidism

BIOCHEMISTRY – WHAT YOU NEED TO KNOW

- In hyponatraemia, an accurate estimation of a patient's volume status is critical.
- SIADH is a diagnosis of exclusion.
- Think about high and low levels of salts under the headings 'intake', 'shifts' and 'losses'.
- Hyperkalaemia is a life-threatening medical emergency and requires urgent action.
- There are many ways to assess kidney function, each with its own pros and cons. Estimated GFR is used most commonly, but in certain circumstances (eg in acute kidney injury, pregnancy, children, amputees), it too can yield unreliable results.
- Calculated osmolality = 2 x (sodium + potassium) + urea + glucose [all in mmol/l]
- If albumin <40 g/l: adjusted calcium (mmol/l) = calcium in mmol/l + 0.02 × (40 – albumin in g/l)
- If albumin >45 g/l: adjusted calcium (mmol/l) = calcium in mmol/l - 0.02 × (albumin in g/l - 45)
- The commonest causes of hypercalcaemia are malignancy and primary hyperparathyroidism.
- In hepatocellular damage, AST and ALT will be raised predominantly.
- In cholestatis, ALP and GGT will be raised predominantly.
- Think about jaundice in terms of the headings 'pre-hepatic', 'hepatic' and 'post-hepatic'.
- When interpreting an ABG, think about oxygenation and acid-base status separately. Adopt a systematic approach to acid-base interpretation.
- The commonest causes of a high anion gap metabolic acidosis are ketoacidosis, lactic acidosis and renal failure.
- There are many causes of a raised troponin other than myocardial infarction.
- For pleural effusions, 30 g/l of protein is the cut-off between exudates and transudates, although using Light's criteria can be more reliable.
- For ascites, 25 g/l of protein is the cut-off between exudates and transudates, but one should always calculate the serum-ascites albumin gradient to characterise fluid with more certainty.

2

THERAPEUTIC DRUG MONITORING AND TOXICOLOGY

Therapeutic drug monitoring

Several drugs in common use have narrow therapeutic windows. This means that there is a relatively small difference between the dose required to produce the desired effects and the dose that causes toxicity. These drugs are often monitored to ensure that a patient is taking the correct dose. It is important that you are aware of the existence of these drugs and some important points relating to when blood samples should be taken. The key facts are listed in the box below.

DRUG	NOTES
Antimicrobials, eg gentamicin, tobramycin, vancomycin, teicoplanin, amikacin	Peak and trough levels often checked until correct dosing regimen established
Anti-rejection drugs, eg ciclosporin, tacrolimus	Overdose can cause adverse effects; underdosing can cause rejection
Anticonvulsants, eg phenytoin	'Trough' level recommended
Digoxin	Sample blood 6–8 h post-dosing
Lithium	Sample blood 12 h post-dosing
Theophylline	Tested less often now

Azathioprine is commonly used as a steroid-sparing drug in patients with autoimmune disease. It is standard practice to measure thiopurine methyltransferase (TMPT) activity before initiating this drug, because, if a patient has inadequate TPMT activity, he or she would be at risk of bone marrow failure if he or she were to take this drug.

Toxicology

Poisoning is one of the most common causes of admission to hospital. It is most often deliberate, but can also be accidental (especially in children), or due to the accumulation of prescribed medications.

The management of a poisoned patient largely involves supportive care, allowing the body to excrete or metabolise a drug naturally. In certain circumstances, antidotes may be necessary along with the use of other methods designed to clear a drug more quickly from the body.

It is important that you are able to assimilate data of a variety of types when treating a poisoned patient.

Paracetamol

Paracetamol (called acetaminophen in the USA) is one of the most common drugs taken in cases of self-poisoning. When taken in overdose quantities, paracetamol metabolites deplete antioxidant stores in hepatocytes and can result in liver damage. If a patient takes a significant quantity of paracetamol and is delayed in their presentation to hospital, the following abnormalities may be apparent:

1. Elevated liver enzymes, particularly aspartate aminotransferase (AST) and alanine aminotransferase (ALT). Bilirubin levels will also rise. These changes occur because of liver cell damage. Further details on liver tests can be found on page 16.
2. Elevated prothrombin time (PT) (and international normalised ratio [INR], because this is calculated from the PT). This occurs because of impaired liver synthesis of clotting factors. Further details on PT and INR can be found on pages 84 and 85.
3. Impaired kidney function (elevated urea and creatinine). This can arise secondary to liver impairment (hepatorenal syndrome) or sometimes as a direct effect of paracetamol metabolites on the kidney.
4. Metabolic acidosis mainly due to liver failure. This will be a high anion gap metabolic acidosis. For further details, refer to page 27.

Administration of an antidote, *N*-acetylcysteine, can help patients after a significant paracetamol overdose. This agent replenishes liver antioxidant stores.

On most occasions in clinical practice, patients present to hospital within a few hours of taking an overdose. Although *N*-acetylcysteine is a fairly safe and effective drug, anaphylaxis has been reported after its administration. It is therefore routine practice to weigh up whether or not a patient requires antidote administration. This is done by measuring blood paracetamol levels and using the nomogram in Fig 2.1 (which can be found in the *British National Formulary*).

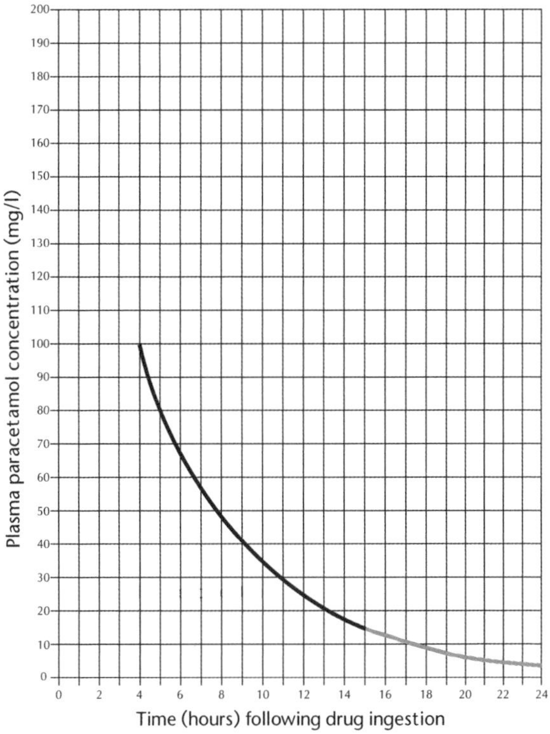

Fig 2.1: Nomogram to assist in deciding who requires treatment in paracetamol poisoning.

Timing of the overdose is critical because blood levels are interpretable only if the time of drug ingestion is known. You will note that the line on the nomogram starts at 4 hours - blood levels taken within 4 hours of ingestion are meaningless because absorption will be incomplete, and levels could rise if blood is re-sampled later. Once timing has been established and the post-4-hour blood levels measured, plot the patient's data on the nomogram. If the patient's level lies above the relevant line at the time point chosen, then they are deemed to be at significant risk of liver injury, and the antidote should be administered. If their level is below the treatment line, the risk of liver damage is small and treatment is not generally required.

As mentioned, knowledge of the time of ingestion is critical. It is, however, acknowledged that it is often extremely difficult to be certain about this, because patients who have taken an overdose are often intoxicated, drowsy or generally uncooperative. One should collect information from every available source, and generally speaking one should have a low threshold for treatment if details are sketchy. Another point of note is that the nomogram curve flattens considerably towards the right side of the chart.

The differences in blood levels between whom to treat and whom not to treat if presentation is delayed are very small, and generally treatment should be instigated in all cases of delayed presentation. Patients who have taken a potentially lethal quantity of paracetamol (>12 g in most circumstances) but who present earlier than 4 hours should generally receive treatment, which can be stopped if their post-4-hour drug level suggests that treatment is not required. In addition, patients who have taken a staggered overdose should generally be treated regardless of the blood level.

DON'T FORGET

Always check plasma paracetamol levels at least 4 h after ingestion.

It used to be standard practice to stratify patients poisoned with paracetamol as at 'normal' risk or 'high' risk of developing problems. This is no longer done - all patients are now considered to be high risk.

Salicylate

Salicylates (such as aspirin) are found in a wide variety of preparations commonly available in households and are therefore taken reasonably commonly in overdose. Two main types of data can be useful in salicylate poisoning:

1. **Salicylate levels:** the higher the level, the greater the likelihood of symptoms and organ damage, and the more likely it will be that specific treatments will be required to increase clearance of salicylate from the body. The absorption of salicylates can be slow. It is therefore good practice to repeat blood levels at intervals until they start to fall.
2. **Abnormalities of acid-base balance:** see page 25 for detailed information about the interpretation of acid-base abnormalities. Significant salicylate overdose produces a characteristic pattern of acid-base disturbance. The respiratory centre in the brain is stimulated, causing patients to hyperventilate and 'blow off' carbon dioxide. The levels of the acidic gas carbon dioxide therefore fall, resulting in a respiratory alkalosis. At the same time, however, a metabolic acidosis develops due to the production of a variety of acids. Levels of bicarbonate fall, and the pH becomes acidic. The overall effect on a particular patient is hard to predict. Either alkalosis or acidosis can predominate, or alternatively the pH can remain neutral due to opposing respiratory and metabolic effects.

Opioids

Significant opioid poisoning will have a variety of effects on the patient. From a data interpretation perspective, however, the one piece of data that can provide a clue to the fact that opioids have been taken is the respiratory rate. Opioids suppress respiratory drive, so, if a patient has taken a cocktail of unknown drugs and the respiratory rate is slow, it would be reasonable to assume that they have taken an opioid and to administer the antidote (naloxone).

Tricyclic antidepressants

Tricyclic antidepressants (TCAs) such as amitriptyline are extremely dangerous when taken in overdose. The two major clinical complications that can arise are:

1. Cardiac toxicity – this can cause hypotension, arrhythmias and cardiac arrest
2. Seizures.

It would seem logical that one should measure blood levels of these drugs to predict which patients are likely to develop problems. This is, however, not part of routine management, and the following two tests are much more useful:

1. An electrocardiograph (ECG). Please see Chapter 12 for more information on ECG interpretation. There are two major signs on the ECG that indicate that a significant TCA overdose has been taken:
   (a) QRS broadening: the normal QRS width is $<$120 ms (three small squares on ECG paper). In the setting of TCA overdose, any QRS widening over 100 ms is significant. The broader the QRS complex, the higher the risk of cardiac arrhythmia and seizure.
   (b) Abnormally tall R wave in lead aVR, as shown in Fig 2.2.

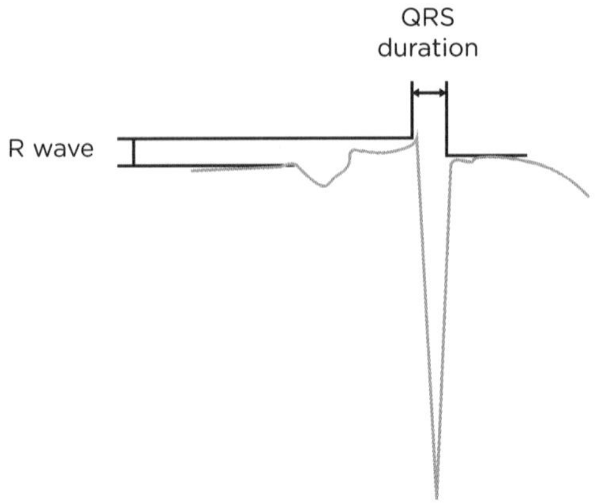

Normal ECG appearance in lead aVR

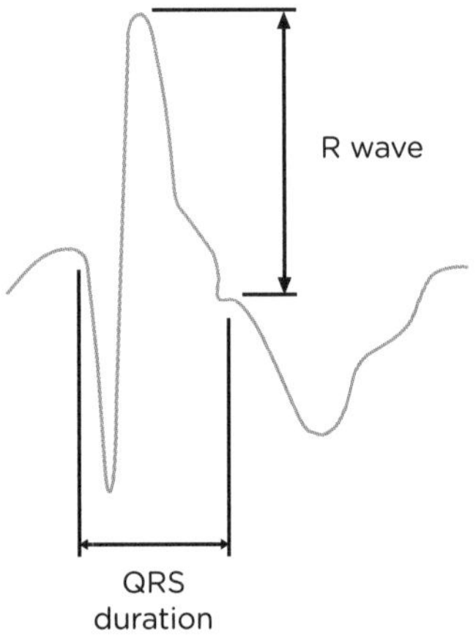

ECG appearance in lead aVR in severe tricyclic antidepressant poisoning

Fig 2.2: ECG Lead aVR changes in tricyclic antidepressant poisoning.

2. Arterial blood gas analysis: a metabolic acidosis can occur in significant TCA overdose and should be treated with sodium bicarbonate. A respiratory acidosis may also occur.

Toxic alcohols

Toxic alcohols include ethylene glycol (antifreeze) and methanol. They can cause a range of problems when ingested, and often antidote therapy and/or dialysis is required to improve the outcome. The two key biochemical abnormalities that are useful in diagnosis are a high anion gap metabolic acidosis (see page 25) and a high osmolar gap (see page 11). It is possible to directly measure toxic alcohols in the laboratory, but this is a very specialised test and may not always be available.

Drugs of abuse

Urine testing for drug metabolites

A number of drugs can be detected in urine. A urine drug screen is often requested when a patient presents with unusual symptoms and there is a suspicion of potential drug use.

TYPICAL COMPONENTS OF URINE 'DRUGS' SCREEN
Amphetamines, barbiturates, benzodiazepines, methadone, cannabinoids, cocaine metabolites, LSD and opiates

THERAPEUTIC DRUG MONITORING AND TOXICOLOGY - WHAT YOU NEED TO KNOW

- Drugs with narrow therapeutic windows tend to have levels checked regularly since there is a fine line between under-dosing (with low efficacy) and over-dosing (with toxicity).
- It is critical that samples are taken at the correct times, or interpretation will be difficult.
- In paracetamol poisoning, blood levels must be taken at least 4 hours post-ingestion to enable correct treatment decisions to be made.
- In salicylate poisoning, patients can have a mixed respiratory alkalosis and metabolic acidosis.
- ECG abnormalities are common in tricyclic antidepressant overdose: QRS broadening and abnormalities of the R wave in aVR.
- Think about toxic alcohol ingestion in a patient with a high anion gap metabolic acidosis and a high osmolar gap.

3

ENDOCRINOLOGY

Endocrine disorders can be divided into primary and secondary disorders. In a primary endocrine gland disorder, the problem lies within the endocrine gland itself. Thus, in primary hyperthyroidism, the principal problem is an overactive thyroid gland. Secondary endocrine diseases arise when there is a problem with the hormones controlling the activity of the target gland, such as the overproduction of a hormone by the pituitary gland.

Interpretation of stimulation and suppression tests in endocrinology necessitates knowledge of the normal range of responses. As cut-off values differ between guidelines and hospitals, none are provided here. Rather, the principles of the tests are explained.

Pituitary disease

Six hormones are released from the anterior pituitary gland (thyroid-stimulating hormone [TSH], adrenocorticotrophic hormone [ACTH], prolactin, growth hormone [GH], luteinising hormone [LH] and follicle-stimulating hormone [FSH]). Two hormones are released from the posterior pituitary gland (ADH and oxytocin).

Pituitary disease can result in hormone deficiency (hypopituitarism) or excess. Hypopituitarism has a range of causes (see box below). Hormone excess is usually caused by a pituitary tumour. The mainstays of pituitary investigations are hormone tests and imaging (usually MRI).

CAUSES OF HYPOPITUITARISM (MNEMONIC – 'VITAMIN')
Vascular – Sheehan syndrome, pituitary apoplexy
Iatrogenic, eg post-surgery or radiotherapy
Trauma
Anorexia nervosa
Miscellaneous causes, eg sarcoidosis, haemochromatosis
Infective, eg tuberculous meningitis
Neoplasia

Thyroid-stimulating hormone

For problems pertaining to TSH, see 'Thyroid hormones' – page 60.

Adrenocorticotrophic hormone

For problems pertaining to ACTH, see 'Adrenal hormones' - page 62.

Prolactin

There are many causes of a raised serum prolactin level (see box below). Very high levels (>5000 mU/l) strongly suggest a prolactin-secreting pituitary tumour.

COMMON CAUSES OF HYPERPROLACTINAEMIA

Physiological:
- Pregnancy
- Lactation

Prolactin-secreting pituitary tumour

Medications:
- Phenothiazine antipsychotics
- Most antiemetics

Polycystic ovarian syndrome

Following a seizure

Primary hypothyroidism

Another cause is so-called 'macro-prolactin'. This is of no known pathological significance and should be identified automatically by modern laboratories.

Growth hormone

Low levels of GH in adults can cause a wide range of non-specific symptoms. Excessive GH in adults results in acromegaly. Measuring the level of GH is not a reliable method of making this diagnosis. Insulin-like growth factor I (IGF-I) concentration can be used as a marker of average GH levels and, if raised, is suggestive of acromegaly. The definitive test for the diagnosis is a glucose tolerance test, exactly like that used in the investigation of hyperglycaemia. The test is performed in the same manner, but GH levels are measured. Failure of the GH level to fall below a defined level is in keeping with a diagnosis of acromegaly.

Luteinising hormone and follicle-stimulating hormone

For problems pertaining to LH and FSH, see 'Gonadal hormones' - page 67.

Antidiuretic hormone

The two major syndromes associated with ADH are: SIADH - ADH excess; and diabetes insipidus (DI) - ADH insufficiency. SIADH is considered on page 5. DI is considered in the box opposite.

Polyuria with polydipsia

The combination of passing excessive volumes of urine (polyuria) with excessive thirst (polydipsia) is a frequently occurring problem. The most common cause is diabetes mellitus, which is considered elsewhere. The water deprivation test is used to differentiate between two major causes - psychogenic polydipsia and diabetes insipidus (DI).

Patients with psychogenic polydipsia simply drink fluid in excess for psychological or psychiatric reasons.

In DI, there is a problem with antidiuretic hormone (ADH). ADH normally acts on the collecting ducts in the kidney to stimulate water reabsorption. If ADH does not function properly, too much urine is passed. In turn the patient becomes relatively dehydrated and drinks to compensate for this.

MEMORY AID

Diuretic medications increase urine volume.

Therefore, antidiuretic hormone (ADH) does the opposite, and acts to conserve water.

There are two forms of DI - cranial and nephrogenic. In cranial DI, there is a problem with the release of ADH from the hypothalamus. Blood levels of ADH are low. In nephrogenic DI, there is sufficient ADH in the system, but it fails to exert its effects on the kidney.

The water deprivation test restricts patients' intake of water. If they have psychogenic polydipsia, reducing water intake will solve their problem and they will gradually return to normal. However, with DI, water restriction will result in a worsening state of dehydration.

The test involves forbidding the patient to drink in a carefully supervised environment. Blood and urine osmolalities are tested each hour for a period of 8 h. In health (or psychogenic polydipsia), one would expect the patient to retain water and to pass increasingly concentrated urine (with a high urine osmolality). In DI, the urine osmolality does not rise, and the patient becomes dehydrated with a rise in serum osmolality.

To differentiate between the two forms of DI, patients are then given a dose of a synthetic ADH compound called desmopressin. This will correct the problem in cranial DI, but will have no effect in nephrogenic DI.

Oxytocin

Oxytocin is seldom measured in clinical practice.

Thyroid hormones

Normally, thyrotropin-releasing hormone (TRH) is released from the hypothalamus and stimulates the pituitary gland to release thyroid-stimulating hormone (TSH). This hormone then acts on the thyroid gland and results in the liberation of thyroxine (T_4) and triiodothyronine (T_3) into the circulation. These hormones exert negative feedback on both the hypothalamus and the pituitary, and result in a reduction in the production of TRH and TSH. Most of the T_3 and T_4 in the body is carried by carrier proteins (principally thyroxine-binding globulin, TBG). A small percentage is present in unbound form, and it is this that is physiologically active. In clinical practice, the commonly measured hormones are TSH, free T_4 and T_3. Total T_4 (ie bound and unbound forms) is sometimes given.

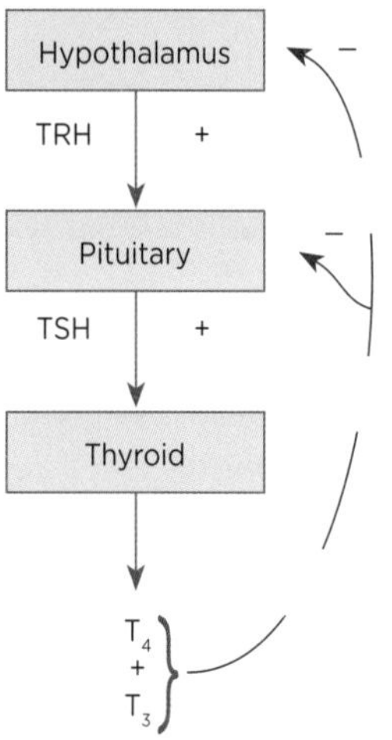

Fig 3.1: Negative feedback loops for thyroid hormone production.

Hyperthyroidism

In primary hyperthyroidism (eg with Graves' disease), the thyroid gland autonomously produces thyroid hormones. The levels of T_3 and T_4 therefore rise. Normal negative feedback continues, and the level of TSH will be low. In T_3 thyrotoxicosis, the T_3 level may be elevated in isolation.

In secondary hyperthyroidism (eg due to a pituitary tumour secreting TSH), the levels of T_3 and T_4 will again be high, but this time the TSH level will be inappropriately normal or high.

A similar picture (high TSH, T_3 and T_4) can also be seen in thyroid hormone resistance, and when there is a problem measuring the hormones due to a technical issue in the laboratory.

DON'T FORGET

The finding of a normal TSH level in the setting of raised T_3 and T_4 should raise suspicions of a pituitary lesion, since in normal circumstances the TSH level will be suppressed.

Hypothyroidism

In primary hypothyroidism the thyroid gland is defective. The levels of T_3 and T_4 are low. As a result of reduced negative feedback, the TSH level will be high.

'Subclinical hypothyroidism' is the term used to describe the situation when T_3 and T_4 are normal but TSH is raised. Treatment with thyroxine is advised in specific circumstances.

In secondary hypothyroidism (eg destructive pituitary tumour), the levels of T_3 and T_4 will again be low, but this is because of low TSH levels.

Sick euthyroid syndrome

Caution should be taken when interpreting thyroid function tests in a patient with an acute illness. This is because thyroid function tests are often abnormal during the acute phase of an illness, but normalise on its resolution. This phenomenon is known as the sick euthyroid syndrome, indicating that the patient is euthyroid (ie normal thyroid function), but that he or she has an intercurrent illness. The common picture in sick euthyroid syndrome is one of low T_3 and T_4 with low or normal TSH.

DON'T FORGET

Be cautious when interpreting thyroid function tests in an acutely unwell patient.

SUMMARY OF HORMONE CHANGES IN VARIOUS THYROID DISEASE STATES

	T_3/T_4	TSH
Primary hyperthyroidism	↑	↓
T_3 thyrotoxicosis	Only T_3 ↑	↓
Secondary hyperthyroidism	↑	N
Primary hypothyroidism	↓	↑
Secondary hypothyroidism	↓	↓
Sick euthyroid syndrome	↓	N

Variations in thyroxine-binding globulin levels

Care must be taken when interpreting free and total T_4 levels. This is because the level of TBG can vary in various states. Always remember that it is the level of free hormone that is important physiologically. Factors influencing the level of TBG are listed below.

INCREASE TBG	DECREASE TBG
High oestrogen states, eg pregnancy, oral contraceptive pill use	High corticosteroid levels
Hypothyroidism	Protein deficiency states: low intake (malnutrition); low synthesis (chronic liver disease); increased losses (nephrotic syndrome)
	Thyrotoxicosis

Adrenal hormones

Normally, corticotrophin-releasing hormone (CRH) is released from the hypothalamus and stimulates the pituitary gland to release adrenocorticotrophic hormone (ACTH). This hormone then acts on the adrenal cortex and results in the release of glucocorticoids. Glucocorticoids exert negative feedback on both the hypothalamus and pituitary, and result in a reduction in the production of CRH and ACTH (Fig 3.2).

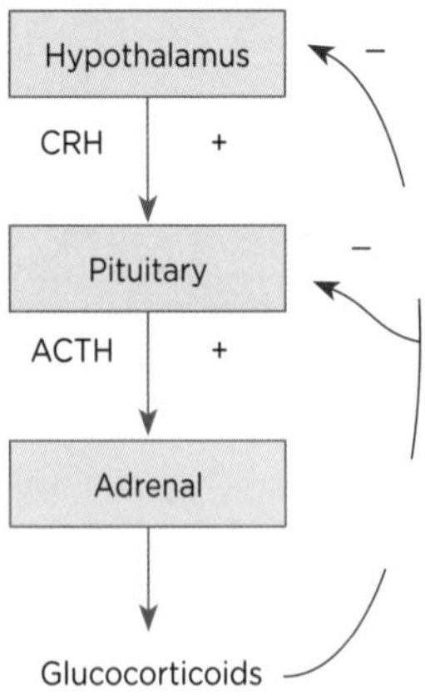

Fig 3.2: Negative feedback loops for adrenal hormone production.

Cushing syndrome

Cushing syndrome results from glucocorticoid excess. It is seen most commonly in patients receiving glucocorticoid treatment, eg for chronic severe asthma. Endogenous forms of Cushing syndrome have several causes which are listed below.

ENDOGENOUS CAUSES OF CUSHING SYNDROME
Primary adrenal disease • Adrenal tumour (adenoma or carcinoma)
ACTH excess • From the pituitary gland (Cushing's disease) • From an ACTH-producing tumour outside the pituitary, eg lung cancer

In primary adrenal disease causing Cushing syndrome, the adrenal gland autonomously produces adrenal hormones. Normal negative feedback continues, and the level of ACTH will be low.

In instances of secondary hyperadrenalism (eg due to a pituitary tumour), the ACTH level will be normal or high.

There are several methods for screening for Cushing syndrome:

1. **Measure free cortisol in a 24-hour urine collection**

   An elevated level of free cortisol in the urine is in keeping with Cushing syndrome. An abnormal test should be followed up by a repeat test in the first instance.

2. **Perform a 1-mg overnight dexamethasone suppression test**

   In healthy individuals, taking 1 mg dexamethasone will have a negative feedback effect on the pituitary gland, thereby decreasing ACTH and hence cortisol production. In patients with Cushing syndrome, cortisol production will not be affected, and hence a cortisol test the morning after dosing will reveal abnormally elevated cortisol levels.

3. **Perform a low-dose dexamethasone suppression test**

   The rationale for this test is similar to that for the overnight suppression test. For this test, however, 0.5 mg dexamethasone is given 6-hourly for 48 hours. A cortisol level taken 6 hours after the last dose will reveal an abnormally elevated level in patients with Cushing syndrome.

Other more specialised tests can also be used to confirm the diagnosis and to help differentiate between the causes of Cushing syndrome.

1. **Perform a high-dose dexamethasone suppression test**

   This is similar to the low-dose test in execution, although 2 mg rather than 0.5 mg of dexamethasone is given 6-hourly. In Cushing's disease (pituitary hypersecretion of ACTH), cortisol will be suppressed, but, in other causes of Cushing syndrome, cortisol secretion will not suppress to the same extent.

2. **Perform a corticotrophin-releasing hormone (CRH) test**

   Exogenous administration of CRH will cause the cortisol level to rise if Cushing's disease is present. No rise is expected with other causes.

3. **Check ACTH levels**

4. **Undertake imaging studies**

   Imaging of the adrenal glands using CT or MRI is often performed. Imaging of other body areas will be necessary if ectopic ACTH secretion is suspected.

5. **Adrenal vein sampling**

   It is possible, although technically challenging, to introduce an intravenous catheter into the veins draining the adrenal glands and sample blood there. Measuring hormone levels in this blood can identify hypersecretion of a hormone and can identify asymmetry of secretion if, for example, there is a tumour in one of the glands.

Nieman LK, Biller BM, Findling JW, et al. The diagnosis of Cushing's syndrome. *J Clin Endocrinol Metab* 2008;**93**:1526–40.

Primary hyperaldosteronism

Patients with this disorder have a tendency to retain sodium and lose potassium. You should consider it in hypertensive patients, especially if they have hypokalaemia.

The measurement of aldosterone and renin levels is important in patients suspected of having primary hyperaldosteronism. In this condition, aldosterone levels are elevated and renin levels are suppressed (due to negative feedback mechanisms). Measuring these hormones is fraught with difficulty because the levels vary depending on posture (lying or standing, for example), and can be affected by a variety of drugs. The particular way in which the hormones are measured and the units of measurement vary between laboratories, so take care when interpreting results that you understand what is being reported.

In order to screen carefully selected patients for the presence of primary hyperaldosteronism, increasing emphasis is being placed on the ratio between aldosterone and renin levels (the aldosterone:renin ratio or ARR). If plasma aldosterone concentration is given in nanograms/decilitre and plasma renin activity in nanograms/millilitre per hour, then one frequently used cut-off for an abnormal ARR is 30. If the ARR is above this level, the patient may well have the condition and further investigations would be warranted.

There are several tests available to confirm or refute the diagnosis in patients with an abnormal ARR. One test that is commonly used is the 'saline suppression test'. The principle of the test is that an intravenous infusion of saline should reduce blood aldosterone levels. Failure of aldosterone levels to suppress after administration of saline makes the diagnosis of primary hyperaldosteronism more likely.

If the diagnosis seems likely, imaging should be performed to visualise the adrenal glands. If unilateral adrenal gland disease appears likely, blood can be sampled from the adrenal veins in an attempt to prove that aldosterone is being produced in excess.

Funder JW, Carey RM, Fardella C, et al. Case detection, diagnosis, and treatment of patients with primary aldosteronism: An Endocrine Society Clinical Practice Guideline. *J Clin Endocrinol Metab* 2010;**93**:3266–81.

Hypoadrenalism

In primary hypoadrenalism (eg Addison's disease), the adrenal gland itself is defective. As a result of reduced negative feedback, the ACTH level will be high.

In secondary hypoadrenalism, ACTH levels will be low. Patients with hypoadrenalism may develop hyponatraemia, hyperkalaemia and hypoglycaemia.

Short Synacthen® test

Synacthen®, or SYNthetic ACTH, is used to stimulate the adrenal gland. Normally, an injection of Synacthen® will result in an increase in circulating cortisol levels. If the patient has hypoadrenalism, the Synacthen® will not have its normal effect, and the rise in cortisol levels will be poor. The Synacthen® test may be normal in cases of secondary hypoadrenalism, but in long-standing disease, the adrenal gland can atrophy, resulting in an abnormal Synacthen® test also.

Insulin tolerance test

This test is used in specialist centres to assess adrenal function as well as to assess for growth hormone deficiency.

Several criteria must be met before this test can be attempted.

CRITERIA TO BE MET BEFORE PERFORMING AN INSULIN TOLERANCE TEST
Cortisol level >100 nmol/l
Normal thyroid function
No cardiovascular disease
No epilepsy or other seizure activity or blackouts

The essence of the test is to induce hypoglycaemia (blood glucose must fall to less than 2.2 mmol/l) in a carefully controlled environment. In a normal patient, a stress response will occur with a rise in cortisol and growth hormone levels.

Phaeochromocytoma

These tumours are associated with excess circulating catecholamines. Diagnosis relies on the demonstration of excessive amounts of catecholamine breakdown products in the plasma (free metanephrines) or urine (fractional metanephrines).

If levels are extremely high, phaeochromocytoma is likely. If levels are only slightly high, a 'clonidine suppression test' can be performed. Plasma free metanephrines are measured after dosing with clonidine, and would be expected to be suppressed in people without a phaeochromocytoma.

If the diagnosis seems likely, an attempt should be made to visualise the tumour. This can be done using MRI or CT. Alternatively, radionuclide scanning or positron emission tomography (PET) may be necessary.

Lenders JW, Eisenhofer G, Mannelli M, Pacak K. Phaeochromocytoma. *Lancet* 2005;**366**:665–75.

Gonadal hormones

The physiology of the gonadal hormone system is reasonably complex, particularly in females because of the menstrual cycle. In essence, however, gonadotrophin-releasing hormone (GRH) is released from the hypothalamus and stimulates the anterior pituitary to produce LH and FSH. In males, LH and FSH act on the testes and result in the formation of testosterone, spermatozoa and various proteins. There is a negative feedback loop in place. In females, LH and FSH production drives ovarian oestrogen production and ovulation. After ovulation, a corpus luteum produces oestradiol and progesterone.

Hypogonadism can be primary, when there is a problem with the testes or ovaries, or secondary, when the problem is due to the hypothalamus or pituitary. In primary hypogonadism, testosterone levels are low in males and oestradiol levels are low in females, whereas LH and FSH will be elevated in both sexes. In secondary hypogonadism, testosterone/oestradiol levels will be low, whereas LH and FSH will be low or inappropriately normal. Primary hypogonadism can result from a genetic problem or damage to the testes/ovaries. In women, a picture of primary hypogonadism is seen after the menopause. Secondary hypogonadism can be due to any of the causes of hypopituitarism (see page 57).

In pregnancy, oestrogen and progesterone levels are high, whereas LH and FSH are suppressed. The β-human chorionic gonadotrophin (β-hCG) is the hormone most frequently tested for in pregnancy tests. In early pregnancy, the level of β-hCG tends to double every 2 days. A failure of β-hCG to double in this way can be a feature of an ectopic pregnancy.

Disorders of glucose metabolism

Diabetes mellitus

The diagnosis of diabetes mellitus and related hyperglycaemic states relies on accurate interpretation of blood glucose readings. A patient's glycaemic status can be classed as one of the following:

- Normal
- Impaired fasting glucose
- Impaired glucose tolerance
- Diabetes mellitus
- Gestational diabetes mellitus.

In some circumstances, diabetes will be suspected clinically, particularly if the patient is symptomatic from hyperglycaemia. In other instances, hyperglycaemia will be detected incidentally when a blood glucose level is checked. Typical symptoms are shown in the box below.

SYMPTOMS OF DIABETES MELLITUS
Polyuria
Polydipsia
Weight loss
Fatigue
Blurring of vision
Symptoms related to a complication of diabetes such as a cutaneous abscess

An oral glucose tolerance test (OGTT) is often used in differentiating between these various states. This test involves giving the patient a 75-g glucose load by mouth, after they have been fasting. The plasma glucose level is measured at baseline and after 2 h.

Diabetes mellitus may be diagnosed in a variety of ways. Any one of the following is sufficient:

1. A single random plasma glucose of more than 11.1 mmol/l in a patient with symptoms
2. Two separate random plasma glucose samples of more than 11.1 mmol/l in a patient without symptoms
3. A single fasting plasma glucose of more than 7.0 mmol/l in a patient with symptoms
4. Two separate fasting plasma glucose samples of more than 7.0 mmol/l in a patient without symptoms
5. A plasma glucose level of 11.1 mmol/l or more 2 h after a glucose load in an OGTT. An OGTT is generally performed only if borderline results are obtained on random or fasting samples.
6. In certain circumstances, an HbA1c (see below) level ≥48 mmol/l is diagnostic of type 2 diabetes in a patient with symptoms.
7. In certain circumstances, two separate HbA1c levels ≥48 mmol/l are diagnostic of type 2 diabetes in an asymptomatic patient.

DON'T FORGET

If a patient is asymptomatic, two blood tests are required before diabetes mellitus can be diagnosed.

Patients with **normoglycaemia** (ie definitely not diabetic) have a fasting plasma glucose of less than 6.1 mmol/l. Two hours following a glucose load in an OGTT, the plasma glucose will be less than 7.8 mmol/l.

'**Impaired fasting glucose**' and '**impaired glucose tolerance**' are terms used to describe states of glycaemic control that lie somewhere between normal and frank diabetes mellitus. The terms are not mutually exclusive. It is therefore possible for a patient to have both impaired fasting glucose and impaired glucose tolerance. Alternatively, they may have one or other of the terms attached to them in isolation. The significance of labelling a patient with one of these terms lies with the fact that such patients have an increased risk of developing diabetes mellitus in the future. The diagnostic criteria are shown in the table below.

	NORMAL	IMPAIRED FASTING	IMPAIRED GLUCOSE TOLERANCE	DIABETES MELLITUS
Fasting plasma glucose (mmol/l)	<6.1	6.1–6.9	Not necessary for diagnosis	≥7.0
Plasma glucose 2 hours after glucose load in OGTT (mmol/l)	<7.8	Not necessary for diagnosis	7.8–11.0	≥11.1

Gestational diabetes mellitus describes diabetes that is of new onset in pregnancy, or that is first noted during pregnancy. The significance of gestational diabetes mellitus relates to the fact that such patients have a reasonable chance of having a 'large-for-dates' fetus, and that they have a chance of developing diabetes mellitus in later life. Gestational diabetes can be diagnosed if the fasting glucose is ≥5.6 mmol/l or if the 2-hour post-OGTT level is ≥7.8 mmol/l.

Glycated haemoglobin

Random blood glucose measurements are useful for monitoring variations on a day-to-day basis; however, the inevitable variation makes interpretation of long-term trends difficult. For this reason measurement of glycated haemoglobin (HbA1 or HbA1c) is often used.

Glycated haemoglobin is the product of the reaction between glucose and haemoglobin A (the main type of haemoglobin in most adults). The higher the average blood glucose level, the higher the glycated haemoglobin level will be. As red blood cells have an average life-span of around 120 days, glycated haemoglobin estimation provides information on the glycaemic control over this time period.

HbA1c can now be used to diagnose type 2 diabetes, with a level >4.8 mmol/mol being in keeping with this diagnosis.

Glycated haemoglobin is reliable only when normal haemoglobin is present in red blood cells that have normal life-spans. If a haemoglobin disorder is present, or in patients who have red cells with shortened life-spans (eg haemolytic anaemia), measurement of fructosamine levels may be used instead to measure glycaemic control. Fructosamine is a glycated plasma protein, and provides information on glucose levels over the previous 1–3 weeks.

Hypoglycaemia

Hypoglycaemia describes a plasma glucose that is lower than normal (less than 3.5 mmol/l). The most common cause is an imbalance between intake and insulin requirements in a patient with type 1 diabetes mellitus (eg the patient who takes their normal insulin without eating lunch). Other causes of hypoglycaemia are listed in the box.

CAUSES OF HYPOGLYCAEMIA
Imbalance between insulin and calorie intake in type 1 diabetes
Excess exogenous insulin administration
As a side effect of anti-hyperglycaemic medication
Insulinoma
Liver failure
Alcohol ingestion
Hypoadrenalism

A fairly common clinical scenario is the patient who presents with hypoglycaemia of unknown cause. Endogenous insulin (ie insulin derived from an insulinoma) can be differentiated easily from exogenous insulin (ie a patient with Munchausen syndrome who administers insulin to themselves in an attempt to seek medical attention) with a little knowledge of insulin physiology.

Normal physiological insulin is manufactured in the body from proinsulin which in turn is derived from pre-proinsulin. Each protein precursor is cleaved to yield its product. This cleavage process generates a 'waste' chain of amino acids called C-peptide.

If hypoglycaemia is due to excess endogenous insulin from an insulinoma, one would expect high insulin and C-peptide levels in a patient who is hypoglycaemic.

Exogenous insulin does not contain C-peptide. Therefore, a hypoglycaemic patient with raised levels of insulin in the blood but normal/low levels of C-peptide is likely to have been given insulin.

ENDOCRINOLOGY - WHAT YOU NEED TO KNOW

- In primary endocrine gland disorders, there is a problem with the gland itself. In secondary disorders, there is a problem with the hormones controlling the gland.
- Very high prolactin levels are strongly suggestive of a pituitary tumour.
- A water deprivation test is used to diagnose diabetes insipidus.
- Beware a normal TSH result in a patient with elevated thyroid hormones. This is abnormal and can indicate pituitary disease.
- Acutely unwell patients often have 'sick euthyroid syndrome', making their thyroid tests difficult to interpret.
- Cushing syndrome is characterised by excessive quantities of glucocorticoids. Diagnosing it relies upon demonstrating elevated levels of glucocorticoids and abnormal responses to suppression tests.
- Consider primary hyperaldosteronism in hypertensive patients with hypokalaemia. Measure the aldosterone to renin ratio first line.
- A short Synacthen® test is useful in diagnosing hypoadrenalism. With normal adrenal glands, the cortisol level should rise significantly after Synacthen® injection.
- Female sex hormone profiles vary considerably depending on the point of the menstrual cycle at which blood is sampled.
- There are many ways to diagnose diabetes mellitus, utilising measures of glucose, HbA1c or an oral glucose tolerance test.

4

HAEMATOLOGY

Full blood picture

The full blood picture (FBP) contains a wealth of information about blood cells. The typical constituent parts of an FBP are as shown in the table.

A TYPICAL FBP COMPRISES THE FOLLOWING TESTS:
Haemoglobin concentration (Hb)
Mean cell volume (MCV)
Mean corpuscular haemoglobin (MCH)
Packed cell volume (PCV)
Red cell distribution width (RDW)
White cell count (WCC) incorporating a differential white cell count
Platelet count

Abnormal red blood cells

Anaemia

Anaemia describes a low level of haemoglobin. It is usually defined by an arbitrary cut-off haemoglobin concentration (eg <130 g/l in men aged >15 years, <120 g/l in non-pregnant women aged >15 years and <110 g/l in pregnant women), below which a patient is deemed to be anaemic.

Before deciding on the particular subtype of anaemia present in a patient, it is worth looking at the other cell types described on the full blood picture. If there are problems with red cells, white cells and platelets, then the major problem is likely to be a disease of the bone marrow, and the test most likely to give the diagnosis would be a bone marrow biopsy.

If the only problem on the full blood picture is low haemoglobin, the next stage is to check the reticulocyte count if available. Reticulocytes are immature red blood cells, and will be found in increased amounts in patients who are bleeding and in those in whom red cells are being destroyed (haemolysis). The history should distinguish between these types. If the reticulocyte count is not elevated, the next step in diagnosis is to look at the size of the red cells.

Anaemia can be split into three big groups by looking at the size of the red blood cells. In microcytic anaemia red cells are small, in normocytic anaemia they are normal size and in macrocytic anaemia they are large. The mean cell volume (MCV) provides an average measurement of red cell size.

TYPE OF ANAEMIA	SIZE OF ERYTHROCYTES
Microcytic	Small
Normocytic	Normal
Macrocytic	Large

Fig 4.1 shows the various causes based on this classification of anaemia.

Note that the MCV provides a measure of average cell size, and this is reliable in most instances. If, however, a patient has two ongoing pathologies, such as iron deficiency and folate deficiency, the MCV can be unreliable. They may have two populations of red cells, one with a low MCV and another with a high MCV. When these measures are averaged, the MCV will be normal. For this reason, the red cell distribution width (RDW) is sometimes measured. This gives an indication of the distribution of red cell sizes. This measure will be raised if two red cell populations are present.

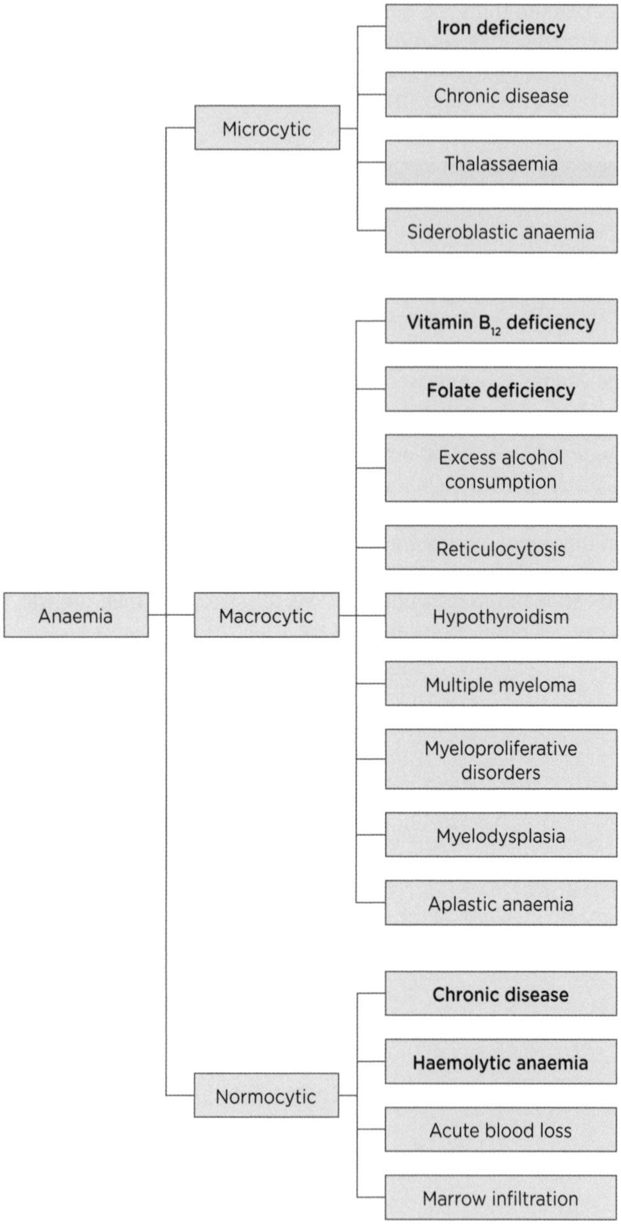

Fig 4.1: The various causes of the major classifications of anaemia.

Haemolytic anaemia

There are many causes of haemolytic anaemia, but in each case there is abnormal destruction of red blood cells.

Evidence of haemolysis

When red blood cells are destroyed, haemoglobin is degraded, and bilirubin liberated. Bilirubin is conjugated in the liver and passes into the bowel in the bile. Here, it is converted into urobilinogen by the action of bowel microbes. Some urobilinogen will be passed in the stools, whereas some will be reabsorbed and excreted in the urine, where it can be detected using a urinalysis strip. In cases of haemolysis, the plasma unconjugated bilirubin will rise, and increased amounts of urobilinogen will be detected in the urine. The level of lactate dehydrogenase (LDH) will also rise because this enzyme is normally found inside red cells and it is released when they are destroyed.

When red cells are destroyed inside blood vessels, haemoglobin is released. Haptoglobin binds to free haemoglobin and escorts it to the liver. However, haptoglobins can become saturated and in such circumstances haemoglobin may be passed in the urine (haemoglobinuria), or converted to haemosiderin which is then passed in the urine (haemosiderinuria). Alternatively, further reactions can occur which result in the presence of methaemalbumin in the circulation.

With excessive red cell destruction, the bone marrow works hard to replace the number of circulating cells. The number of primitive red cells (reticulocytes) in the circulation therefore increases.

INTRAVASCULAR HAEMOLYSIS IS SUGGESTED BY

- anaemia
- elevated bilirubin
- elevated LDH
- low haptoglobins
- elevated reticulocyte count

The causes of haemolytic anaemia are illustrated in Fig 4.2.

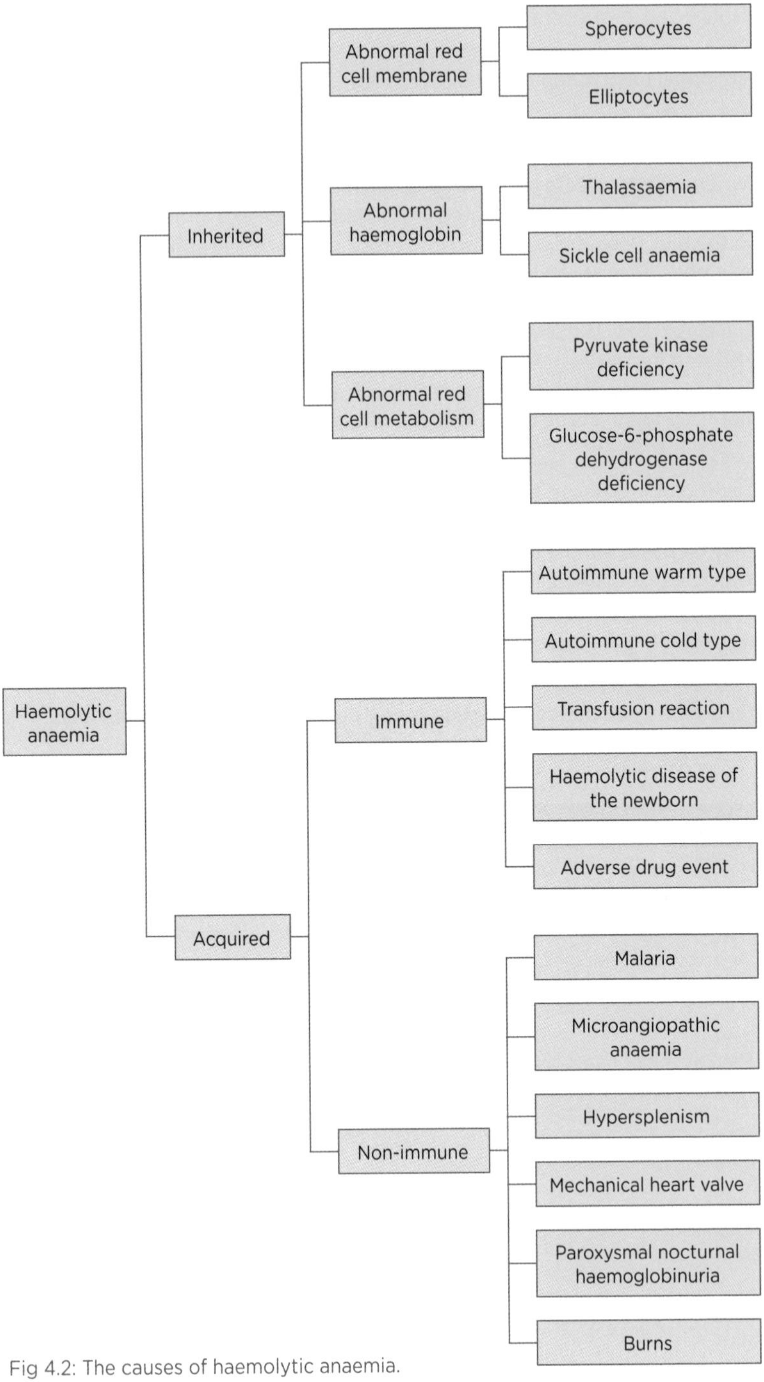

Fig 4.2: The causes of haemolytic anaemia.

Osmotic fragility test

Hereditary spherocytosis is a condition associated with an abnormal red blood cell membrane where red cells become spherical in shape. These cells are less resilient to damage than normal. This can be assessed using an osmotic fragility test. Spherocytes have increased osmotic fragility.

Direct antiglobulin test

In autoimmune haemolytic anaemias, antibodies attack red cells and cause their destruction. The main laboratory test for autoimmune haemolytic anaemia is the direct antiglobulin test (DAT or Coombs' test). In this test, antibodies to human immunoglobulin are added to a sample of red cells from the patient. If the red cells are coated in antibodies (ie if the patient has an autoimmune haemolytic anaemia), they will agglutinate.

World Health Organization. *Worldwide Prevalence of Anaemia, 1993–2005*. Geneva: WHO, 2008.

Polycythaemia

Polycythaemia is defined as a packed cell volume (PCV) greater than 0.51 in males or greater than 0.48 in females.

POLYCYTHAEMIA
Males - PCV >0.51 Females - PCV >0.48

Red cell mass

In order to distinguish between true and apparent polycythaemia, the red cell mass must be measured. In true polycythaemia, the red cell mass is raised. Apparent polycythaemia is due to a reduction in plasma volume rather than an increase in red cell mass.

Red cell mass is measured by labelling red cells with a radioactive isotope. A predicted red cell mass can be calcuated based on the patient's height and weight. True polycythaemia is diagnosed if the red cell mass is more than 25% higher than that predicted.

To distinguish between causes of true polycythaemia, further tests should be arranged. These usually include:

- arterial blood gas analysis (to look for hypoxia)
- erythropoietin level (to detect inappropriately high levels)
- an ultrasound of the abdomen (to detect structural renal or hepatic disease and to visualise the spleen)
- further investigations depending on the most likely cause.

The causes of polycythaemia are shown in Fig 4.3.

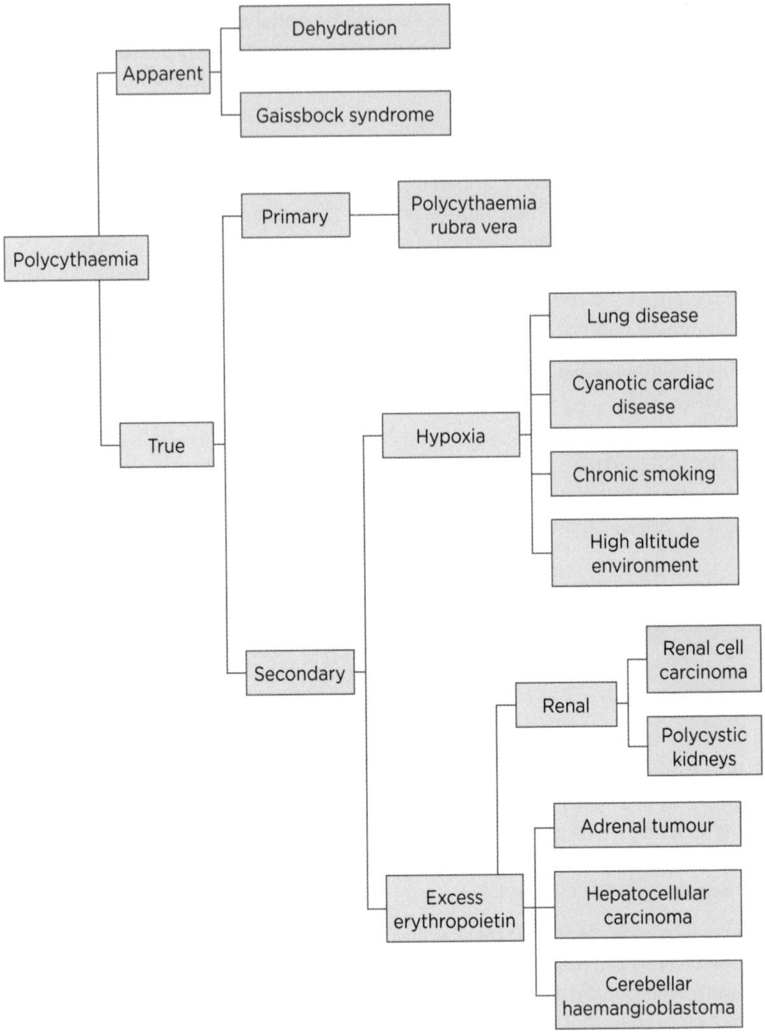

Fig 4.3: Causes of polycythaemia.

Haemoglobinopathies

Haemoglobin electrophoresis can be used to diagnose a variety of diseases in which the structure of haemoglobin is abnormal. The most common diseases of this type are sickle cell disease and the thalassaemias. In sickle cell disease, haemoglobin electrophoresis shows the presence of HbS.

Abnormal white blood cells

There are five subtypes of white blood cells: neutrophils, lymphocytes, monocytes, eosinophils and basophils. Abnormalities are common. The most frequently occurring abnormalities are listed in the boxes below with common causes.

COMMON CAUSES OF NEUTROPHILIA (NEUTROPHILS >7.5 x 10^9/l)	
Bacterial infections	Malignancy
Inflammation	Myeloproliferative disorders
Necrosis, eg after myocardial infarction	Metabolic disorders, eg renal failure
	Treatment with corticosteroids

COMMON CAUSES OF NEUTROPENIA (NEUTROPHILS <2.0 x 10^9/l)
Post-chemotherapy
Post-radiotherapy
Adverse drug reactions, eg clozapine, carbimazole
Viral infection
Felty syndrome

COMMON CAUSES OF LYMPHOCYTOSIS (LYMPHOCYTES >3.5 x 10^9/l)
Viral infections
Chronic infections, eg TB
Chronic lymphocytic leukaemia
Lymphomas

COMMON CAUSES OF EOSINOPHILIA (EOSINOPHILS >0.5 x 10^9/l)	
Allergic disorders	Skin diseases, eg eczema
Parasite infection	Malignancy, eg Hodgkin's disease
Hypereosinophilic syndrome	Allergic bronchopulmonary aspergillosis

Abnormal platelets

Thrombocytosis

Thrombocytosis describes a high platelet count (>400 x 10^9/l). The common causes are shown in the box below.

COMMON CAUSES OF THROMBOCYTOSIS

Primary haematological diseases:
- Essential thrombocythaemia and other myeloproliferative disorders
- Chronic myeloid leukaemia
- Myelodysplasia

Reactive thrombocytosis secondary to:
- Infection
- Inflammation
- Malignancy
- Bleeding
- Pregnancy
- Post-splenectomy

Thrombocytopenia

Thrombocytopenia describes a low platelet count (<150 x 10^9/l). The common causes are shown in the box below.

CAUSES OF THROMBOCYTOPENIA

Reduced platelet production due to bone marrow failure:
- Infections (particularly viral, eg infectious mononucleosis)
- Drug induced, eg penicillamine
- Leukaemia
- Aplastic anaemia
- Myelofibrosis (later stages)
- Bone marrow replacement with tumour, eg myeloma or metastases
- Myelodysplasia
- Megaloblastic anaemia

Increased platelet destruction:
- Immune-mediated platelet destruction
  - Autoimmune idiopathic thrombocytopenic purpura (AITP)
  - Drug induced, particularly heparin-induced thrombocytopenia (HIT)
- Hypersplenism, eg in liver cirrhosis
- Thrombotic thrombocytopenic purpura/haemolytic uraemic syndrome
- Disseminated intravascular coagulation (DIC)
- After a massive red cell transfusion

PLATELET CLUMPING

This is a relatively common cause for an apparently low platelet count. If a blood sample is sent to the laboratory in a tube containing citrate anticoagulant clumping will not occur and the true platelet count will be apparent. It is therefore always worth sending a 'citrated' sample for a platelet count if unexpected thrombocytopenia is found.

Pancytopenia

Pancytopenia is the term used to describe the pattern present when there are low levels of red blood cells, white blood cells and platelets in the circulation. There is a wide variety of causes, the most common of which are shown in the box.

COMMON CAUSES OF PANCYTOPENIA

- Aplastic anaemia
- Bone marrow infiltration, eg with tumour
- Hypersplenism
- Megaloblastic anaemia
- Sepsis
- Systemic lupus erythematosus (SLE)

Erythrocyte sedimentation rate

The erythrocyte sedimentation rate (ESR) measures how rapidly red blood cells form sediment when a column of blood is kept upright for 1 hour. The further the red cells sink in the hour, the higher the ESR.

The ESR is a non-specific marker of disease. In inflammatory processes, raised levels of plasma proteins result in red blood cells forming clumps called rouleaux. These clumps of cells sink more easily than single cells, and thus, in the presence of such proteins, the ESR is high.

The ESR normally rises with advancing age, but levels of more than 35 mm/h should raise the suspicion of a disease process in any age group. Common causes of a high ESR are listed in the box.

COMMON CAUSES OF A RAISED ESR

- Infectious disease
- Neoplastic disease (particularly multiple myeloma)
- Connective tissue disease (particularly giant cell arteritis and polymyalgia rheumatica)
- Anaemia
- Renal disease

Blood film interpretation

Examination of a peripheral blood film can aid or clinch a diagnosis in a range of clinical scenarios. Correct identification of various cell types requires significant training, but knowledge of the different terminology used can greatly aid interpretation of blood film reports. The following abnormal cell types are among those most commonly seen.

Abnormal red blood cells

Colour or shape

ABNORMALITY	MEANING	FOUND IN
Hypochromic cells	Pale red cells	Iron deficiency or defective haemoglobin synthesis
Microcytosis	Small cells	Iron deficiency or defective haemoglobin synthesis
Macrocytosis	Large cells	Megaloblastic anaemia, high alcohol intake, liver disease
Pencil cells	Pencil-shaped cells	Iron deficiency
Spherocytes	Spherical cells	Hereditary spherocytosis, haemolytic anaemia, burns
Elliptocytes	Elliptical cells	Hereditary elliptocytosis, thalassaemia major, iron deficiency
Acanthocytes	Spiky-appearing cells	Abetalipoproteinaemia, post-splenectomy, liver disease
Target cells	Target-like cells	Thalassaemia, iron deficiency, post-splenectomy, liver disease

ABNORMALITY	MEANING	FOUND IN
Stomatocytes	Cells with mouth-shaped area of pallor	Hereditary stomatocytosis, high alcohol intake, liver disease
Ecchinocytes	Also known as burr cells – less spiky than acanthocytes	Post-splenectomy, liver disease, uraemia
Sickle cells	Sickle shaped	Sickle cell anaemia (homozygous HbS disease)
Fragmented cells	Broken pieces of cell	Microangiopathic haemolytic anaemia, haemolytic uraemic syndrome, thrombotic thrombocytopenic purpura, mechanical heart valves, disseminated intravascular coagulation
Tear cells (dacryocytes)	Tear-shaped cells	Myelofibrosis and other causes of extramedullary haematopoiesis
Poikilocytosis	Abnormal shapes of red cells	Iron deficiency
Anisochromia	Varying shades of colour	Iron deficiency

Intracellular abnormalities

ABNORMALITY	FOUND IN
Heinz bodies	Unstable haemoglobin states
Howell–Jolly bodies	Hyposplenism, post-splenectomy
Pappenheimer bodies	Post-splenectomy, haemolytic anaemia, sideroblastic anaemia
Basophilic stippling	Lead poisoning, thalassaemia, myelodysplasia
Cabot rings	Myelodysplasia, megaloblastic anaemia

Abnormal white blood cells

ABNORMALITY	FOUND IN
Hypersegmented neutrophils	Megaloblastic anaemias, chronic infections
Toxic granulation of neutrophils	Bacterial infection, poisoning, burns, chemotherapy
Auer rods	Acute myeloid leukaemia
Smear cells	Chronic lymphocytic leukaemia

Leukoerythroblastic blood film

This is a term used to describe the overall appearance of a blood film in which immature red and white blood cells are seen in peripheral blood. There are several causes.

CAUSES OF A LEUKOERYTHROBLASTIC BLOOD FILM
• Bone marrow infiltration, eg with tumour • Idiopathic myelofibrosis • Severe sepsis • Haemolysis

Disorders of coagulation

Haemostasis (the process of stopping bleeding) is a complex process. It involves the interplay of blood vessel walls, platelets and clotting factors. The common tests used to assess coagulation are as follows:

COMMON TESTS OF COAGULATION
• Prothrombin time (PT) • International normalised ratio (INR) • Activated partial thromboplastin time (APTT) • Bleeding time

Prothrombin time

The PT is dependent on clotting factors I, II, V, VII and X. In clinical practice, it is most commonly measured to assess the synthetic function of the liver (eg in liver failure), or to monitor the effects of warfarin therapy.

International normalised ratio

To allow comparison of coagulation results between laboratories, the PT is often converted to the INR, by applying a correction factor. This takes into account differences in laboratory methods, and means that the patient's INR should be the same regardless of the laboratory used to measure it.

The INR is the parameter most commonly used to monitor the effects of warfarin. In a patient with normal coagulation, the INR will be close to 1.0 before warfarin is commenced. As warfarin is introduced, the INR rises. The higher the INR, the less coagulable the blood becomes (ie the more difficult it will be for the blood to clot). Target INRs are set, and warfarin dosing must be adjusted to aim for these targets.

DISEASE	TARGET INR
Deep venous thrombosis (DVT)	2.5
Pulmonary embolism (PE)	2.5
Atrial fibrillation	2.5
Mechanical prosthetic heart valve	2.5
Recurrent DVT/PE in a patient with a therapeutic INR	3.5

The essence of warfarin prescribing involves increasing the dose if the INR is too low, reducing the dose if the INR is too high, and omitting it if the INR is dangerously high or the patient is bleeding. An example of a warfarin prescribing chart is shown on page 396.

Activated partial thromboplastin time

The APTT depends on all clotting factors except factor VII. In clinical practice, the APTT is used most commonly in patients receiving an infusion of heparin. The APTT is monitored frequently, and the rate of the heparin infusion adjusted to achieve the desired level of anticoagulation. With the common prescribing of low-molecular-weight heparin, in preference to unfractionated heparin, this process is now performed infrequently. A frequent cause of concern relates to elevated APTTs in patients with central venous catheters. The proximal end of such catheters is often filled with heparin to keep the lumen patent when they are not being used. A spuriously high APTT will be obtained if blood is withdrawn from one such lumen. If the APTT is tested on a sample of blood tested peripherally, the true value will be obtained.

Coagulation correction testing

In cases of deranged coagulation, laboratories will often perform a coagulation correction test. This is performed to detect problems in coagulation arising because of a low level of a particular clotting factor. Essentially, normal plasma (containing normal clotting factors) is mixed with the patient's sample. If the patient is deficient in clotting factors, a deranged coagulation profile would be expected to normalise. There will be no change, however, if an inhibitor of coagulation is present. Specialised assays for individual clotting factors are also available.

Bleeding time

Bleeding time is measured directly at the bedside. A sphygmomanometer cuff is inflated around the patient's arm to 40 mmHg. A specially designed blade is then used to make a small puncture in the arm. Blood is removed from the area at fixed time intervals (eg 15 s) using a piece of filter paper to soak it up. The time taken for bleeding to stop is recorded. Elevated bleeding times indicate defective platelet function or low platelet numbers. This test should not be performed if the patient is known to have severe thrombocytopenia.

Bear in mind that patients with abnormal numbers or deranged function of platelets may also have abnormal bleeding. Patients with von Willebrand's disease may have normal coagulation profiles.

DON'T FORGET

Patients with von Willebrand's disease may have normal coagulation profiles.

Disseminated intravascular coagulation

Disseminated intravascular coagulation (DIC) is a disease of two apparently conflicting problems. On the one hand, fibrin deposition in various organs results in areas of micro-infarction. On the other hand, the body's supplies of clotting factors become used up because of all the clotting, leaving the patient prone to bleeding.

DISSEMINATED INTRAVASCULAR COAGULATION

A disease in which clotting and bleeding cause problems simultaneously.

Typical laboratory findings in DIC are as follows:

Raised PT and APTT	Since clotting factors are reduced
Reduced fibrinogen	Due to widespread fibrin formation
Raised D-dimer	Due to the body's attempt to break down the excess fibrin deposits

D-dimer

D-dimer is the most commonly measured fibrinogen/fibrin degeneration product. It is detected following clot formation in the vasculature, as the body's fibrinolytic system attempts to break the clot down. D-dimer levels are often tested in cases of suspected deep venous thrombosis and pulmonary embolism, and in the majority of cases will be raised. However, D-dimer levels are also raised in many other conditions, and a raised level should always be interpreted in light of the clinical scenario.

Laboratory findings in bleeding disorders

	PT	APTT	FIBRINOGEN
Warfarin treatment	Increased	Normal (or increased)	Normal
Heparin treatment	Normal (or increased)	Increased	Normal
Haemophilia A or B	Normal	Increased	Normal
Liver disease	Increased	Increased	Normal
DIC	Increased	Increased	Reduced

Multiple myeloma and similar disorders

Diseases of plasma cells are common, and their investigation is often a cause for confusion. They represent a spectrum of disorders, with multiple myeloma being the most important at the undergraduate level, and monoclonal gammopathy of unknown significance (MGUS) being the most common. The hallmark of these conditions is that plasma cells secrete abnormal protein in excess. The effects of multiple myeloma can be far-reaching, and can lead to the following features:

- Anaemia
- Renal impairment
- Low levels of normal immunoglobulins with resultant infections
- Bone involvement, causing bony pain, hypercalcaemia, lytic lesions and problems if bones collapse
- Hyperviscosity of the blood.

The conditions should be suspected if any of the following abnormalities are present:

- Elevated ESR
- Hypercalcaemia
- Anaemia
- Renal impairment
- Abnormal M-protein detected on plasma protein electrophoresis
- Abnormal quantities of immunoglobulin light chains in the serum (with an abnormal $\kappa:\lambda$ ratio)
- Low levels of immunoglobulins
- Lytic lesions on radiograph of bones
- Detection of Bence Jones protein in the urine (this represents immunoglobulin light chains)
- Abnormal plasma cells seen on bone marrow biopsy
- Elevated β_2-microglobulin.

See pages 33–34 for further details on analytical issues relating to these conditions.

HAEMATOLOGY – WHAT YOU NEED TO KNOW

- Classify anaemia into microcytic, normocytic or macrocytic when thinking about a cause.
- Classically, iron deficiency causes microcytic anaemia, vitamin B_{12}/folate deficiency causes macrocytic anaemia, and normocytic anaemia is caused by chronic disease or haemolytic anaemia.
- In intravascular haemolysis, elevated bilirubin, LDH and reticulocytes might be seen, whereas haptoglobin will be reduced.
- Polycythaemia can be apparent or true and, if true, can be primary or secondary. Secondary polycythaemia can be due to hypoxia or excess erythropoietin.
- Learn causes for abnormal numbers of neutrophils, lymphocytes, eosinophils and platelets.
- ESR is a non-specific marker of disease.
- Inspection of a blood film can be very helpful in making a diagnosis.
- A prolonged prothrombin time can be seen in liver failure and with warfarin therapy.
- D-dimer is a non-specific test that should be interpreted with caution. An abnormal D-dimer concentration does not necessarily mean that a patient has a blood clot.
- Multiple myeloma can cause a wide variety of blood test abnormalities, and should always be considered as a possible diagnosis, particularly in older individuals with test abnormalities.

5

MICROBIOLOGY

Infections account for a wide spectrum of human illness. Bacteria and viruses predominate in clinical medicine in the UK, but one should bear in mind that other organisms (eg fungi, protozoa, helminths and arthropods) can all cause problems. Infections that are rare in clinical practice in the UK should be borne in mind when patients have been travelling or are from endemic regions. In addition, patients who are immunocompromised are prone to infections that are not normally seen in individuals with healthy immune systems.

If treatment is required for an infection, a drug must be chosen that has activity against the pathogen causing the problem. Often, a 'best guess' at treatment is made. For example, an antibiotic called trimethoprim is often given to patients with symptoms of a urinary tract infection because the bacteria that are responsible for most urinary tract infections are likely to be targeted by this drug. In many cases, however, it is appropriate to collect samples from the patient so that an attempt can be made to accurately identify the organism that is causing the infection. It is the results from the analysis of such samples that are considered further here.

To have the best chance of identifying a causative organism, samples should normally be taken from the body site that is affected. Common samples include sputum, urine, faeces, synovial fluid, swabs from mouth, skin or genitals, pus from any site, cerebrospinal fluid and biopsy samples. On occasion, organisms can move from the site of origin into the bloodstream causing septicaemia. Thus, blood is often cultured in addition to material from the likely focus of infection.

Bacterial infection

Infections with bacteria tend to predominate in undergraduate assessments because they are the infections that most commonly cause serious disease in the UK. Once a sample containing bacteria has been collected, there are two basic methods for identifying the organism. First, the sample can be examined using light microscopy with a stain applied. The stain normally used first is the Gram stain. Organisms that stain blue are termed 'Gram positive' and those that stain pink are termed 'Gram negative'. Bacteria can then be described using their shape. 'Bacilli' are rod shaped whereas 'cocci' are spherical. Thus, very quickly one can have a fair idea of the likely organism contained in a sample. Common organisms characterised by staining characteristics and shape are listed in the box on page 91. 'Aerobes' grow best in oxygen-rich environments, whereas 'anaerobes' grow best in oxygen-poor environments. This will become apparent during culture.

Another staining technique, Ziehl-Neelsen staining, can be used to detect mycobacteria (responsible for tuberculosis).

EXAMPLES OF COMMON ORGANISMS		
Aerobes	**Gram-positive cocci**	*Staphylococcus aureus* *Streptococcus pyogenes* *Streptococcus pneumoniae* *Enterococcus faecalis*
	Gram-positive bacilli	*Listeria monocytogenes* *Bacillus anthracis*
	Gram-negative cocci	*Moraxella catarrhalis* *Neisseria meningitidis*
	Gram-negative bacilli	*Escherichia coli* *Pseudomonas aeruginosa*
Anaerobes	**Cocci**	Peptococci Peptostreptococci
	Bacilli	*Bacteroides fragilis* *Clostridium difficile*

The second method for organism identification is culture. Samples are placed on growth media and given time for the organisms to multiply. After multiplication has taken place, microbiologists use a range of techniques for identifying the particular type of bacteria present. This takes time – several days for most bacteria. The identification of tuberculosis can take weeks, however. The payoff for waiting is that the exact species of organism can usually be identified after culturing. Once a bacterium is cultured, its sensitivity to a batch of suitable common antimicrobial agents is tested. There are three outcomes to this testing: sensitive (S), intermediately sensitive (I) and resistant (R). A typical culture and antibiotic sensitivity report might look like this:

Urine culture	
>10^5 organisms/ml *Proteus* species	
Co-amoxiclav	R
Ampicillin	S
Ciprofloxacin	S
Cefotaxime	S
Nitrofurantoin	I
Tazocin	S
Trimethoprim	R
Cephalexin	S

In this example, the patient's urinary tract infection appears to have been caused by the Gram-negative bacillus *Proteus* species. If treatment is deemed necessary, it would be most appropriate to prescribe one of the drugs shown as sensitive (S), because this would be expected to have the highest likelihood of killing the microorganism in question.

MINIMUM INHIBITORY CONCENTRATION (MIC) AND MINIMUM BACTERICIDAL CONCENTRATION (MBC) TESTING

Occasionally it is desirable to have more information about an organism's sensitivity to a particular antimicrobial agent rather than a simple yes/no answer. This is commonly the case for infections that are difficult to treat or that require prolonged courses of antibiotics, eg infective endocarditis. In such circumstances detailed testing can be performed to work out the minimum concentration of antibiotic necessary to stop bacterial growth (MIC) and the minimum concentration of antibiotic necessary to kill the bacteria (MBC). These data can then be translated into the most appropriate dose and duration for drug prescription purposes.

Staphylococcus aureus requires special mention for two reasons:

1. If resistant to meticillin, it is deemed meticillin-resistant *Staphylococcus aureus* (MRSA). This is highly important because different antibiotics are required to treat this particular type of bacterium.
2. It is a reasonably common finding to isolate 'coagulase-negative' *Staphylococcus aureus* on blood cultures. Laboratories often test staphylococci for their production of coagulase. Staphylococci that normally colonise skin (such as *S. epidermidis*) do not produce coagulase. The identification of these organisms on blood cultures usually reflects the fact that the skin surface was inadequately sterilised before blood was drawn.

Other methods are available for detecting certain bacteria, but the clinician must actually have the knowledge to suspect a likely organism and request the appropriate test. In patients presenting with pneumonia, for example, urine is often tested for the presence of antigens to *Streptococcus pneumoniae* and *Legionella* species. In patients with diarrhoea, faecal samples are often tested for the presence of *Clostridium difficile* toxin. Genetic testing can also be carried out to look for the presence of bacterial DNA or RNA in a sample. Polymerase chain reaction (PCR) techniques can be used to assist in this process.

Finally, it is possible to perform serological tests to detect antibodies to various organisms in a patient's blood. Immunoglobulin type M (IgM) levels tend to rise early in a disease course, with IgG levels rising later. If IgM is detected to a particular bacterium, it is likely that this is the cause of the illness. The IgG level is more difficult to interpret, however, because the IgG antibody level would be expected to be elevated if a patient has either had a particular illness previously or been immunised against it. It is thus difficult to distinguish between current infection and previous exposure based on a single measure of IgG. The best use of serological testing is in the measurement of acute and convalescent levels of IgG, ie measure the level during the acute illness and again once the patient has recovered. If there has been a significant rise in the antibody levels to a particular microorganism during the patient's recovery, it is probable that the organism suspected was the likely pathogen. The disadvantage with serological tests is the inevitable time lag in making the diagnosis, and the fact that treatment decisions must therefore be made without confirmation of the pathogen.

Tests for *Helicobacter pylori*

The Gram-negative bacillus *H. pylori* can infect the stomach and predispose to the development of peptic ulcer disease. Testing for the presence of the organism should be carried out in all patients with a peptic ulcer, and eradication should be attempted in affected individuals.

There are several methods that can be used to test for the presence of *H. pylori*.

Breath testing

This test relies on the fact that *H. pylori* organisms produce urease, an enzyme that breaks down urea to form ammonia and carbon dioxide. The ammonia produced raises the pH and helps the organism survive the acidic environment in the stomach.

In a *H. pylori* breath test, the patient is given a tablet containing radiolabelled urea ([^{13}C]urea). If infection is present, the organisms act on the urea to liberate radiolabelled carbon dioxide ($^{13}CO_2$). A sample of breath is collected (eg in a tube or balloon), and analysed for the presence of $^{13}CO_2$. If this is detected, the test is positive and the patient can be assumed to be infected.

This test rapidly becomes negative if *H. pylori* is eradicated.

Detection of *H. pylori* antibodies

A sample of blood can be tested for the presence of IgG antibodies to *H. pylori*. The test can remain positive for up to a year after eradication therapy, and so it is not a particularly useful way of testing for clearance.

Campylobacter-like organism (CLO) test

This test also requires a biopsy sample obtained at oesophagogastro-duodenoscopy (OGD). The sample of tissue is placed into a medium that contains urea and phenol red. Phenol red is a dye that turns red in alkaline conditions. If *H. pylori* is present in the biopsy sample, its urease enzyme will liberate ammonia from the urea in the medium, causing the pH to rise. The colour of the medium will therefore turn red (Fig 5.1).

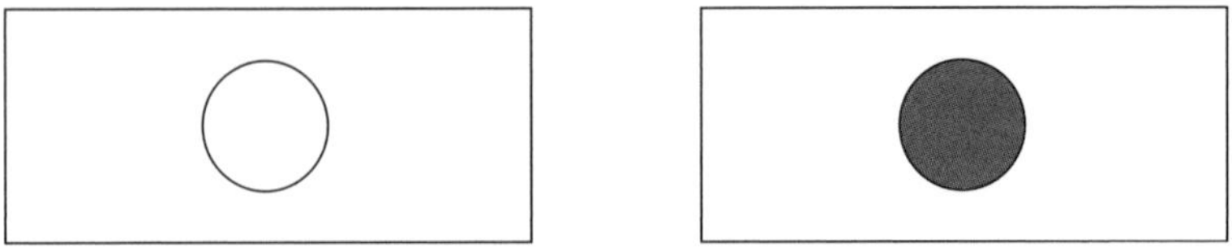

CLO test negative *CLO test positive (red circle)*

Fig 5.1

Tissue histology

A stomach biopsy sample can be stained and examined under a microscope. This may reveal curved organisms at the mucosal surface.

Tissue culture

A biopsy sample obtained at OGD can be cultured to look for the presence of offending organisms.

Infections with other organisms

The principles for the detection of other microorganisms are similar to those used for bacteria. Light microscopy can be useful in detecting fungi (eg in skin scraping samples), parasites (eg in faecal samples) and protozoa (eg malaria in blood). Electron microscopy can be used to identify certain viruses. Pathogen antigen testing can be attempted with certain organisms also (eg hepatitis B surface antigen). Genetic testing employing PCR techniques is being increasingly used for the rapid detection of viruses. An example would be the rapid testing of cerebrospinal fluid for herpes simplex virus in patients with suspected encephalitis (viral brain infection). Fungi can be cultured similarly to bacteria, but culture of viruses and other organisms is time-consuming and difficult because they must be grown in cell or tissue preparations. Serological testing is the method most useful in clinical practice for confirming infection with a virus.

It should be apparent that the difficulty with microbiological investigations for a clinician lies with knowing which test to request. Thanks to the efforts of highly skilled laboratory technicians, the interpretation of test results is generally relatively straightforward.

Interpretation of drug levels

Drug treatment of patients with infections sometimes requires the use of drugs with 'narrow therapeutic ratios' (see page 49). Use too low a dose, and the infection may not be adequately treated. Use too high a dose, and you will put the patient at risk of an adverse drug reaction. It is possible to measure a peak drug level in the blood (sample taken shortly after drug administration) or a trough level (taken just before the next dose being administered). Target ranges for peak and/or trough levels are listed in drug formularies. Generally, if levels are lower than required, dosing is increased. If levels are too high, the drug is omitted until the level returns to a safe level before a modified dosing regimen is re-started.

Bedside testing for urinary tract infection

Urine samples can be quickly analysed using a reagent strip that is dipped into the urine. Typical strips allow for the estimation of a range of substances in the urine (see page 344 for more details) Substances that are useful in the detection of urinary tract infection (UTI) include leukocyte esterase, nitrites, protein and blood. Urinalysis can only at best point towards the diagnosis of UTI - culture is necessary for a definitive diagnosis. The sensitivity and specificity of abnormalities in each of the parameters mentioned have been published with regard to diagnosing a UTI, but a good rule of thumb is to say that, if urinalysis is totally normal, then a UTI is unlikely. If it is abnormal in any way, a UTI is a possibility and culture should be performed if there is clinical suspicion.

Simerville JA, Maxted WC, Pahira JJ. Urinalysis: a comprehensive review. *Am Fam Physician* 2005;**71**:1153-62.

6

IMMUNOLOGY

Interpretation of autoantibodies is often difficult. This is because of the degree of overlap in the presence of antibodies between various disease states. For example, rheumatoid factor can be found in well over a dozen diseases. Furthermore, certain autoantibodies may be found in healthy people, and the absence of an autoantibody may not rule out a particular disease. Therefore, always bear in mind that the presence of an autoantibody does not necessarily mean that a patient has a particular disease.

DON'T FORGET

A disease may be present without the typical autoantibody profile.

For the purpose of undergraduate examinations, the classic autoantibody associations will be tested. These are listed in the box below. Those tested commonly in examinations are in bold type.

DISEASE	AUTOANTIBODIES
Addison's disease	Anti-21-hydroxylase
Anti-phospholipid syndrome	**Anti-cardiolipin** **Lupus anticoagulant antibodies**
Autoimmune haemolytic anaemia	**Red blood cell autoantibodies** (this disease can be classified into warm and cold, depending on the temperature at which the antibodies best attach to red cells)
Autoimmune hepatitis	**Anti-nuclear** **Anti-smooth muscle** **Anti-liver/kidney microsomal-I** Myeloperoxidase anti-nuclear cytoplasmic antibody (MPO-ANCA), also called perinuclear ANCA (pANCA)
Churg–Strauss syndrome	**MPO-ANCA**
Coeliac disease	**Anti-tissue transglutaminase** Anti-endomysial Anti-reticulin Anti-gliadin

DISEASE	AUTOANTIBODIES
Diffuse cutaneous scleroderma	**Anti-ScL-70** **Polymerase 1, 2 and 3** Rheumatoid factor Anti-nuclear
Goodpasture syndrome	**Anti-glomerular basement membrane**
Graves' disease	**Anti-TSH receptor** Anti-peroxidase
Hashimoto's thyroiditis	**TSH-receptor-blocking antibodies** Anti-peroxidase
Lambert-Eaton myasthenic syndrome	Anti-P/Q-type voltage-gated calcium channels
Limited cutaneous scleroderma	**Anti-centromere** Rheumatoid factor Anti-nuclear
Mixed connective tissue disease (overlap syndrome)	Anti-U1-RNP
Myasthenia gravis	**Anti-acetylcholine receptor antibodies** Anti-nuclear
Paraneoplastic conditions	Anti-YO Anti-Hu Anti-Ri Anti-MA Anti-CV2/CRMP5 Anti-amphiphysin
Pernicious anaemia	**Anti-parietal cell** **Anti-intrinsic factor**
Polyarteritis nodosa	**MPO-ANCA**
Polymyositis/ dermatomyositis	**Anti-Jo-1** Anti-nuclear Rheumatoid factor
Primary biliary cirrhosis	**Anti-mitochondrial** (more particularly against pyruvate dehydrogenase complex type E2- and/ or E3-binding protein)
Rheumatoid disease	**Rheumatoid factor** **Anti-CCP** Anti-nuclear

DISEASE	AUTOANTIBODIES
Sjögren syndrome	**Anti-Ro (SS-A)** **Anti-La (SS-B)** Rheumatoid factor Anti-nuclear
Systemic lupus erythematosus	**Anti-double-stranded DNA** Rheumatoid factor Anti-nuclear Anti-Ro (SS-A) Anti-Sm Anti-U1-RNP Anti-cardiolipin
Wegener syndrome	**Proteinase 3 anti-nuclear cytoplasmic antibody** (PR3-ANCA), also called cytoplasmic ANCA (cANCA)

CELLULAR PATHOLOGY

This chapter lists typical pathological findings for a range of disease states. It is not by any means comprehensive, but includes most of the classic abnormalities that are commonly tested in general medical examinations. Further reading will be required when preparing for pathology examinations.

DISEASE	TYPICAL PATHOLOGICAL CHANGES
Gastroenterology	
Barrett's oesophagus	Lower oesophageal epithelium undergoes metaplasia to become gastric or intestinal-type epithelium
Coeliac disease	Total or subtotal villous atrophy in the small bowel Crypt hyperplasia with inflammatory cells in the mucosa
Crohn's disease	Can affect any part of the gastrointestinal tract *Macroscopically*: skip lesions (ie lengths of normal bowel between diseased segments); cobblestone appearance with fissured ulcers *Microscopically*: thickened wall with transmural inflammation; granulomas
Ulcerative colitis	Affects large bowel only Affects mucosa and submucosa only Crypt abscesses and superficial ulcers
Chronic cholecystitis	Chronic inflammatory changes Rokitansky–Aschoff sinuses
Hepatology	
Acute viral hepatitis	Swelling of hepatocytes with spotty necrosis Councilman's bodies
Alcoholic hepatitis	Fatty accumulation in cytoplasmic vacuoles, necrosis, Mallory's hyaline material
Chronic active hepatitis	Piecemeal necrosis
Autoimmune hepatitis	Interface hepatitis, portal plasma cell infiltration
Haemochromatosis	Excessive hepatic iron (shows up blue on Perl's stain)
Primary biliary cirrhosis	Portal hepatitis and granulomatous destruction of bile ducts. Later, periportal hepatitis and bile duct proliferation

DISEASE	TYPICAL PATHOLOGICAL CHANGES
Liver cirrhosis	*Macroscopically*: macronodular or micronodular *Microscopically*: fibrous tissue (shows up red on van Gieson's stain)
Respiratory	
Diffuse alveolar damage (DAD) which can lead to adult respiratory distress syndrome (ARDS)	Alveolar hyaline membranes and thickened alveolar walls
Previous asbestos exposure	Asbestos bodies in lung
Pulmonary fibrosis	Proliferation of type II pneumocytes with thickening of the alveolar walls
Nephrology	
Malignant hypertension	Renal arteriole fibrinoid necrosis
Diabetic glomerulosclerosis	Kimmelstiel-Wilson nodules, thickened capillary basement membranes with hyalinisation of arterioles
Haematology	
Hodgkin's disease	Reed-Sternberg cells Abnormal lymph node architecture Nodular sclerosing type has fibrous tissue
Myelofibrosis	Bone marrow fibrosis secondary to fibroblast proliferation
Multiple myeloma	Plasma cell proliferation in bone marrow
Rheumatology	
Temporal arteritis	Temporal artery biopsy may be normal Alternatively, plasma cells, lymphocytes and multinucleate giant cells can be present
Polymyositis	Muscle fibre necrosis Lymphocyte infiltration
Endocrinology	
Pituitary tumours	Acromegaly is associated with acidophil macroadenomas (somatotroph adenomas) Hyperprolactinaemia is associated with chromophobe adenomas ACTH excess is associated with basophil microadenomas (corticotroph adenomas)

DISEASE	TYPICAL PATHOLOGICAL CHANGES
Neurology	
Alzheimer's disease	*Macroscopically*: thinning of gyri *Microscopically*: neurofibrillary tangles; plaques
Parkinson's disease and dementia with Lewy bodies	Lewy bodies (inclusions inside neurons)
Obstetrics and gynaecology	
Ovarian endometriosis	*Macroscopically*: chocolate cyst

8

GENETICS

Pedigree interpretation

In clinical practice, pedigrees (family trees with genetic information superimposed) are often recorded when there is a suspicion that a disease may have a familial element.

To the untrained eye, interpretation of these can seem like a daunting process, and many students resort to guessing what the inheritance pattern might be. However, if a few simple rules are borne in mind, interpretation can be made fairly simple. Being able to work out the expected inheritance patterns for the common mendelian disorders from first principles is a good way to check that your answer is correct.

Work through the various inheritance patterns for the common mendelian disorders below, and attempt to reproduce the information for yourself. This will be much easier to remember than if you simply learn off a list of rules.

The two main classes of conditions that are inherited in a mendelian manner are:

- autosomal conditions (affecting the autosomes, ie chromosomes 1 to 22)
- sex chromosomal conditions (affecting the sex chromosomes, ie X and Y).

Genotype refers to the genetic code.

Phenotype refers to the actual manifestation of the genetic code.

Autosomal conditions

Autosomal dominant inheritance

There are usually two copies of each chromosome in each cell, each carrying copies of the same genes. In autosomal dominant conditions, inheritance of one faulty gene is sufficient to give rise to the disorder. Thus one chromosome in the pair will be normal; the other will carry the faulty gene.

In the following diagram, the letter 'a' is used to denote a normal chromosome. The capital letter 'A' represents a chromosome with an abnormal gene. Thus an individual with two 'a' chromosomes will be normal. Someone with one 'a' chromosome and one 'A' chromosome will have the disorder, since only one faulty gene is needed for the condition to be manifest. If both parents are affected, it would also be possible for offspring to have two 'A' chromosomes.

Since 50% of the offspring's genetic code comes from one parent and 50% from the other, there is a 50% chance that either chromosome will be passed on.

		Mother	
		a	a
Father	a	aa	aa
	A	Aa	Aa

In the example, the father has an autosomal dominant condition, and therefore has one normal chromosome (a) and one abnormal chromosome (A). The mother has two normal chromosomes. There are four possible ways that the genes can be passed on to the offspring (aa, aa, Aa and Aa).

Thus for autosomal dominant conditions:

- both males and females can be affected
- if one parent is affected, there will be a 50% chance that a child will also be affected.

Autosomal recessive inheritance

For an autosomal recessive disorder to be manifest, both chromosomes in a pair must carry the abnormal gene. One abnormal gene must therefore be passed on from each parent.

If a person has one normal and one abnormal chromosome, he or she is a termed 'a carrier' and does not usually exhibit any features of the disorder, and therefore will appear normal (ie normal phenotype).

The inheritance pattern for one carrier parent and one normal parent will be as follows (remember 'a' is the normal chromosome, and 'A' the abnormal).

		Mother	
		a	a
Father	a	aa	aa
	A	Aa	Aa

For autosomal recessive conditions with one carrier parent:

- both male and female offspring can be carriers
- 50% of the offspring will be carriers.

		Mother	
		a	A
Father	a	aa	aA
	A	Aa	AA

For autosomal recessive conditions with two carrier parents:

- both male and female offspring can be carriers or be affected
- 50% of the offspring will be carriers
- 25% of the offspring will be normal (ie not carriers)
- 25% of the offspring will have the condition.

The inheritance pattern for one affected parent will be as follows.

		Mother	
		a	a
Father	A	Aa	Aa
	A	Aa	Aa

For autosomal recessive conditions with an affected parent:

- both male and female offspring can be carriers
- all offspring will be carriers.

Sex chromosomal conditions

X-linked recessive inheritance

X-linked disorders involve faulty genes found on the X chromosome. Since females have two X chromosomes, having one faulty chromosome is of minor consequence with a recessive disorder, because the other X chromosome is normal. Males, however, have only one X (but also one Y) chromosome. A faulty X chromosome in a male will therefore result in phenotypical effects.

If a female has one abnormal X chromosome, she is termed 'a carrier' and generally does not exhibit any features of the disorder. Occasionally mild signs of disease may be present.

The inheritance pattern for a carrier mother and a normal father will be as follows (X = normal chromosome, **X** = abnormal chromosome):

		Mother	
		X	**X**
Father	X	XX	X**X**
	Y	YX	Y**X**

For X-linked recessive disorders with a carrier mother:

- only males can be affected
- 50% of male offspring will have the disorder
- 50% of female offspring will be carriers
- 50% of all offspring will be normal.

The inheritance pattern for an affected father and a normal mother will be as follows:

		Mother	
		X	X
Father	**X**	**X**X	**X**X
	Y	YX	YX

For X-linked recessive disorders with an affected father:

- no offspring will be affected
- all daughters will be carriers
- all sons will be normal.

X-linked dominant inheritance

In these disorders, only one faulty X chromosome is necessary for the disease to be manifest. Thus, diseases can occur in both males and females.

The inheritance pattern for an affected mother and a normal father will be as follows:

		Mother	
		X	X
Father	X	XX	XX
	Y	YX	YX

For X-linked dominant disorders with an affected mother:

- both males and females can be affected
- 50% of male offspring will have the disorder
- 50% of female offspring will have the disorder.

The inheritance pattern for an affected father and a normal mother will be as follows:

		Mother	
		X	X
Father	X	XX	XX
	Y	YX	YX

For X-linked dominant disorders with an affected father:

- only female offspring can be affected
- all daughters will have the disorder
- all sons will be normal.

Other modes of inheritance

Mitochondrial inheritance

Mitochondria are cellular organelles that have a major role in energy production. They have their own DNA, which may undergo mutations. Diseases caused by mitochondrial genetic problems have an interesting inheritance pattern resulting from the fact that female ova all contain mitochondria; however, male sperm do not. Therefore, mitochondrial disorders can be passed on only by females. To summarise:

- both males and females can be affected
- affected females can pass on the disorder to all offspring
- affected males cannot pass on the disorder.

Genetic imprinting

This phenomenon relates to the fact that certain genes are expressed only if inherited from a particular parent. This can best be explained by looking at two conditions - Prader-Willi and Angelman syndromes. For Prader-Willi syndrome, only the paternal gene is important. Failure to inherit the paternal copy will therefore result in the syndrome. Angelman syndrome results from failure to inherit the maternal gene. The disorders may result from gene deletion mutations, where the gene from a particular parent is deleted. Alternatively, they may arise when two chromosomes are inherited from one parent rather than one from each. This is known as uniparental disomy.

MEMORY AID

In **P**rader-Willi syndrome - the **P**aternal gene is inactive

In Angel**m**an syndrome - the **M**aternal gene is inactive

Other points

Variable expression relates to the fact that a person may carry the necessary genetic make-up for a condition, but not exhibit all the phenotypical features. At the extreme of this is 'non-penetrance' where the person has no features of the condition.

Genetic disorders may appear to arise out of the blue, with no family members being affected. This is most commonly due to a new genetic mutation, but can also result from gonadal mosaicism where a parent carries the mutated genes only in the germ cells.

When faced with a family tree, and asked to comment on inheritance patterns, the flow diagram below should be helpful.

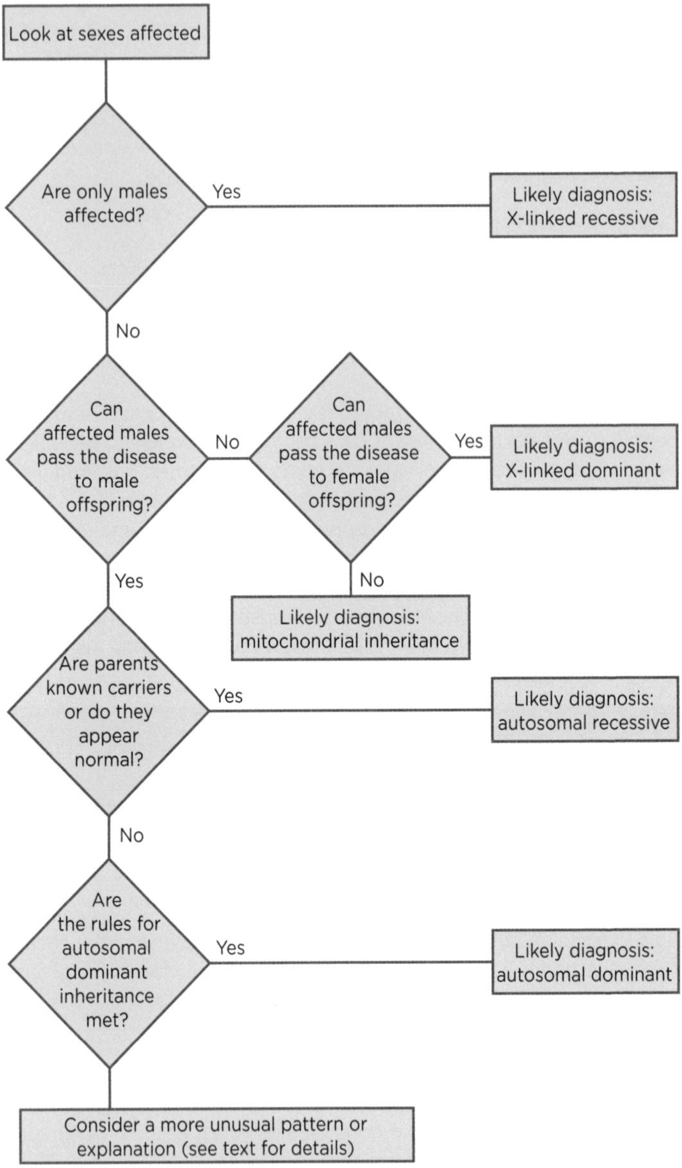

Fig 8.1: Interpreting genetic pedigrees.

Examples of genetic conditions with different inheritance patterns

Those most commonly tested in undergraduate examinations are highlighted in bold in the following table.

MODE OF INHERITANCE	EXAMPLES
Autosomal dominant	Achondroplasia **Adult polycystic kidney disease** **Dystrophia myotonica** Ehlers–Danlos syndrome Familial adenomatous polyposis **Familial hypercholesterolaemia** Hereditary haemorrhagic telangiectasia **Huntington's disease** **Marfan syndrome** **Neurofibromatosis** Noonan syndrome Osteogenesis imperfecta Otosclerosis **Tuberous sclerosis**
Autosomal recessive	Albinism Congenital adrenal hyperplasia **Cystic fibrosis** Friedreich's ataxia Galactosaemia Glycogen storage diseases **Hereditary haemochromatosis** Hurler syndrome Oculocutaneous albinism Phenylketonuria **Sickle cell disease** Tay–Sachs disease Thalassaemia Wilson's disease
X-linked dominant	Vitamin D-resistant rickets
X-linked recessive	Alport syndrome Becker muscular dystrophy **Duchenne muscular dystrophy** **Fragile X syndrome** Glucose-6-phosphate dehydrogenase deficiency **Haemophilia A** **Haemophilia B** Hunter syndrome
Mitochondrial	Leber hereditary optic neuropathy

Karyotype analysis

The following table lists the common chromosomal abnormalities that you would be expected to recognise.

CHROMOSOMAL ABNORMALITY	CONDITION
Trisomy 21	Down syndrome
Trisomy 18	Edward syndrome
Trisomy 12	Patau syndrome
45, XO	Turner syndrome
47, XXY	Klinefelter syndrome
47, XXX	Triple X syndrome
47, XXY	Associated with behavioural problems
5p-	Cri-du-chat syndrome
Microdeletion at 22q11	DiGeorge syndrome
Microdeletion at 7q11	Williams syndrome

Common mutations

DISEASE	COMMON MUTATION
Cystic fibrosis	ΔF508 mutation on long arm of chromosome 7. This codes for the cystic fibrosis transmembrane conductance regulator
Haemochromatosis	C282Y mutation on the *HFE* gene on the short arm of chromosome 6. The H63D mutation can also be found

INTERPRETING LABORATORY RESULTS: CASES

1

Adrenal hormones	1.17, 1.41
Analysis of peritoneal fluid	1.27, 1.45, 1.46, 1.56
Analysis of pleural fluid	1.9, 1.18, 1.43, 1.44, 1.58
Analysis of synovial fluid	1.16
Arterial blood gas analysis	1.8, 1.49, 1.50, 1.52, 1.77, 1.78, 1.79, 1.80, 1.85
Blood film interpretation	1.81
Bone profile and magnesium	1.11, 1.21, 1.30, 1.32, 1.59, 1.66, 1.74, 1.82
Cardiac biomarkers	1.48, 1.51, 1.53
Disorders of coagulation	1.10, 1.28, 1.29, 1.90
Disorders of glucose metabolism	1.42
Endocrinology	1.3, 1.57, 1.60, 1.84
Erythrocyte sedimentation rate	1.19, 1.35
Examination of urine	1.35
Full blood picture	1.2, 1.4, 1.7, 1.12, 1.15, 1.25, 1.32, 1.35, 1.37, 1.54, 1.53, 1.62, 1.64, 1.69, 1.73, 1.76, 1.81, 1.86, 1.88
Genetics	1.1, 1.47, 1.68, 1.89
Immunology	1.15
Liver function tests	1.14, 1.22, 1.31, 1.32, 1.33, 1.34, 1.38, 1.70, 1.71
Markers of nutrition	1.1, 1.4, 1.62, 1.64, 1.75
Other common tests	1.16, 1.24
Osmolality	1.71, 1.79, 1.83
Pituitary disease	1.40, 1.42
Plasma proteins and enzymes	1.2, 1.12, 1.31, 1.36
Thyroid hormones	1.6, 1.89
Toxicology	1.8, 1.63, 1.67, 1.70, 1.72, 1.79
Tumour markers	1.13, 1.23, 1.26, 1.37, 1.38, 1.39,
Urea and electrolyte profile	1.3, 1.5, 1.8, 1.12, 1.20, 1.32, 1.35, 1.37, 1.54, 1.61, 1.63, 1.65, 1.67, 1.69, 1.70. 1.72, 1.77, 1.80, 1.83

Case 1.1

You review a 45-year-old man at the diabetes clinic. He has recently started insulin with good effect, but complains of excessive tiredness that seems out of proportion to what might be expected from the diabetes alone. You suspect that he might be anaemic and request the following tests:

Hb	146 g/l	(130–180 g/l males)
MCV	87 fl	(76–96 fl)
WCC	6.6×10^9/l	(4.0–11.0×10^9/l)
Platelets	420×10^9/l	(150–400×10^9/l)
Vitamin B_{12}	588 ng/l	(191–663 ng/l)
Folate	7.6 µg/l	(>2 µg/l)
Iron	28 µmol/l	(11–32 µmol/l)
Ferritin	2783 µg/l	(12–200 µg/l)
Transferrin saturation	86%	

1. **What is the most likely unifying diagnosis?**
2. **What other tests would be useful?**
3. **What will be the mainstay of his treatment?**

➥ **answer on page 164**

Case 1.2

A 65-year-old woman presents with generalised lethargy with aches and pains. There are no features in the history that point towards blood loss. She eats a healthy diet, and does not report haematuria or vaginal bleeding. The following investigations are organised.

Hb	86 g/l		(120–160 g/l females)
MCV	101 fl		(76–96 fl)
WCC	5.6×10^9/l		(4.0–11.0×10^9/l)
Platelets	320×10^9/l		(150–400×10^9/l)
Vitamin B_{12}	487 ng/l		(191–663 ng/l)
Folate	5.6 µg/l		(>2 µg/l)
Ferritin	498 µg/l		(12–200 µg/l)
Immunoglobulins		normal	
Serum protein electrophoresis		normal	
Free light chains:	κ 60.1 mg/l		(3.3–19.4 mg/l)
	λ 6.3 mg/l		(5.7–26.3 mg/l)
	ratio κ:λ 9.54		(0.26–1.65)

1. **What is the likely diagnosis?**
2. **What other investigations are necessary?**

➥ **answer on page 164**

Case 1.3

A 25-year-old woman is referred to her GP after having her BP measured at a medical check-up arranged by her employer. She is asymptomatic, and there is no significant family history. Her BP at the surgery is 162/104 mmHg. On examination, she is of normal appearance with a body mass index of 23.2 kg/m². There are no cardiac murmurs, and peripheral pulses are normal. She is on no prescribed medication. The following results are returned:

Na^+	142 mmol/l	(135–145 mmol/l)
K^+	2.8 mmol/l	(3.5–5.0 mmol/l)
Cl^-	89 mmol/l	(95–105 mmol/l)
HCO_3^-	28 mmol/l	(24–30 mmol/l)
Urea	4.2 mmol/l	(2.5–6.7 mmol/l)
Creatinine	68 μmol/l	(79–118 μmol/l)
eGFR	>60 ml/min per 1.73 m²	(>60 ml/min per 1.73 m²)
Urinalysis:	normal	

1. **What secondary cause for hypertension requires exclusion first?**
2. **What tests would you request to further investigate this situation?**
3. **What pathological abnormalities can underlie this condition?**

➥ **answer on page 165**

Case 1.4

A 48-year-old retired civil servant is concerned with her pale colour and feelings of faintness that have occurred over the past 4 weeks. She had felt well before this and enjoyed regular trips to southern France. Brief clinical examination reveals pallor. Her blood tests come to your attention.

Hb	87 g/l	(120–160 g/l females)
MCV	64.5 fl	(76–96 fl)
Platelets	556 x 10^9/l	(150–400 × 10^9/l)
WCC	7.7 x 10^9/l	(4.0–11.0 × 10^9/l)
Iron	6 μmol/l	(11–32 μmol/l)
Ferritin	10 μg/l	(12–200 μg/l)
TIBC	90 μmol/l	(42–80 μmol/l)
Vitamin B_{12}	221 ng/l	(191–663 ng/l)
Folate	8.2 μg/l	(>2 μg/l)

1. **How would you interpret these results?**
2. **How would you investigate?**

➥ **answer on page 165**

Case 1.5

A 22-year-old university student is trapped in her house during a fire and when rescued by firefighters has developed substantial burns to the arms and chest. She is admitted to the burns unit. U+Es on her third day are shown.

Na^+	150 mmol/l	(135–145 mmol/l)
K^+	3.6 mmol/l	(3.5–5.0 mmol/l)
Urea	3.2 mmol/l	(2.5–6.7 mmol/l)
Creatinine	62 μmol/l	(79–118 μmol/l)
Cl^-	96 mmol/l	(95–105 mmol/l)
HCO_3^-	25 mmol/l	(24–30 mmol/l)

What is the main biochemical problem and name some of its causes?

➥ **answer on page 165**

Case 1.6

A 64-year-old woman is admitted with palpitations. She feels that these have been intermittent over the last month. Examination reveals an anxious woman with an irregularly irregular pulse at 120 beats/min. ECG confirms the suspicions of atrial fibrillation. As part of her initial investigations, the following blood test is returned.

Free T_4	70 pmol/l	(7.6–19.7 pmol/l)
TSH	<0.01 mU/l	(0.4–4.5 mU/l)

What is the underlying cause of the atrial fibrillation?

➥ **answer on page 166**

Case 1.7

A 55-year-old woman with essential hypertension attends the medical clinic. Her blood pressure remains elevated despite treatment with four drugs. Her consultant commences her on methyldopa. Four weeks later she attends the accident and emergency department feeling generally unwell. The A&E doctor sends off a variety of blood tests, which are shown here.

Hb	92 g/l	(120–160 g/l females)
MCV	93.4 fl	(76–96 fl)
Platelets	376 x 10^9/l	(150–400 × 10^9/l)
WCC	7.2 x 10^9/l	(4.0–11.0 × 10^9/l)
Iron	25 μmol/l	(11–32 μmol/l)
Ferritin	154 μg/l	(12–200 μg/l)
TIBC	65 μmol/l	(42–80 μmol/l)
Vitamin B_{12}	423 ng/l	(191–663 ng/l)
Folate	6.5 μg/l	(>2 μg/l)
Total bilirubin	45 μmol/l	(3–17 μmol/l)
AST	25 U/l	(5–35 U/l)
ALT	22 U/l	(5–35 U/l)
GGT	15 U/l	(7–33 U/l female)
ALP	98 U/l	(30–150 U/l)

She is admitted to the medical unit, and several other tests are requested.

Urinary urobilinogen	Positive
Blood film	Large numbers of reticulocytes
Direct antiglobulin test	Positive

1. **Interpret the results above**
2. **What is the likely diagnosis?**

➥ **answer on page 166**

Case 1.8

A 20-year-old law student attends A&E feeling unwell after a car journey back to Belfast from Dublin, having been to visit his girlfriend over the weekend. He has a headache and informs you that he had great difficulty concentrating on the final part of his trip. He does admit to having a 'big weekend' while in Dublin. On examination his pulse is bounding in character.

His various investigations are shown. The arterial blood gas was sampled with the patient breathing room air.

Na^+	140 mmol/l	(135–145 mmol/l)
K^+	4.2 mmol/l	(3.5–5.0 mmol/l)
Urea	4.8 mmol/l	(2.5–6.7 mmol/l)
Creatinine	76 μmol/l	(79–118 μmol/l)
Cl^-	105 mmol/l	(95–105 mmol/l)
HCO_3^-	23 mmol/l	(24–30 mmol/l)
pH	7.41	(7.35–7.45)
PaO_2	13.8 kPa	(11–13 kPa)
$PaCO_2$	4.3 kPa	(4.7–6.0 kPa)
HCO_3^-	24.3 mmol/l	(24–30 mmol/l)
Carboxyhaemoglobin	17%	(0.5–1.5% of total haemoglobin in non smokers)
Alcohol	nil	
Urine - trace of cannabinoids		

Describe the abnormalities seen and explain the cause of this man's symptoms.

➥ **answer on page 166**

Case 1.9

A 36-year-old man is admitted with shortness of breath and a cough productive of green sputum. He is feverish and complains of left-sided pleuritic chest discomfort. He has no significant past medical history. He is a smoker of 10 pack-years. On examination a pleural effusion is noted on the left side to the mid-zone. This finding is confirmed on chest radiography.

The effusion is aspirated at ward level and sent for analysis.

Pleural fluid sample	
Total protein	35 g/l
WCC	19/mm^3
LDH	230 U/l
pH	7.36
Microbiology	Nil noted

Describe the findings and the likely cause of the pleural effusion.

➥ **answer on page 167**

Case 1.10

A patient attends the emergency department because of a swollen leg on the right side. He has a history of dementia, and is unsure for how long the leg has been swollen. On inspection, the right calf is 0.3 cm larger than the left, there is no erythema and the calf is non-tender. You order a blood test to help with management.

D-dimer	0.12 mg/l	(<0.5 mg/l)

How would you proceed?

➥ **answer on page 167**

Case 1.11

A 69-year-old retired nurse complains of generalised aches and pains for the past 5 weeks, sometimes preventing her from sleeping at night. Her past medical history includes hypothyroidism, hypertension and a mastectomy 2 years ago for breast carcinoma. She is a very active member of the Women's Institute and feels less able to complete her daily tasks of late.

Blood tests included a bone profile. Liver function tests were normal.

Adjusted Ca^{2+}	2.34 mmol/l	(2.10–2.65 mmol/l)
Phosphate	0.91 mmol/l	(0.8–1.45 mmol/l)
ALP	215 U/l	(30–150 U/l)
Albumin	38 g/l	(35–50 g/l)

Describe the findings on the bone profile and give an explanation.

➥ **answer on page 167**

Case 1.12

A 77-year-old patient with dementia was admitted generally unwell. No history was obtained. He was pyrexic and appeared a little short of breath. Examination was difficult, although there was the impression of reduced breath sounds at the right lung base. Urinalysis was normal. Blood tests were taken.

Hb	139 g/l	(130-180 g/l males)
MCV	95.5 fl	(76-96 fl)
Platelets	188 x 10^9/l	(150-400 × 10^9/l)
WCC	9.7 x 10^9/l	(4.0-11.0 × 10^9/l)
Na^+	142 mmol/l	(135-145 mmol/l)
K^+	4.4 mmol/l	(3.5-5.0 mmol/l)
Urea	4.6 mmol/l	(2.5-6.7 mmol/l)
Creatinine	75 μmol/l	(79-118 μmol/l)
Cl^-	100 mmol/l	(95-105 mmol/l)
HCO_3^-	24 mmol/l	(24-30 mmol/l)
CRP	156 mg/l	(<10 mg/l)

How do these tests help in the management of this patient?

➥ **answer on page 168**

Case 1.13

A 55-year-old senior civil servant plucks up the courage to attend his GP after complaints of a poor urinary stream, frequency and nocturia. He is concerned as his father had 'prostate problems', On rectal examination an enlarged prostate was felt. Later that week his renal function and prostate-specific antigen tests come back.

Na^+	139 mmol/l	(135-145 mmol/l)
K^+	4.3 mmol/l	(3.5-5.0 mmol/l)
Urea	5.1 mmol/l	(2.5-6.7 mmol/l)
Creatinine	67 μmol/l	(79-118 μmol/l)
Cl^-	104 mmol/l	(95-105 mmol/l)
HCO_3^-	25 mmol/l	(24-30 mmol/l)
PSA	2.2 ng/ml	(<3.5 ng/ml 50-59 years)

Does this patient have anything to worry about?

➥ **answer on page 168**

Case 1.14

A 32-year-old man is recalled by his occupational health department following a recent 'medical' before transfer to an overseas operation within the company. He is teetotal. He cannot understand what all the fuss is about as he feels fine.

The blood results of concern are shown.

Total bilirubin	11 μmol/l	(3-17 μmol/l)
AST	188 U/l	(5-35 U/l)
ALT	197 U/l	(5-35 U/l)
ALP	45 U/l	(30-150 U/l)
GGT	57 U/l	(11-58 U/l males)
Albumin	39 g/l	(35-50 g/l)

1. **What pattern of LFTs is demonstrated?**
2. **What further blood tests may help in coming to a diagnosis?**

➥ **answer on page 168**

Case 1.15

A 57-year-old woman attends her GP complaining of tiredness. The GP knows her medical history well as she also suffers from Graves' disease. A full blood picture was analysed as well as haematinics.

Hb	99 g/l	(120-160 g/l females)
MCV	104.5 fl	(76-96 fl)
Platelets	199 x 10^9/l	(150-400 × 10^9/l)
WCC	6.7 x 10^9/l	(4.0-11.0 × 10^9/l)
Iron	21 μmol/l	(11-32 μmol/l)
Ferritin	50 μg/l	(12-200 μg/l)
TIBC	60 μmol/l	(42-80 μmol/l)
Vitamin B_{12}	22 ng/l	(191-663 ng/l)
Folate	9.8 μg/l	(>2 μg/l)

1. **Interpret these blood results.**

Following these results the GP also requests another test shown below.

Anti-parietal cell antibody	Titre 1:220
Anti-intrinsic factor antibody	Positive

2. **What is the diagnosis?**

➥ **answer on page 169**

Case 1.16

A 34-year-old woman with acute lymphoblastic leukaemia (ALL) is receiving chemotherapy within the haematology suite of the hospital. Several days into treatment she complains of an intensely sore right knee. On examination there is an effusion and she is unable to extend the knee fully due to pain. She has no pre-existing joint disease. Fluid was aspirated from the knee and sent for analysis along with blood samples.

Na^+	143 mmol/l	(135–145 mmol/l)
K^+	4.1 mmol/l	(3.5–5.0 mmol/l)
Urea	5.8 mmol/l	(2.5–6.7 mmol/l)
Creatinine	79 μmol/l	(79–118 μmol/l)
Cl^-	97 mmol/l	(95–105 mmol/l)
HCO_3^-	25 mmol/l	(24–30 mmol/l)
Urate	0.88 mmol/l	(0.15–0.50 mmol/l)

Synovial fluid analysis
Negatively birefringent needle-shaped crystals on polarised light microscopy

Interpret these results.

➥ **answer on page 169**

Case 1.17

A patient is reviewed at the chest clinic. He was treated over 1 year ago for pulmonary tuberculosis. He now complains of lethargy. Clinical examination reveals no chest abnormalities, but he is found to have significant postural hypotension. A urea and electrolyte (U+E) blood test is sent and, on the basis of the results, the following test is arranged.

Time (min)	0	30
Cortisol (nmol/l)	140	150

1. **What is the test, and what does it demonstrate in this case?**
2. **What were the likely abnormalities on the U+E that raised suspicions of this disorder?**
3. **What is the likely underlying disease?**

➥ **answer on page 169**

Case 1.18

A 65-year-old retired headmaster presents with progressive shortness of breath and swelling of the feet. Nine years ago he sustained an anterior myocardial infarction and has had subsequent problems with angina requiring coronary artery stenting. He also suffers from hypertension and gout. Following a recent flare of gout his GP prescribed a short course of ibuprofen. Examination reveals pitting oedema to the mid-calves bilaterally and a jugular venous pulse (JVP) raised by 3 cm. The bases of both lungs are dull to percussion. Breath sounds are reduced and vocal resonance is decreased over these areas.

After some initial treatment these examination findings remain and a decision is made to carry out pleural aspiration: 30 ml was aspirated from the right hemithorax and sent for analysis.

Pleural fluid sample	
Total protein	21 g/l
LDH	140 U/l
pH	7.36
Microbiology	Nil noted

Describe the findings and likely cause.

➥ answer on page 170

Case 1.19

A 74-year-old man presents to the A&E department after a 5-minute episode of loss of vision affecting the right eye. Further questioning revealed that the patient had a similar episode 2 days previously. On each occasion the vision was lost rapidly, 'like a curtain being drawn' over the visual field. Direct questioning revealed that he had been lethargic for several weeks, and experienced some pain in his jaw on chewing. Initial blood tests revealed the following:

Hb	142 g/l	(130–180 g/l males)
MCV	81 fl	(76–96 fl)
Platelets	212 x 10^9/l	(150–400 × 10^9/l)
WCC	10.2 x 10^9/l	(4.0–11.0 × 10^9/l)
ESR	132 mm/h	(0–15 mm/h males)

1. **What is the likely diagnosis?**
2. **What treatment would you prescribe immediately?**

➥ answer on page 170

Case 1.20

A 76-year-old woman is admitted unwell with vomiting and is found to have a low blood pressure. She had recently been given diclofenac following a complaint of back pain. Her initial blood results included U+E.

Na^+	137 mmol/l	(135–145 mmol/l)
K^+	6.7 mmol/l	(3.5–5.0 mmol/l)
Urea	22.3 mmol/l	(2.5–6.7 mmol/l)
Creatinine	609 μmol/l	(79–118 μmol/l)
Cl^-	95 mmol/l	(95–105 mmol/l)
HCO_3^-	24 mmol/l	(24–30 mmol/l)

1. **What has happened to this patient?**
2. **What immediate treatment is indicated?**

➥ **answer on page 170**

Case 1.21

A 55-year-old woman is admitted with a fractured neck of femur after a minor trip in the car park of her local supermarket. Looking back through her old records, the admitting doctor notices the following bone profile taken 2 weeks previously.

Adjusted Ca^{2+}	2.31 mmol/l	(2.10–2.65 mmol/l)
Phosphate	0.87 mmol/l	(0.8–1.45 mmol/l)
ALP	69 U/l	(30–150 U/l)
Albumin	39 g/l	(35–50 g/l)

What bone disease might you suspect?

➥ **answer on page 171**

Case 1.22

A 68-year-old woman was admitted with itch, lethargy and discoloration of the skin over the past month. On examination she is icteric and cachexic. There are no stigmata of chronic liver disease. Nursing staff indicate that there is discoloration of her urine.

Her admission bloods include LFTs.

Total bilirubin	78 μmol/l	(3–17 μmol/l)
AST	35 U/l	(5–35 U/l)
ALT	39 U/l	(5–35 U/l)
ALP	156 U/l	(30–150 U/l)
GGT	176 U/l	(7–33 U/l females)
Albumin	39 g/l	(35–50 g/l)

1. **Outline the abnormalities seen on the liver function tests.**
2. **What would be your next choice of investigation?**
3. **What are the potential causes of these results?**

➥ **answer on page 171**

Case 1.23 +

A 44-year-old reformed intravenous drug user with known hepatitis C is well known to the local hepatologists. He has been attending on a regular basis and is enrolled in the hepatocellular carcinoma surveillance programme. Below are an overview of his blood tests.

Date	α-Fetoprotein (kU/l)
04/01/2004	6
05/06/2004	8
12/12/2004	7
14/01/2005	16
05/06/2005	57
01/09/2005	27
03/12/2005	8

(Age-appropriate reference range: <10 kU/l)

What may explain the pattern in these results?

➥ **answer on page 171**

Case 1.24

A 58-year-old man complains of an exquisitely tender great toe. It is red, swollen and impossible to examine fully because of pain. No other joints are affected. He has a history of hypertension and a previous myocardial infarction at 49 years of age. He drinks 14 units of alcohol a week. To his knowledge he does not have any kidney problems. Blood tests are shown.

Na^+	141 mmol/l	(135–145 mmol/l)
K^+	4.4 mmol/l	(3.5–5.0 mmol/l)
Urea	5.6 mmol/l	(2.5–6.7 mmol/l)
Creatinine	99 μmol/l	(79–118 μmol/l)
Cl^-	98 mmol/l	(95–105 mmol/l)
HCO_3^-	24 mmol/l	(24–30 mmol/l)
Urate	0.78 mmol/l	(0.15–0.50 mmol/l)

Does this man have gout? Justify your answer.

➥ **answer on page 172**

Case 1.25

You see a 64-year-old woman in A&E. She has severe chronic obstructive pulmonary disease (COPD), and has been an inpatient on several occasions in the past year. She appears short of breath, and complains of a worsening cough productive of green sputum. This has become worse over the last 3 days. Part of her admission blood tests are shown.

Hb	162 g/l	(120–160 g/l females)
PCV	0.53	(0.37–0.47 females)
MCV	84.6 fl	(76–96 fl)
Platelets	398 x 10^9/l	(150–400 × 10^9/l)
WCC	16.5 x 10^9/l	(4.0–11.0 × 10^9/l)
Neutrophils	14.1 x 10^9/l	(2.0–7.5 × 10^9/l)
Lymphocytes	2.2 x 10^9/l	(1.5–4.0 × 10^9/l)

Outline the abnormalities shown, and discuss their most likely causes.

➥ **answer on page 172**

Case 1.26

A 55-year-old woman is admitted under the care of the surgical team with a distended abdomen. She admits that it has become increasingly large over the past few weeks, but was scared to come to hospital. She has no complaints of abdominal pain and her bowel habit is normal. The enthusiastic junior doctor who admitted the patient included in the notes that she has sent blood for CEA, CA-125 and CA-19-9.

CEA	3.4 ng/ml
CA-125	599 U/ml
CA-19-9	32 U/ml

What do these blood results tell you?

➥ answer on page 172

Case 1.27

A 42-year-old salesman with established alcoholic liver cirrhosis is a known patient to the ward. He has been admitted on multiple previous occasions and continues to drink heavily. On this admission he is a little confused and tremulous. On examination, ascites is present along with small bilateral pleural effusions. His abdomen is mildly tender throughout. Bowel sounds are present.

The on-call doctor performs a diagnostic peritoneal aspiration. One hour later, the laboratory technician phones with the report below.

Analysis of peritoneal fluid		
WCC	322 cells/mm^3 - predominantly neutrophils	
Albumin	16 g/l	(35–50 g/l)
Amylase	92 U/l	(25–125 U/l)
Microscopy	Gram-negative bacilli seen on Gram stain	

His blood albumin level is 29 g/l.

What is the diagnosis, and how should the patient be treated?

➥ answer on page 173

Case 1.28

A 58-year-old patient with immunodeficiency is admitted to the intensive care unit with severe pneumonia. Despite aggressive antibiotic therapy, his condition does not improve. On his third day in the unit, the nurses report that he is beginning to bleed around the sites of his indwelling venous lines. The doctor in charge requests a coagulation profile. The blood is taken from a peripheral vein.

PT	29.5 s	(12–16 s)
APTT	66 s	(24–38 s)
Fibrinogen	0.35 g/l	(2–4 g/l)
D-dimer	>20 mg/l	(<0.5 mg/l)

What is the likely diagnosis?

➥ answer on page 173

Case 1.29

A 62-year-old woman is admitted with septic arthritis of the knee. A D-dimer blood test is sent in error, but comes back as follows:

D-dimer	1.2 mg/l	(<0.5 mg/l)

Would you arrange investigations to test for thromboembolic disease?

➥ answer on page 174

Case 1.30

A 72-year-old former engine driver attends his GP complaining of generalised aches and pains. During the consultation you have to speak loudly to be understood. As part of your investigations you request a bone profile. Liver function tests were normal.

Adjusted Ca^{2+}	2.45 mmol/l	(2.10–2.65 mmol/l)
Phosphate	0.84 mmol/l	(0.8–1.45 mmol/l)
ALP	178 U/l	(30–150 U/l)
Albumin	42 g/l	(35–50 g/l)

On the basis of this test he received a course of treatment. Following treatment his bone profile is repeated and is as follows.

Adjusted Ca^{2+}	2.42 mmol/l	(2.10–2.65 mmol/l)
Phosphate	0.79 mmol/l	(0.8–1.45 mmol/l)
ALP	76 U/l	(30–150 U/l)
Albumin	41 g/l	(35–50 g/l)

1. **What bone disease does this patient have?**
2. **What treatment is he likely to have received to explain the change in his bone profile?**

➥ **answer on page 174**

Case 1.31 ✚

A 34-year-old labourer is admitted with right upper quadrant discomfort, fever and sweats. He returned from a project overseas 3 weeks earlier. On examination he is tender to palpitation over the right hypochondrium making complete examination difficult. A spiking fever pattern is seen on his observation chart. His LFTs are as follows.

Total bilirubin	51 μmol/l	(3–17 μmol/l)
AST	46 U/l	(5–35 U/l)
ALT	76 U/l	(5–35 U/l)
ALP	10 U/l	(30–150 U/l)
GGT	87 U/l	(11–58 U/l males)
Albumin	42 g/l	(35–50 g/l)
CRP	142 mg/l	(<10 mg/l)

1. **What investigation does this patient need as soon as possible based on his clinical history and blood tests?**
2. **What is the likely diagnosis?**

➥ **answer on page 174**

Case 1.32 +

A 37-year-old manual worker is admitted with generalised abdominal discomfort, vomiting and shakiness. On examination there is a 4-cm mildly tender hepatomegaly. He is sweaty to the touch. Some blood tests are requested.

Hb	134 g/l	(130–180 g/l males)
MCV	105.6 fl	(76–96 fl)
Platelets	124 x 10^9/l	(150–400 × 10^9/l)
WCC	5.6 x 10^9/l	(4.0–11.0 × 10^9/l)
Na^+	142 mmol/l	(135–145 mmol/l)
K^+	3.4 mmol/l	(3.5–5.0 mmol/l)
Urea	2.1 mmol/l	(2.5–6.7 mmol/l)
Creatinine	58 μmol/l	(79–118 μmol/l)
Cl^-	105 mmol/l	(95–105 mmol/l)
HCO_3^-	26.7 mmol/l	(24–30 mmol/l)
Mg^{2+}	0.42 mmol/l	(0.7-1.0 mmol/l)
PO_4^{3-}	0.32 mmol/l	(0.8–1.45 mmol/l)
Adjusted Ca^{2+}	2.36 mmol/l	(2.10–2.65 mmol/l)
Total bilirubin	14 μmol/l	(3–17 μmol/l)
AST	32 U/l	(5–35 U/l)
ALT	33 U/l	(5–35 U/l)
ALP	67 U/l	(30–150 U/l)
GGT	145 U/l	(11–58 U/l males)
Albumin	30 g/l	(35-50 g/l)

1. **Outline the abnormalities on this set of blood results.**
2. **Explain the likely cause of the LFT abnormalities given the abnormalities in the other results.**

➥ **answer on page 175**

Case 1.33 +

A 44-year-old woman with primary biliary cirrhosis has been attending hepatology outpatients for many years. Over the past 18 months she has been feeling less well in herself and her frequency of attendance for review has increased at the insistence of her physician. On examination she is jaundiced and her abdomen is mildly distended with a 3-cm hepatomegaly.

Her recent blood results are shown.

Date	04/04	06/04	10/04	02/05	05/05	08/05	12/05
Total bilirubin (μmol/l)	14	15	17	25	41	49	69
AST (U/l)	45	46	48	45	51	54	59
ALT (U/l)	46	48	49	55	48	51	53
ALP (U/l)	166	188	203	278	398	487	603
GGT (U/l)	88	94	96	95	99	101	101
Albumin (g/l)	37	36	33	32	32	30	28

(Reference ranges: Total bilirubin 3-17 μmol/l, AST 5-35 U/l, ALT 5-35 U/l, ALP 30-150 U/l, GGT 7-33 U/l, Albumin 35-50 g/l)

Give a summary of the findings.

➥ **answer on page 175**

Case 1.34 +

A patient is referred to a psychiatrist for investigation of bizarre thoughts. She has occasional involuntary movements. The psychiatrist requests a series of blood tests as part of her initial screening tests, and the following results are obtained.

Total bilirubin	15 μmol/l	(3-17 μmol/l)
AST	82 U/l	(5-35 U/l)
ALT	78 U/l	(5-35 U/l)
ALP	72 U/l	(30-150 U/l)
GGT	112 U/l	(7-33 U/l females)
Albumin	46 g/l	(35-50 g/l)

What disease could account for the presentation and the blood test abnormalities? How would you investigate it further?

➥ **answer on page 175**

Case 1.35

A 38-year-old woman complains of a rash over her face and nose that has been present for several weeks and a recent problem with pain and swelling in the joints of her hands. She is married but without children. A number of blood tests were sent - some of which are shown below.

Hb	110 g/l	(120–160 g/l females)
MCV	94.4 fl	(76–96 fl)
Platelets	128 x 10^9/l	(150–400 × 10^9/l)
WCC	2.7 x 10^9/l	(4.0–11.0 × 10^9/l)
ESR	77 mm/h	(0–22 mm/h females)
Na^+	136 mmol/l	(135–145 mmol/l)
K^+	4.4 mmol/l	(3.5–5.0 mmol/l)
Urea	4.9 mmol/l	(2.5–6.7 mmol/l)
Creatinine	64 μmol/l	(79–118 μmol/l)
Cl^-	99 mmol/l	(95–105 mmol/l)
HCO_3^-	26 mmol/l	(24–30 mmol/l)
CRP	7 mg/l	(<10 mg/l)
Urinalysis	Protein ++	

1. **Summarise the results shown.**
2. **Using the clinical information what is the most likely diagnosis?**

➥ **answer on page 176**

Case 1.36

A 32-year-old woman with diabetes is admitted for treatment of a large abscess. The patient is reluctant to undergo surgical intervention and medical treatment is pursued initially. Four days into her care she becomes more unwell and her treatment is changed. A further 3 days on, when her condition remains poor, she agrees to surgical intervention. Below is a chart of her CRP throughout this period.

Day	1	2	3	4	5	6	7	8	9	10	11
CRP (mg/l)	356	345	387	444	467	499	550	422	302	143	121

Try to explain the trend in the results.

➥ **answer on page 176**

Case 1.37 +

A 67-year-old man attends outpatients with a complaint of constipation and vague abdominal discomfort. Abdominal examination and proctoscopy were normal. Imaging investigations and endoscopy have been arranged. CEA levels were also requested, along with routine blood tests.

Hb	91 g/l	(130-180 g/l males)
MCV	71.2 fl	(76-96 fl)
Platelets	199 x 10^9/l	(150-400 × 10^9/l)
WCC	5.6 x 10^9/l	(4.0-11.0 × 10^9/l)
Na^+	139 mmol/l	(135-145 mmol/l)
K^+	4.2 mmol/l	(3.5-5.0 mmol/l)
Urea	4.5 mmol/l	(2.5-6.7 mmol/l)
Creatinine	87 µmol/l	(79-118 µmol/l)
Cl^-	104 mmol/l	(95-105 mmol/l)
HCO_3^-	26 mmol/l	(24-30 mmol/l)
CEA	81 ng/ml	(<10 ng/ml)

What underlying diagnosis unites all the abnormalities observed?

➥ **answer on page 176**

Case 1.38 +

A 55 year old with haemophilia attends her routine 6-monthly review at hepatology outpatients. She has been attending for several years after contracting hepatitis C from a blood transfusion. The doctor notes that she has not attended for 8 months, and requests a number of blood tests.

Total bilirubin	8 µmol/l	(3-17 µmol/l)
AST	111 U/l	(5-35 U/l)
ALT	121 U/l	(5-35 U/l)
ALP	76 U/l	(30-150 U/l)
GGT	37 U/l	(7-33 U/l females)
Albumin	26 g/l	(35-50 g/l)
α-Fetoprotein	9 kU/l	(<15 kU/l 50-70 years)

What would you infer from these results?

➥ **answer on page 177**

Case 1.39

A 28-year-old media studies student attends A&E with a swollen left testicle. He is sexually active, with multiple sexual partners in the last 6 months. The A&E officer is concerned, and arranges admission. Ultrasound of the scrotum and blood tests were requested.

α-Fetoprotein	140 kU/l	(<10 kU/l <50 years)
β-Human chorionic gonadotrophin	220 U/l	(<5 U/l)

Can these results be explained by a diagnosis of epididymo-orchitis?

→ **answer on page 177**

Case 1.40

A patient is referred to the endocrine clinic complaining of excess thirst and of passing excessive amounts of urine. A random blood glucose level is 4.2 mmol/l. He is admitted to hospital and a water deprivation test is arranged. The results are shown.

Time (h)	Plasma osmolality (mosmol/kg)	Urine osmolality (mosmol/kg)
0	297	115
1	300	117
2	305	115
3	309	115
4	316	114
5	324	113
6	326	115
7	332	116
8	336	115
Following desmopressin injection		750

(Reference range: Plasma osmolality 280–300 mosmol/kg)

1. **What is your interpretation of the blood glucose level?**
2. **What is the diagnosis?**

→ **answer on page 177**

Case 1.41

A 57-year-old man is referred to the hypertension clinic. Two tests are performed in order to screen for an endocrine cause of hypertension.

Urine volume	1825 ml
Urinary normetanephrine	1772 nmol/24h (440-2960)
Urinary metanephrine	273 nmol/24h (141-1289)
Blood cortisol	225 nmol/l at 9.00am following 1 mg dexamethasone at 11.00pm the evening before

How would you interpret these results?

➥ **answer on page 178**

Case 1.42

A patient is referred to the endocrine clinic after having been assessed in the eye A&E. The registrar arranges for a glucose tolerance test to be carried out.

Time (min)	0	120
Glucose (mmol/l)	6.5	15.2
Growth hormone (mU/l)	12	11

1. **What two diagnoses can be made on the basis of this test?**
2. **Why do you think the patient was seen in the eye A&E?**

➥ **answer on page 178**

Case 1.43

As the medical junior doctor on-call you are asked by your surgical colleagues to see a 45-year-old overweight housewife. She was admitted with abdominal pain 2 days ago and an ultrasound scan of the abdomen showed gallstones with extrahepatic bile duct dilatation. Bowel gas obscured visualisation of the pancreas. Your opinion is sought as the patient is short of breath and complains of left-sided pleuritic chest discomfort. On examination you detect a left-sided pleural effusion which is confirmed on chest radiography. You decide to perform a diagnostic pleural aspiration.

Pleural fluid sample	
Total protein	38.6 g/l
LDH	332 U/l
pH	7.36
Microbiology	Nil seen
Glucose	4.9 mmol/l
Amylase	10 321 U/l

What is your interpretation of this result?

→ answer on page 178

Case 1.44

A 33-year-old secretary presents with malaise, joint discomfort and by her own admission generally feeling 'out of sorts'. She was diagnosed with Graves' disease 3 years ago and has been rendered euthyroid (normal thyroid function). She has also suffered from coeliac disease since her teens. She has no respiratory complaints. As part of her investigative work-up a chest radiograph is taken, which to the medical team's surprise shows a right-sided pleural effusion of moderate size.

Pleural aspiration is performed.

Pleural fluid sample	
Total protein	33.2 g/l
LDH	287 U/l
pH	7.36
Microbiology	Nil seen
Glucose	2.2 mmol/l
Amylase	65 U/l
Rheumatoid factor	556 IU/ml

What is the cause of her effusion?

→ answer on page 179

Case 1.45 +

A frail 88-year-old nursing home resident is brought to hospital because of abdominal pain. Her nurse is also concerned about the progressive increase in her abdominal girth over the past 6 weeks. She has a history of vascular dementia. On examination there is a grossly distended abdomen, with shifting dullness and a fluid thrill. A CT scan of the abdomen and pelvis demonstrated a massive mixed solid–cystic lesion in the pelvis and gross ascites.

Peritoneal aspiration was performed for diagnostic purposes and symptomatic benefit: 9500 ml was drained and sent for analysis. The results are shown.

Analysis of peritoneal fluid	
WCC	25 cells/mm^3 - mixed leukocytes
Albumin	28 g/l
Microscopy	No organisms seen
Cytology	Tumour cells seen - in keeping with adenocarcinoma

Her blood albumin level is 29 g/l.

Provide a diagnosis and explain your reasoning.

→ **answer on page 179**

Case 1.46 +

A 36-year-old banker attends A&E complaining of recurrent bouts of intense abdominal discomfort. He has been reluctant to present previously for fear of admission. He admits to being a heavy drinker, but his family and colleagues are not aware of his problem. On examination there is distension of the abdomen with ascites present, tenderness in the upper abdomen and a faint upper midline incision.

You are concerned about his level of abdominal pain. He agrees to peritoneal aspiration, but does not wish to be admitted.

Analysis of peritoneal fluid	
WCC	147 cells/mm^3 - predominantly neutrophils
Albumin	29 g/l
Amylase	894 U/l
Microscopy	No organisms seen

The patient's blood albumin level is 32 g/l.

Give a diagnosis and list useful further investigations.

→ **answer on page 179**

Case 1.47

What is the inheritance pattern in the following family tree?

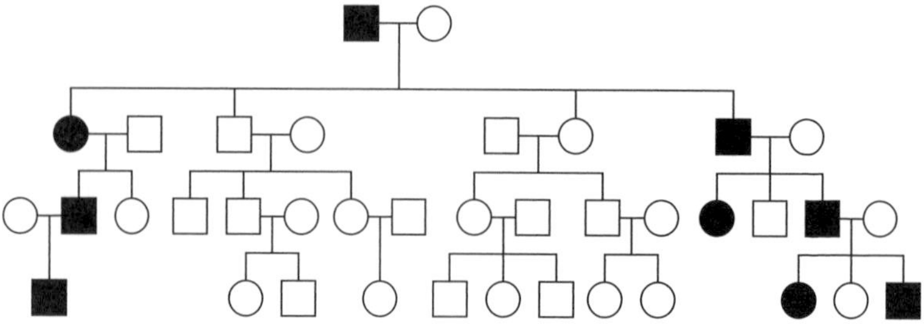

Key

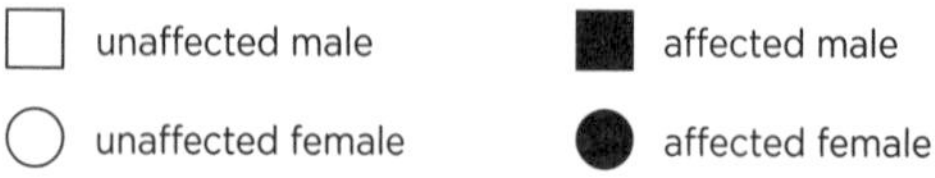

➥ **answer on page 180**

Case 1.48

You assess an elderly man who complains of shortness of breath on exertion. He has fine crepitations on auscultation of both lung bases, and you suspect cardiac failure as a possible diagnosis. On review of his blood tests, you note that a colleague requested the following test 1 month ago.

N-terminal pro-BNP	51 ng/l (<125 ng/l)

Should you order an echocardiogram?

➥ **answer on page 180**

Case 1.49

A 57-year-old man is medically retired from his former job in the local shipyard. For the past 6 years his health has deteriorated with an exercise tolerance now reduced to 10 metres on the flat. He is a life-long non-smoker. A recent high-resolution CT scan of the chest demonstrated diffuse bibasal interstitial changes. His ABG was taken on room air without any intercurrent illness.

pH	7.43	(7.35–7.45)
PaO_2	6.9 kPa	(11–13 kPa)
$PaCO_2$	4.9 kPa	(4.7–6.0 kPa)
HCO_3^-	25.7 mmol/l	(24–30 mmol/l)
BE	1.7 mmol/l	(–2 to +2 mmol/l)

1. **Outline the abnormalities seen.**
2. **What are the likely causes for an ABG such as this?**
3. **What long-term therapy might be considered?**

➥ **answer on page 180**

Case 1.50

The blood gas below was taken following admission of an elderly patient to the acute medical unit. He was breathing room air.

pH	7.55	(7.35–7.45)
PaO_2	9.2 kPa	(11–13 kPa)
$PaCO_2$	5.7 kPa	(4.7–6.0 kPa)
HCO_3^-	35.7 mmol/l	(24–30 mmol/l)
Base excess (BE)	13.8 mmol/l	(–2 to +2 mmol/l)

1. **Outline the abnormalities on this ABG.**
2. **What are the likely causes for these abnormalities?**

➥ **answer on page 180**

Case 1.51

A 55-year-old man who smokes and has a strong family history of coronary heart disease presents 14 h after a 30-min episode of central crushing chest pain. He was afraid to come to hospital at the time. He is currently pain free, and his ECG was normal. The A&E officer requests the following test:

High sensitivity troponin T	1512 ng/l	(<14 ng/l)

Where should this patient be managed?

➥ **answer on page 181**

Case 1.52

An anxious 27-year-old student was admitted with shortness of breath and tingling in her hands. On examination, she had a respiratory rate of 28 breaths per minute. Chest examination was unremarkable. Chest radiograph and routine blood tests were normal. An ECG showed sinus tachycardia. An ABG was taken on 35% oxygen.

pH	7.52	(7.35-7.45)
PaO_2	28 kPa	(11-13 kPa)
$PaCO_2$	2.0 kPa	(4.7-6.0 kPa)
HCO_3^-	18.7 mmol/l	(24-30 mmol/l)
BE	+6 mmol/l	(-2 to +2 mmol/l)

1. **Outline the abnormalities on this ABG.**
2. **What is the likely cause?**
3. **How might one treat this woman?**

➥ **answer on page 181**

Case 1.53

You assess a patient after a short-lived episode of central chest pain. His medical history includes chronic kidney disease, not requiring dialysis at present. A 12-lead ECG is normal. Blood is sampled 12 hours after the onset of pain.

Na^+	143 mmol/l	(135–145 mmol/l)
K^+	4.6 mmol/l	(3.5–5.0 mmol/l)
Urea	13.8 mmol/l	(2.5–6.7 mmol/l)
Creatinine	355 μmol/l	(79–118 μmol/l)
eGFR	25 ml/min per 1.73 m^2	(>60 ml/min per 1.73 m^2)
High sensitivity troponin T	27 ng/l	(<14 ng/l)

Has the patient suffered a myocardial infarction?

➥ **answer on page 181**

Case 1.54 ++

An 82-year-old man undergoes an elective total hip replacement for osteoarthritis. Blood tests around the time of the operation are as follows:

	Preoperative	Day 1 postoperative	Day 2 postoperative
Hb (g/l)	142	96	92
WCC (× 10^9/l)	4.5	11.5	11.3
Platelets (× 10^9/l)	210	160	155
Na^+ (mmol/l)	136	130	127
K^+ (mmol/l)	4.2	3.8	3.6
Cl^- (mmol/l)	89	85	82
HCO_3^-	25	24	25
Urea (mmol/l)	2.4	3.2	4.0
Creatinine (μmol/l)	75	82	85

(Reference ranges: Hb 130–180 g/l, WCC 4.0–11.0 × 10^9/l, Platelets 150–400 × 10^9/l, Na^+ 135–145 mmol/l, K^+ 3.5–5.0 mmol/l, Cl^- 79–118 μmol/l, HCO_3^- 24–30 mmol/l, Urea 2.5–6.7 mmol/l, Creatinine 79–118 μmol/l)

1. **Discuss the blood results.**
2. **How would you approach the management of this sodium disorder?**
3. **The urinary sodium is reported as <20 mmol/l. There is no evidence of fluid overload clinically. What treatment is required?**

➥ **answer on page 182**

Case 1.55 ++

A 50-year-old man is referred to the medical outpatient clinic on account of the finding of abnormal aminotransferases in his liver function tests. He is a successful businessman who often travels. He would never drink alcohol to the extent that he becomes intoxicated, and has never used recreational drugs. He has no medical history of note, and is on no regular medication. Examination is unremarkable, with the exception of mild bilateral gynaecomastia. His FBP is as follows:

Hb	132 g/l	(130–180 g/l males)
MCV	104 fl	(76–96 fl)
WCC	6.8 × 10^9/l	(4.0–11.0 × 10^9/l)
Platelets	76 × 10^9/l	(150–400 × 10^9/l)
Vitamin B_{12}	527 ng/l	(191–663 ng/l)
Folate	6.6 μg/l	(>2 μg/l)

Describe and account for the abnormalities in his blood results.

➥ **answer on page 182**

Case 1.56 ++

An attempt is made to insert a suprapubic urinary catheter into a patient with ascites due to liver cirrhosis. The operator is unsure whether the catheter has entered the bladder, and hence whether the fluid draining is urine or ascites. A sample is sent to the lab, and the results are shown:

Creatinine	12 mmol/l	(79–118 μmol/l)

Is the urinary catheter in the correct place?

➥ answer on page 183

Case 1.57 ++

A couple in their 30s attend an infertility clinic because they are having difficulties conceiving. Blood tests are returned as follows.

Male partner		
Testosterone	3.2 nmol/l	(11.4–27.9 nmol/l)
LH	17.5 U/l	(1.7–8.6 U/l)
FSH	21.2 U/l	(1.5–12.4 U/l)
Female partner		
Testosterone	1.2 nmol/l	(0.28–1.7 nmol)
Oestradiol	610 pmol/l	Depends on mentrual status
Progesterone	51 nmol/l	Depends on mentrual status
LH	5.2 U/l	Depends on mentrual status
FSH	4.5 U/l	Depends on mentrual status
Prolactin	1496 mU/l	(102–496 mU/l)
Mono-prolactin	110 mU/l	(102–496 mU/l)

1. **Which partner's samples suggest an abnormality that could account for the difficulty conceiving?**
2. **What are the possible causes for this presentation?**

➥ answer on page 183

Case 1.58 ++

A patient develops a pleural effusion 2 days after thoracic surgery. Pleural fluid is drained, and the following results are returned after analysis:

Pleural fluid:		
Total protein	41 g/l	
LDH	225 U/l	
Cholesterol	3.2 mmol/l	
Triglyceride	2.9 mmol/l	(<2.2 mmol/l)
Serum:		
Total protein	70 g/l	(60–80 g/l)
LDH	240 U/l	(70–250 U/l)
Cholesterol	4.8 mmol/l	(<5.0 mmol/l)
Triglyceride	1.8 mmol/l	(<2.2 mmol/l)

1. **Interpret these results and state the most likely classification for the pleural effusion.**
2. **What is the most likely overall cause for the effusion?**

➥ **answer on page 183**

Case 1.59 ++

A 72-year-old woman is brought to A&E with facial grimacing and spasms affecting her hands and feet. Her past medical history includes hypertension, peptic ulcer disease, thyroidectomy and osteoporosis. She is on the following medication: amlodipine, atenolol, omeprazole, levothyroxine and risedronate. The following results are returned:

Na^+	142 mmol/l	(135–145 mmol/l)
K^+	4.4 mmol/l	(3.5–5.0 mmol/l)
Cl^-	96 mmol/l	(95–105 mmol/l)
HCO_3^-	24 mmol/l	(24–30 mmol/l)
Urea	3.9 mmol/l	(2.5–6.7 mmol/l)
Creatinine	58 μmol/l	(79–118 μmol/l)
eGFR	>60 ml/min per 1.73 m^2	(>60 ml/min per 1.73 m^2)
Adjusted Ca^{2+}	1.55 mmol/l	(2.10–2.65 mmol/l)
Phosphate (PO_4^{3-})	1.50 mmol/l	(0.8–1.45 mmol/l)
Mg^{2+}	0.68 mmol/l	(0.7–1.0 mmol/l)

What electrolyte disturbance is responsible for her presentation, and what is the most likely underlying cause?

➥ **answer on page 184**

Case 1.60 ++

A patient undergoes a series of tests in the department of endocrinology. The results are as follows:

24-hour urine collection for free cortisol:
699 nmol/24 h (reference range <210 nmol/24 h).

Low-dose dexamethasone suppression test:

Time	Cortisol (nmol/l)
9am before test	733
After 48 h of treatment	602

High-dose dexamethasone suppression test:

Time	Cortisol (nmol/l)
9am before test	652
After 48 h of treatment	103

CRH test:

Time (min)	ACTH (ng/l)	Cortisol (nmol/l)
−15	38	810
0	36	802
5	70	1450
10	76	1585
15	80	1720
30	74	1801
45	72	1879
60	72	1852

1. **What is the precise diagnosis suggested by these results?**
2. **What other test could be carried out to back up this diagnosis?**

➥ **answer on page page 184**

Case 1.61 ++

A 49-year-old missionary is brought to your hospital by his wife. He has been vomiting for the past 24 h. He is now very weak. He last ate 2 days previously and has struggled to keep down any liquids since. On examination his mouth is dry, his abdomen is generally uncomfortable and he has reduced skin turgor. After taking his routine blood tests, a 0.9% saline drip is erected before any results are checked. A short time later the following result is available.

Na^+	130 mmol/l	(135-145 mmol/l)
K^+	2.8 mmol/l	(3.5-5.0 mmol/l)
Urea	10.6 mmol/l	(2.5-6.7 mmol/l)
Creatinine	79 μmol/l	(79-118 μmol/l)
Cl^-	97 mmol/l	(95-105 mmol/l)
HCO_3^-	24 mmol/l	(24-30 mmol/l)

1. **Outline the abnormalities on this blood result.**

After noting the above results, his intravenous fluid prescription is changed to 1 litre of 0.9% saline containing 40 mmol/l of potassium chloride, to be infused over 6 h.

Two hours later, his U+E is repeated, and is shown below.

Na^+	149 mmol/l	(135-145 mmol/l)
K^+	5.7 mmol/l	(3.5-5.0 mmol/l)
Urea	9.6 mmol/l	(2.5-6.7 mmol/l)
Creatinine	69 μmol/l	(79-118 μmol/l)
Cl^-	96 mmol/l	(95-105 mmol/l)
HCO_3^-	25 mmol/l	(24-30 mmol/l)

The ward doctor is concerned, and a further sample is taken.

Na^+	133 mmol/l	(135-145 mmol/l)
K^+	3.8 mmol/l	(3.5-5.0 mmol/l)
Urea	8.9 mmol/l	(2.5-6.7 mmol/l)
Creatinine	71 μmol/l	(79-118 μmol/l)
Cl^-	94 mmol/l	(95-105 mmol/l)
HCO_3^-	24 mmol/l	(24-30 mmol/l)

2. **How would you account for the discrepancy between these two blood tests?**

➥ **answer on page 185**

Case 1.62 ++

A 49-year-old woman with systemic sclerosis complains of malaise and palpitations. Her disease has been quiescent for 2 years and she is not on any immunosuppressant medications. She has a balanced diet and has had no previous surgery. Her rheumatologist requests the following tests:

Hb	82 g/l	(120–160 g/l females)
MCV	109.4 fl	(76–96 fl)
Platelets	169 x 10^9/l	(150–400 × 10^9/l)
WCC	6.2 x 10^9/l	(4.0–11.0 × 10^9/l)
Iron	23 μmol/l	(11–32 μmol/l)
Ferritin	49 μg/l	(12–200 μg/l)
TIBC	62 μmol/l	(42–80 μmol/l)
Vitamin B_{12}	31 ng/l	(191–663 ng/l)
Folate	>10 μg/l	(>2 μg/l)
Anti-parietal cell antibody		Titre <1:120
Anti-intrinsic factor antibody		Negative

Schilling test
Without oral intrinsic factor: 0.03 μg radioactive vitamin B_{12} in 24-h urine sample (3% of oral dose)
With oral intrinsic factor: 0.03 μg radioactive vitamin B_{12} in 24-h urine sample (3% of oral dose)

Hydrogen breath test
Early peak in hydrogen excretion

1. **What would you infer from these results?**
2. **What is the reason for performing a hydrogen breath test?**

→ **answer on page page 186**

Case 1.63 ++

A 72-year-old woman is admitted complaining of poor appetite, nausea and vomiting. She also complains of intermittent palpitations and visual disturbance. She had a stomach upset one week previously and had been off her food and consumed little fluid. Her medical history includes hypertension, atrial fibrillation and vertigo. She is unable to recall her medications. An ECG was reported as having ST-segment abnormalities, but the house officer did not feel that this was significant.

Hb	125 g/l	(120–160 g/l females)
MCV	95.7 fl	(76–96 fl)
Platelets	293 x 10^9/l	(150–400 × 10^9/l)
WCC	6.7 x 10^9/l	(4.0–11.0 × 10^9/l)
Na^+	139 mmol/l	(135–145 mmol/l)
K^+	3.1 mmol/l	(3.5–5.0 mmol/l)
Urea	15.6 mmol/l	(2.5–6.7 mmol/l)
Creatinine	298 μmol/l	(79–118 μmol/l)
Cl^-	104 mmol/l	(95–105 mmol/l)
HCO_3^-	27 mmol/l	(24–30 mmol/l)
Digoxin level	2.9 μg/l	(0.8–2.0 μg/l)

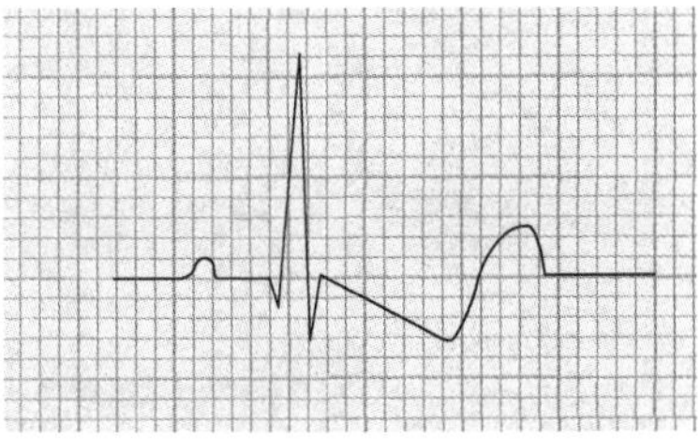

Explain the full significance of these results.

➥ **answer on page 187**

Case 1.64 ++

A 34-year-old accountant with a 15-year history of Crohn's disease attends for outpatient review. He feels reasonable, although has not yet been able to hold down full employment after numerous hospital admissions and surgery over the past 10 years. His last surgery involved small bowel resection and anastomosis after further failure of medical therapy. The doctor in the clinic requests the following tests.

Hb	89 g/l	(130–180 g/l males)
MCV	94.5 fl	(76–96 fl)
Platelets	399 x 10^9/l	(150–400 × 10^9/l)
WCC	9.7 x 10^9/l	(4.0–11.0 × 10^9/l)
RDW	20%	(12–15%)
Iron	9 μmol/l	(11–32 μmol/l)
Ferritin	10 μg/l	(12–200 μg/l)
TIBC	80 μmol/l	(42–80 μmol/l)
Vitamin B_{12}	12 ng/l	(191–663 ng/l)
Folate	1.8 μg/l	(>2 μg/l)

What is your interpretation of these tests?

➥ **answer on page page 187**

Case 1.65 ++

A 46-year-old diplomat is transferred to your care following medical evacuation from Nigeria. In his transfer correspondence it indicates that he has developed renal impairment which as yet has not been investigated in depth.

His U+E is shown, along with a 24-h urine collection for creatinine clearance.

Na^+	139 mmol/l	(135–145 mmol/l)
K^+	5.9 mmol/l	(3.5–5.0 mmol/l)
Urea	27.9 mmol/l	(2.5–6.7 mmol/l)
Creatinine	690 μmol/l	(79–118 μmol/l)
Cl^-	93 mmol/l	(95–105 mmol/l)
HCO_3^-	22 mmol/l	(24–30 mmol/l)
24-h urine collection		
Volume	1543 ml	
Creatinine	8 mmol/l	

Calculate his creatinine clearance.

➥ **answer on page 188**

Case 1.66 ++

A 45-year-old teacher has been complaining of aches and pains for several months. Her colleagues have said that she has not been herself recently, appearing 'under the weather' and sad. She is still menstruating regularly. Among the blood tests requested by her GP was a bone profile.

Adjusted Ca^{2+}	2.99 mmol/l	(2.10–2.65 mmol/l)
Phosphate	0.44 mmol/l	(0.8–1.45 mmol/l)
ALP	156 U/l	(30–150 U/l)
Albumin	41 g/l	(35–50 g/l)

A further blood test, of great importance in diagnosis, was sent the following day.

1. **What is the additional test likely to be?**
2. **What is the likely diagnosis?**

➥ **answer on page 188**

Case 1.67 ++

A 25-year-old shop assistant is brought to hospital by her colleague at 16:30 hours after she admitted to taking an overdose of paracetamol. She regrets the incident and is able to tell you clearly that she has taken one packet of 16 tablets during her lunch break between 12:00 and 12:30 hours. She feels fine and wishes to go home. No other medications or alcohol was taken. She has no health problems and is on no prescribed medications except the oral contraceptive pill. Blood tests taken on arrival at the hospital are shown.

Na^+	136 mmol/l	(135–145 mmol/l)
K^+	3.9 mmol/l	(3.5–5.0 mmol/l)
Urea	5.4 mmol/l	(2.5–6.7 mmol/l)
Creatinine	66 μmol/l	(79–118 μmol/l)
Cl^-	103 mmol/l	(95–105 mmol/l)
HCO_3^-	24 mmol/l	(24–30 mmol/l)
Paracetamol	155 mg/l	(Nil)
Alcohol	Nil	(Nil)
Salicylates	Nil	(Nil)
Liver function tests	Normal	

Would you treat this patient? Detail the logic for your decision.

➥ **answer on page 189**

Case 1.68 ++

Some members of the following family suffer from a rare bone disease. What is the inheritance pattern?

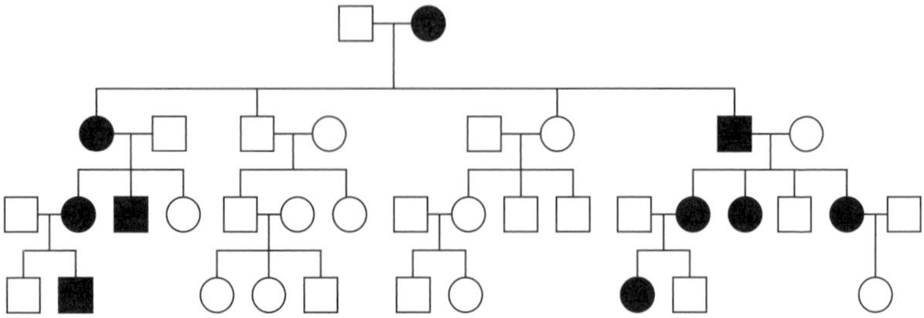

Key

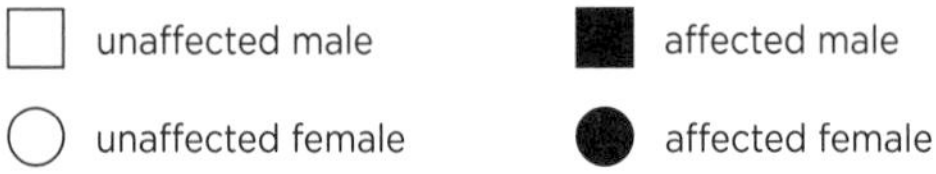

➥ **answer on page 190**

Case 1.69 ++

A 34-year-old man is admitted with epigastric discomfort and a single episode of vomiting following a week-long binge of alcohol. His vital signs are within the normal range. Blood tests were taken at the time of admission.

Hb	109 g/l	(130–180 g/l males)
MCV	100.4 fl	(76–96 fl)
Platelets	499 x 10^9/l	(150–400 × 10^9/l)
WCC	11.2 x 10^9/l	(4.0–11.0 × 10^9/l)
Na^+	141 mmol/l	(135–145 mmol/l)
K^+	4.2 mmol/l	(3.5–5.0 mmol/l)
Urea	13.9 mmol/l	(2.5–6.7 mmol/l)
Creatinine	64 μmol/l	(79–118 μmol/l)
Cl^-	95 mmol/l	(95–105 mmol/l)
HCO_3^-	23 mmol/l	(24–30 mmol/l)

Explain the elevated urea in the context of the other haematological results.

➥ **answer on page 190**

Case 1.70 ++

A 33-year-old single mother attends A&E with her neighbour who found that she had taken an overdose when she came round to visit. The patient is a difficult historian but does indicate that she took about 30–50 tablets from the cupboard during the midday news. It is now 19:15 hours. The neighbour indicates that the woman has a history of epilepsy and she is on medication for this. Blood tests were taken on arrival.

Na^+	139 mmol/l	(135–145 mmol/l)
K^+	3.7 mmol/l	(3.5–5.0 mmol/l)
Urea	5.1 mmol/l	(2.5–6.7 mmol/l)
Creatinine	56 μmol/l	(79–118 μmol/l)
Cl^-	106 mmol/l	(95–105 mmol/l)
HCO_3^-	24 mmol/l	(24–30 mmol/l)
Paracetamol	80 mg/l	(Nil)
Alcohol	25 mmol/l	(Nil)
Salicylates	1.45 mmol/l	(Nil)
Bilirubin	12 μmol/l	(3–17 μmol/l)
AST	78 U/L	(5–35 U/l)
ALT	65 U/L	(5–35 U/l)
ALP	67 U/L	(30–150 U/l)
GGT	100 U/L	(7–33 U/l females)

State what treatment this woman might need and justify your answer.

→ answer on page 190

Case 1.71 ++

A 47-year-old woman is referred to the regional hepatology outpatient clinic by her GP. She attended her GP on several occasions complaining of tiredness, low mood, altered bowel habit and more recently of itch. On examination a 4-cm smooth hepatomegaly is noted, with xanthelasmata around her eyes.

The referral letter contains the following LFTs:

Total bilirubin	13 μmol/l	(3–17 μmol/l)
AST	35 U/l	(5–35 U/l)
ALT	34 U/l	(5–35 U/l)
ALP	180 U/l	(30–150 U/l)
GGT	30 U/l	(7–33 U/l)
Albumin	39 g/l	(35–50 g/l)

A blood test taken at the clinic revealed the following:

Anti-mitochondrial antibody titre	1:140

1. **Interpret these results.**
2. **Suggest a further investigation.**

➥ **answer on page 191**

Case 1.72 ++

A 41-year-old patient with bipolar disorder presents to A&E indicating that she has taken an overdose of her prescribed lithium. She is subdued and states that she had been feeling low at the time. Her examination is normal and she does not have any direct complaints. Blood tests are shown.

Na^+	145 mmol/l	(135–145 mmol/l)
K^+	3.4 mmol/l	(3.5–5.0 mmol/l)
Urea	6.4 mmol/l	(2.5–6.7 mmol/l)
Creatinine	87 μmol/l	(79–118 μmol/l)
Paracetamol	<10 mg/l	(Nil)
Alcohol	10 mmol/l	(Nil)
Salicylates	Nil	(Nil)
Lithium	1.96 mmol/l	(0.5–1.5 mmol/l)

Explain the treatment options in lithium overdose with specific reference to this patient.

➥ **answer on page 192**

Case 1.73 ++

An elderly patient is admitted to the rehabilitation ward 4 weeks after having surgery to repair a fractured neck of femur. Her postoperative course was complicated by pneumonia and renal failure, both of which have been treated successfully. She has not been out of bed since the operation. You review her recent full blood pictures:

	14/06/16	28/06/16	01/07/16	15/07/16	10/07/16
Hb	116 g/l	122	118	124	121
MCV	80 fl	81	79	79	81
Platelets	227 x 10^9/l	264	90	32	8
WCC	5.4 x 10^9/l	4.5	4.7	4.9	4.5

(Reference ranges: Hb 120–160 g/l, MCV 76–96 fl, Platelets 150–400 × 10^9/l, WCC 4.0–11.0 × 10^9/l)

What is the major problem, and name one possible drug-induced cause?

➥ **answer on page 192**

Case 1.74 ++

A 46-year-old office clerk attends a private health clinic complaining of aches in his bones and tenderness over his muscles. This has been troubling him for some time and he is no longer able to walk to work. He has suffered from coeliac disease for many years, but by his own confession finds it hard at times to stick to his gluten-free diet. A 'screen' of tests is taken, some of which are shown below.

Adjusted Ca^{2+}	2.31 mmol/l	(2.10–2.65 mmol/l)
Phosphate	0.42 mmol/l	(0.8–1.45 mmol/l)
ALP	201 U/l	(30–150 U/l)
Albumin	39 g/l	(35–50 g/l)

What is the likely diagnosis?

➥ **answer on page 192**

Case 1.75 ++

A 39-year-old man with a history of Crohn's disease and previous extensive small bowel resection is admitted with anorexia and weight loss. His GP is very concerned that he now weighs only 39 kg and has not been able to tolerate much in the way of oral foods for several months. In hospital, attempts were made to start nasogastric feeding, but it could not be tolerated. Total parenteral nutrition (TPN) was therefore commenced. The following table shows his U+Es and nutritional profile over several days following commencement of parenteral feeding.

		Date			
	Reference ranges	14/02	15/02	16/02	17/02
Na^+ (mmol/l)	(135–145)	135	135	134	136
K^+ (mmol/l)	(3.5–5.0)	3.3	3.4	3.4	3.7
Urea (mmol/l)	(2.5–6.7)	2.1	2.2	2.2	2.3
Creatinine (μmol/l)	(79–118)	44	49	47	45
Cl^- (mmol/l)	(95–105)	94	94	93	93
HCO_3^- (mmol/l)	(24–30)	23	22	23	23
Mg^{2+} (mmol/l)	(0.7–1.0)	0.39	0.37	0.38	0.51
PO_4^{3-} (mmol/l)	(0.8–1.45)	0.70	0.61	0.41	0.40
Adjusted Ca^{2+} (mmol/l)	(2.10–2.65)	2.32	2.05	2.12	2.22
Albumin (g/l)	(35–50)	33	32	33	32

Comment on these results.

➥ **answer on page 193**

Case 1.76 ++

A 24-year-old woman from the Maldives is in Ireland on honeymoon. She attends the emergency department after falling and spraining her wrist. The doctor is concerned about the results of her full blood picture:

Hb	108 g/l	(120–160 g/l females)
MCV	53 fl	(76–96 fl)
Platelets	325 x 10^9/l	(150–400 × 10^9/l)
WCC	5.3 x 10^9/l	(4.0–11.0 × 10^9/l)

What is the most likely diagnosis and what test(s) would you arrange?

➥ **answer on page 193**

Case 1.77 ++

A 32-year-old French tourist is brought to A&E feeling generally unwell. No history is available. He appears dehydrated and has a respiratory rate of 22 breaths per minute. The following ABG and biochemical profile are taken on admission, breathing room air.

pH	7.26	(7.35-7.45)
PaO_2	11.5 kPa	(11-13 kPa)
$PaCO_2$	2.9 kPa	(4.7-6.0 kPa)
HCO_3^-	12.6 mmol/l	(24-30 mmol/l)
BE	-15.8 mmol/l	(-2 to +2 mmol/l)
Na^+	131 mmol/l	(135-145 mmol/l)
K^+	4.5 mmol/l	(3.5-5.0 mmol/l)
Urea	8.8 mmol/l	(2.5-6.7 mmol/l)
Creatinine	130 μmol/l	(79-118 μmol/l)
Cl^-	96.1 mmol/l	(95-105 mmol/l)
HCO_3^-	15 mmol/l	(24-30 mmol/l)

1. **Outline the abnormalities seen.**
2. **What tests should you request?**
3. **Which drugs or substances taken in overdose could give a similar pattern?**

➥ **answer on page page 193**

Case 1.78 ++

A 68-year-old man with a 40-pack-year smoking history was admitted short of breath and with a cough productive of green sputum. On examination he was tachypnoeic and using his accessory muscles of respiration. Auscultation of his chest revealed widespread expiratory wheeze with bibasal coarse crepitations. He was placed on 28% oxygen and his initial ABG is shown below.

pH	7.28	(7.35–7.45)
PaO_2	7.8 kPa	(11–13 kPa)
$PaCO_2$	6.7 kPa	(4.7–6.0 kPa)
HCO_3^-	35.4 mmol/l	(24–30 mmol/l)
BE	-5 mmol/l	(-2 to +2 mmol/l)

1. **Outline the abnormalities on this ABG.**
2. **What is the likely diagnosis?**
3. **What type of assisted ventilation could be considered in the management of this condition?**

➥ **answer on page 194**

Case 1.79 +++

An elderly woman is found lying in the street and is brought to the hospital. She is drowsy and refuses to answer your questions. Physical examination reveals tachypnoea, but is otherwise unremarkable. There are no lateralising neurological signs. Capillary blood glucose is 6.5 mmol/l. Investigations show the following:

Na^+	139 mmol/l	(135–145 mmol/l)
K^+	3.9 mmol/l	(3.5–5.0 mmol/l)
Urea	2.2 mmol/l	(2.5–6.7 mmol/l)
Creatinine	46 µmol/l	(79–118 µmol/l)
Cl^-	85 mmol/l	(95–105 mmol/l)
HCO_3^-	8 mmol/l	(24–30 mmol/l)
eGFR	>60 ml/min per 1.73 m^2	(>60 ml/min per 1.73 m^2)
Ethanol	15 mmol/l	(Nil)
Serum osmolality	352 mosmol/kg	(280–300 mosmol/kg)

Urinalysis:
no evidence of blood, protein, glucose, nitrites or ketones

Arterial blood gas analysis breathing room air:		
pH	7.15	(7.35-7.45)
PaO_2	13.4 kPa	(11-13 kPa)
$PaCO_2$	2.2 kPa	(4.7-6.0 kPa)
HCO_3^-	7 mmol/l	(24-30 mmol/l)

What is the most likely diagnosis, and what treatment would you recommend?

➥ **answer on page 195**

Case 1.80 +++

A 62-year-old woman is sent to the accident and emergency department by her GP, after the results of blood tests are phoned urgently by the laboratory. She had been complaining of generalised fatigue and grittiness of the eyes, and her doctor had organised blood tests that are shown below.

Hb	101 g/l	(120-160 g/l females)
WCC	6.4×10^9/l	(4.0-11.0×10^9/l)
Platelets	259×10^9/l	(150-400×10^9/l)
Na^+	136 mmol/l	(135-145 mmol/l)
K^+	2.4 mmol/l	(3.5-5.0 mmol/l)
Urea	3.2 mmol/l	(2.5-6.7 mmol/l)
Creatinine	48 μmol/l	(79-118 μmol/l)
Cl^-	110 mmol/l	(95-105 mmol/l)
HCO_3^-	14 mmol/l	(24-30 mmol/l)
eGFR	>60 ml/min per 1.73 m^2	(>60 ml/min per 1.73 m^2)

The A&E doctor organises an arterial blood gas (ABG) analysis while the patient is breathing room air:

pH	7.20	(7.35-7.45)
PaO_2	12.5 kPa	(11-13 kPa)
$PaCO_2$	3.75 kPa	(4.7-6.0 kPa)
HCO_3^-	14 mmol/l	(24-30 mmol/l)

1. **What is the most life-threatening biochemical disturbance listed?**
2. **Characterise the acid-base disturbance.**
3. **What is the most likely unifying diagnosis, and how would you investigate this further?**

➥ **answer on page 195**

Case 1.81 +++

A 75-year-old man has a full blood picture performed as part of a private medical check-up. He is told to bring the results of the test to his GP. Below are the results of the test, and a representative image from a blood film that the GP arranges.

Hb	131 g/l	(130–180 g/l males)
WCC	28×10^9/l	($4.0–11.0 \times 10^9$/l)
Platelets	213×10^9/l	($150–400 \times 10^9$/l)

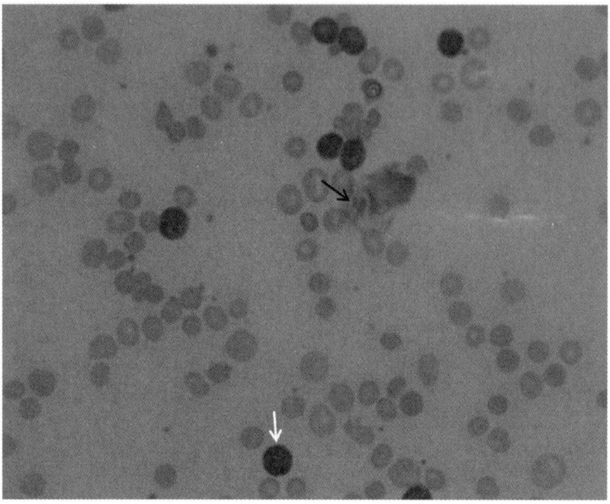

What is the most likely diagnosis?

➥ **answer on page 196**

Case 1.82 +++

A 55-year-old man gives a 1-month history of intermittent spasms. His past medical history includes type 2 diabetes, gout, hypertension, gastritis and osteoarthritis of the knee. You observe occasional twitching of his limbs while taking his history. He takes the following medication: metformin, allopurinol, amiloride, omeprazole and diclofenac. Blood testing reveals the following:

Hb	152 g/l	(130–180 g/l males)
WCC	4.3 × 10^9/l	(4.0–11.0 × 10^9/l)
Platelets	223 × 10^9/l	(150–400 × 10^9/l)
Na^+	135 mmol/l	(135–145 mmol/l)
K^+	3.9 mmol/l	(3.5–5.0 mmol/l)
Urea	4.2 mmol/l	(2.5–6.7 mmol/l)
Creatinine	82 μmol/l	(79–118 μmol/l)
Cl^-	93 mmol/l	(95–105 mmol/l)
HCO_3^-	25 mmol/l	(24–30 mmol/l)
Albumin	35 g/l	(35–50 g/l)
Calcium	2.03 mmol/l	(2.10–2.65 mmol/l)
Mg^{2+}	0.19 mmol/l	(0.7–1.0 mmol/l)

1. **What is the biochemical explanation for his symptoms?**
2. **What is the most likely underlying cause?**

↪ **answer on page 196**

Case 1.83 +++

A 74-year-old man is admitted with severe abdominal pain and shock. His initial blood results show the following:

Na^+	116 mmol/l	(135–145 mmol/l)
K^+	4.9 mmol/l	(3.5–5.0 mmol/l)
Urea	11.2 mmol/l	(2.5–6.7 mmol/l)
Creatinine	148 μmol/l	(79–118 μmol/l)
Cl^-	90 mmol/l	(95–105 mmol/l)
HCO_3^-	18 mmol/l	(24–30 mmol/l)
eGFR	43 ml/min per 1.73 m^2	(>60 ml/min per 1.73 m^2)
Serum osmolality	290 mosmol/kg	(280–300 mosmol/kg)
Urine osmolality	654 mosmol/kg	(250–1250 mosmol/kg)

1. **Describe the abnormalities observed.**
2. **What is the most likely cause for the man's presentation?**

↪ **answer on page 196**

Case 1.84 +++

A 37-year-old man attends a 'well-man clinic' run by a private healthcare company. He elects to pay for a check of his thyroid function, because his sister was recently diagnosed with hyperthyroidism. He receives the following results, and asks for your help in interpreting them:

Free T_4	34 pmol/l	(7.6–19.7 pmol/l)
TSH	20.1 mU/l	(0.4–4.5 mU/l)

You examine him and find no clinical evidence of thyroid disease. You decide to repeat the test, and the following results are returned:

Free T_4	18 pmol/l	(7.6–19.7 pmol/l)
TSH	2.5 mU/l	(0.4–4.5 mU/l)

1. **Which set of results is most probably correct?**
2. **Account for the discrepancy between the two sets of results.**

➥ **answer on page 197**

Case 1.85 +++

A 64-year-old woman was seen at a general surgical clinic. Six months before the appointment, she had undergone a significant small bowel resection after an episode of ischaemia. She was left with a short section of proximal small bowel, terminating in a stoma. Her remaining distal small bowel was left *in situ*, and it was hoped that an anastomosis could be fashioned in the future. She was receiving parenteral nutrition at home, the feeds being handled by a district nursing team. Her medication comprised: lansoprazole, codeine sulfate and loperamide. Her nurse reported that she could, on occasions, be a little drowsy and confused. Investigations at the clinic revealed the following:

Na^+	138 mmol/l	(135–145 mmol/l)
K^+	3.5 mmol/l	(3.5–5.0 mmol/l)
Urea	4.2 mmol/l	(2.5–6.7 mmol/l)
Creatinine	51 μmol/l	(79–118 μmol/l)
Cl^-	94 mmol/l	(95–105 mmol/l)
HCO_3^-	16 mmol/l	(24–30 mmol/l)
eGFR	>60 ml/min per 1.73 m²	(>60 ml/min per 1.73 m²)
Glucose	4.5 mmol/l	(4.0–8.0 mmol/l)
Venous pH	7.29	(7.35–7.45)
Lactate	1.2 mmol/l	(0.5–2.0 mmol/l)

1. Comment on the blood results.
2. What specialist investigation would you request to confirm the most likely diagnosis?

➥ **answer on page 197**

Case 1.86 +++

When on elective in Malawi, you are asked to see a patient. He is 35 years old and complains of anorexia and abdominal discomfort. Examination is unremarkable. A full blood picture is requested.

Hb	135 g/l	(130–180 g/l males)
MCV	89.6 fl	(76–96 fl)
Platelets	189 x 10^9/l	(150–400 × 10^9/l)
WCC	13.2 x 10^9/l	(4.0–11.0 × 10^9/l)
Neutrophils	7.4 x 10^9/l	(2.0–7.5 × 10^9/l)
Lymphocytes	2.5 x 10^9/l	(1.5–4.0 × 10^9/l)

What is the likely diagnosis?

➥ **answer on page 198**

Case 1.87 +++

A 21-year-old woman is referred to the medical clinic because of abnormal thyroid function results noted by her GP. There is no personal or family history of thyroid disease, and she is on no medication, but the GP requested the test because the patient had been feeling generally unwell recently. Clinical examination is unremarkable. The thyroid function tests are repeated and the following results are obtained.

Total T_4	175 nmol/l	(70–140 nmol/l)
TSH	3.2 mU/l	(0.4–4.5 mU/l)

1. How would you interpret these tests?
2. What two tests should be ordered?

➥ **answer on page 198**

Case 1.88 +++

A 45-year-old man with a history of asthma is admitted with symptoms and signs in keeping with cardiac failure. There are no risk factors for ischaemic heart disease. The cause for the cardiac failure remains uncertain until a junior doctor reviews his FBP and suggests the correct diagnosis.

Hb	138 g/l	(130–180 g/l males)
MCV	84 fl	(76–96 fl)
Platelets	225 x 10^9/l	(150–400 × 10^9/l)
WCC	15.2 x 10^9/l	(4.0–11.0 × 10^9/l)
Neutrophils	3.4 x 10^9/l	(2.0–7.5 × 10^9/l)
Lymphocytes	2.8 x 10^9/l	(1.5–4.0 × 10^9/l)

What is the rare disease that the junior doctor suspected?

➥ **answer on page 199**

Case 1.89 +++

Some family members have a rare genetic disorder. This is their family tree. What is the likely inheritance pattern?

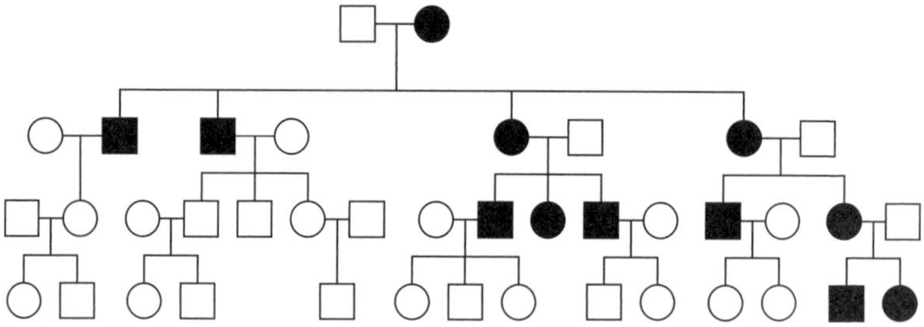

Key

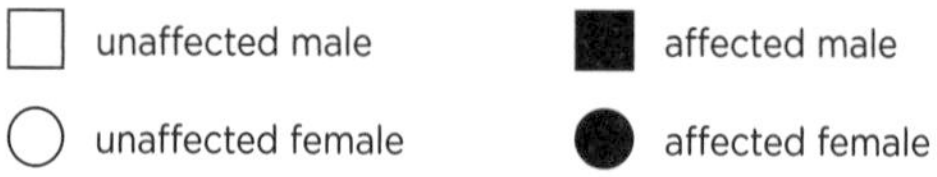

➥ **answer on page 199**

Case 1.90 +++

You are the junior doctor on the vascular surgical unit. One of your patients, a 75-year-old man with peripheral vascular disease, is due to undergo bypass vascular surgery on his legs. You request a battery of preoperative blood tests. The following results give the nursing staff some concern.

PT	12.3 s	(12–16 s)
APTT	60 s	(24–38 s)
Fibrinogen	3.12 g/l	(2–4 g/l)
Na^+	142 mmol/l	(135–145 mmol/l)
K^+	4.6 mmol/l	(3.5–5.0 mmol/l)
Urea	15.3 mmol/l	(2.5–6.7 mmol/l)
Creatinine	376 μmol/l	(79–118 μmol/l)
Cl^-	95 mmol/l	(95–105 mmol/l)
HCO_3^-	24.2 mmol/l	(24–30 mmol/l)

What should you do next?

➥ **answer on page 199**

INTERPRETING LABORATORY RESULTS: ANSWERS

1

Answer 1.1

➥ case on page 112

1. This man's iron profile is highly abnormal, reflecting iron overload. Genetic haemochromatosis could account for this, and may also explain the diabetes mellitus.
2. It would be useful to repeat the iron studies in the fasted state, after the patient had been abstaining from alcohol. Genetic tests for mutations in the *HFE* gene would be helpful. MRI of the liver can be used to estimate the degree of iron overload. The iron content of liver tissue can also be measured in a biopsy specimen. Given that haemochromatosis is an inherited condition, it is good practice for family members to have their iron profiles checked.
3. Venesection is an effective means of depleting body iron stores, and can help prevent some of the problems associated with iron overload.

Answer 1.2

➥ case on page 112

1. This patient has a macrocytic anaemia that does not appear to be due to vitamin B_{12} or folate deficiency. The serum free light chain analysis gives the diagnosis - light chain myeloma. Most patients with multiple myeloma have a monoclonal proliferation of plasma cells which produce IgG, IgM or IgA. In these cases, the diagnosis is usually apparent on serum protein electrophoresis. In a smaller percentage of patients, the abnormal plasma cells secrete immunoglobulin light chains only. These can be detected in the serum (as in this case, with an abnormal ratio of κ and λ light chains pointing to the diagnosis) or the urine (where they are called Bence Jones protein).
2. Other investigations that should be considered include: U+E, calcium, β_2-microglobulin, urinary Bence Jones protein and a bone marrow examination.

Answer 1.3

➥ case on page 113

1. This young woman has hypertension and hypokalaemia. This combination raises the possibility of hyperaldosteronism. There are no physical features to suggest Cushing syndrome (other than the BP), so primary hyperaldosteronism is more likely.
2. The U+E should be repeated to ensure that the hypokalaemia is genuine. The most useful next-line investigation would be a paired renin and aldosterone measurement. In primary hyperaldosteronism, there is autonomous secretion of aldosterone. Renin production shuts off appropriately due to negative feedback. One would therefore expect to find an abnormally high renin:aldosterone ratio.
3. Primary hyperaldosteronism can be due to bilateral adrenal hyperplasia, an adrenal adenoma or adrenal carcinoma.

Answer 1.4

➥ case on page 113

1. This patient has a microcytic anaemia (low Hb, low MCV). Her iron profile is in keeping with iron deficiency with a low iron, low ferritin and high TIBC. There is a mild thrombocytosis which may indicate active bleeding.
2. The most common cause for these findings in young women is menorrhagia. In an older female or male of any age, investigations should be carried out to exclude a sinister cause – in particular an occult gastrointestinal tract malignancy. Investigations should begin with a thorough history and clinical examination which should include rectal examination. The next line of investigation usually involves gastrointestinal tract endoscopy.

Answer 1.5

➥ case on page 114

Hypernatraemia is present. Other components of the U+E are normal. She has lost excessive amounts of fluid through her burnt skin. Consequently, the sodium concentration has risen.

Other causes of hypernatraemia are listed on page 6.

Answer 1.6

➥ case on page 114

This woman has primary hyperthyroidism. Her overactive thyroid gland is producing thyroid hormones in excess. Normal negative feedback mechanisms still function, however, so the TSH level is suppressed.

It is not uncommon for atrial fibrillation to be the only evidence of hyperthyroidism, so always remember to check thyroid function in such patients.

Answer 1.7

➥ case on page 115

1. This patient has a normocytic anaemia. Her haematinics are normal. She has a raised blood bilirubin level and urobilinogen in the urine which would be in keeping with haemoglobin breakdown. Her blood film shows a reticulocytosis indicating that the bone marrow is working hard to make new red blood cells. The direct antiglobulin test is positive indicating that the patient's red cells are coated with antibodies.
2. The patient has an autoimmune haemolytic anaemia, which is most likely to be an adverse effect of treatment with methyldopa.

Answer 1.8

➥ case on page 116

On first inspection, one might suspect that illicit drug use could provide the explanation for this patient's symptoms. However, another diagnosis may be more likely - carbon monoxide poisoning. This student developed symptoms following a car journey of several hours. Typically, students, elderly people and socially deprived people are most susceptible to exposure to carbon monoxide from poorly maintained fires and motor cars. Carbon monoxide poisoning can be diagnosed by measuring carboxyhaemoglobin in an arterial blood gas sample. This patient's carboxyhaemoglobin is elevated, in keeping with the clinical suspicion. It is entirely appropriate that a urine drug screen has been performed, although the patient should be informed if this is being sent. A trace of cannabinoids suggests recent use of cannabis. This is, however, unlikely to be the explanation for this recent onset of symptoms.

Answer 1.9

➥ case on page 116

This patient has symptoms suggestive of a bacterial pneumonia. He is otherwise healthy and there is little to suspect an underlying sinister or chronic disease. A proportion of bacterial pneumonias will present with a pleural effusion. Pleural fluid is produced in excess in reaction to the local irritation of the pleura from the surrounding infection.

The findings from the simple pleural fluid analysis are in keeping with this clinical suspicion. It is an exudate (total protein >30 g/l) and the lactate dehydrogenase level is high.

This patient has a parapneumonic pleural effusion. Treatment consists of antibiotics for the pneumonia, with the effusion expected to resolve over several weeks. The patient should have a repeat chest radiograph 6 weeks after treatment to ensure resolution of the effusion. If the patient's condition were to deteriorate one would have to consider the development of an empyema (pus collection in the pleural space).

Answer 1.10

➥ case on page 117

This patient gives an unconvincing history for deep venous thrombosis (DVT), and there is very little clinical evidence for it. A normal D-dimer in this situation, when the pre-test probability for the condition is low, is helpful in making DVT extremely unlikely in this man. The patient can be reassured that it is extremely unlikely that he has a clot in his leg.

Answer 1.11

➥ case on page 117

The ALP is significantly raised. The rest of the bone profile is normal. ALP may be high in a number of conditions. It is important to exclude liver disease, but we are told here that the rest of her liver function tests were normal.

Bearing in mind the clinical history, a particular concern in this woman would be bony metastases from breast carcinoma. This can occur a considerable time after treatment of the primary tumour. The calcium may be normal or elevated in the presence of bony metastases. Vitamin D and PTH should also be checked here to exclude vitamin D deficiency and mild hyperparathyroidism.

Answer 1.12

➥ case on page 118

Establishing a diagnosis in elderly people can be difficult by clinical assessment alone, especially when no history is available. It is often necessary to place greater emphasis on investigations. Although, in this case, the FBP and U+Es are normal, the CRP is significantly raised. In the presence of infection one might expect the WCC to be raised too, but this is not always the case. An infection is likely to be the cause of the patient's illness. A urinary tract infection and pneumonia are the most common causes of these findings in clinical practice. Given the normal urinalysis and abnormal examination findings in the chest, pneumonia is the most likely diagnosis.

Answer 1.13

➥ case on page 118

Of all the tumour markers available, probably the most commonly requested is the PSA. It is sometimes used in an attempt to identify the presence of prostatic carcinoma, but more usefully in monitoring the disease and treatment response. This patient has obstructive urinary symptoms and an enlarged prostate, but this does not mean that he has prostate cancer. Likewise a normal PSA does not exclude the presence of this tumour. However, this man most likely has benign prostatic hypertrophy. There are a number of causes of a raised PSA, as shown below.

CAUSES OF RAISED PSA
Prostate carcinoma
Instrumentation of prostate (including urinary catheterisation)
Urinary tract infection
Recent ejaculation

Answer 1.14

➥ case on page 119

1. This patient has a parenchymal LFT derangement. Both the ALT and AST are markedly elevated.
2. A set of 'screening' investigations should be performed next to further investigate the situation. See page 18 for details.

This patient had hepatitis C. Not infrequently hepatitis C is diagnosed incidentally when LFTs are checked for some other reason.

Answer 1.15

➥ case on page 119

1. The haemoglobin is low with an elevated mean cell volume. This patient has a macrocytic anaemia. Haematinics show a low vitamin B_{12} level. Iron studies and folate level are within normal limits.
2. The positive antibodies to gastric parietal cells and intrinsic factor indicate that the likely underlying cause of the anaemia is pernicious anaemia. (See Chaoter 6 for details of immunological testing.) You will note that the patient was already known to have an autoimmune disease - Graves' disease. Always remember that patients with one autoimmune disease are prone to developing another.

Answer 1.16

➥ case on page 120

Hyperuricaemia may occur due to excess purine metabolism. This includes those suffering from haematological malignancies in which there is increased cell turnover, especially following cell lysis from chemotherapy.

The presence of negatively birefringent crystals from the joint aspiration confirms gout.

Answer 1.17

➥ case on page 120

1. This is a short Synacthen® test. The cortisol level fails to rise significantly 30 min after injection with Synacthen®. A normal response might be a rise of >500 nmol/l - the precise value will depend on the laboratory. This indicates primary hypoadrenalism (ie a problem with the adrenal gland itself).
2. A low sodium and raised potassium level are commonly found. The glucose level may also be low.
3. The underlying disease is primary hypoadrenalism, probably due to autoimmune adrenalitis or tuberculosis affecting the adrenal gland.

Answer 1.18

➥ case on page 121

The clinical features of this patient suggest a diagnosis of congestive cardiac failure (CCF). The prescription of a non-steroidal anti-inflammatory drug (NSAID) for acute gout has caused fluid retention, leading to worsening of the underlying cardiac failure. The effusions are bilateral, which suggests that they are likely to be transudative. The pleural fluid sample confirms this suspicion with a total protein content of only 21 g/l and an LDH of 140 U/l. Of all the causes of transudate pleural effusions, cardiac failure best fits in this case.

Answer 1.19

➥ case on page 121

1. The episode of loss of vision is typical of amaurosis fugax. Taken together with the history of lethargy and jaw pain on eating (jaw claudication), the clinical suspicion must be of temporal arteritis. Such patients are at high risk of complications, including blindness. The extremely high ESR measured here would support this diagnosis. Temporal arteritis is one of the few causes of an ESR greater than 100 mm/h.

2. Treatment should be given rapidly, and should comprise high-dose prednisolone (eg 60–80 mg orally immediately), followed by a reducing dose regimen.

Answer 1.20

➥ case on page 122

1. The urea and creatinine are both grossly elevated indicating that this patient has renal failure. Comparison with previous blood tests would indicate whether this is acute or chronic. As a consequence of the renal failure, serum potassium is dangerously elevated. The rising potassium is a reflection of the failing tubular function of the kidney. In this case it would appear that the use of a non-steroidal anti-inflammatory drug (diclofenac) and vomiting are the causes of an acute deterioration in renal function.

2. Hyperkalaemia can cause fatal dysrhythmias, including cardiac arrest. This requires immediate treatment. Conventional treatment employs insulin and dextrose. Insulin drives potassium into the cells, whereas glucose prevents hypoglycaemia. Calcium gluconate should be given first to stabilise the myocardium.

   The ultimate treatment is to identify the cause of the renal failure and support the kidneys until function is restored.

Answer 1.21

➥ case on page 122

You should suspect osteoporosis given the history of fracture after minimal trauma, and a previously normal bone profile. Osteoporosis is the most common form of metabolic bone disease. It is predominantly found in postmenopausal women and is considered a silent disease. First presentation is often with a low trauma fracture as in this clinical scenario.

Diagnosis of osteoporosis is usually made using dual energy X-ray absorptiometry (DXA) scan.

Answer 1.22

➥ case on page 122

1. The LFTs show an elevated bilirubin with cholestatic LFTs.
2. An ultrasound scan of the abdomen is the next most important investigation. This will confirm the presence of obstruction and may identify the underlying cause. This can then act as a guide for further investigations.
3. The causes of cholestatic jaundice are listed on page 17.

Answer 1.23

➥ case on page 123

One important role of α-FP measurement is demonstrated well in this patient with hepatitis C. It is one of the more specific tumour markers and can be used with some degree of confidence to monitor patients with liver cirrhosis who have a substantially increased risk of developing hepatocellular carcinoma (HCC). Identifying a patient who has developed HCC early may allow successful treatment to be instigated. The level in January 2005 is higher than 6 months previously but is not dramatically elevated. However, 6 months later it has increased substantially. This suggests the development of HCC, and ultrasound and/or other cross-sectional imaging would be merited. The encouraging downward trend in the following 6 months would indicate that the tumour has been successfully treated.

Answer 1.24

➥ case on page 124

The clinical history is one of podagra (gout of the great toe). The elevated urate in the blood supports this diagnosis. Definitive diagnosis of gout depends on the detection of crystals of sodium urate in synovial fluid (see page 45). However, not all joints with acute gout are amenable to aspiration and one must rely on a clinical impression and supportive blood tests. Remember that the serum urate level can be normal in acute gout.

This patient may well be taking a thiazide diuretic for hypertension. This would place him at higher risk for gout.

Answer 1.25

➥ case on page 124

The first abnormality relates to the raised packed cell volume (PCV) indicating polycythaemia. The most likely cause in this case is a true polycythaemia secondary to chronic hypoxia resulting from COPD. Useful tests to confirm this would be an estimation of red cell mass to confirm true polycythaemia (although this would not normally be done in practice), and an arterial blood gas sample to demonstrate hypoxaemia.

The second abnormality relates to the elevated white cell count. Note that the neutrophil count is markedly elevated, and that the sum of the neutrophil and lymphocyte counts almost adds up to the total white cell count. The small discrepancy is due to the presence of a small number of other white blood cells (eosinophils, monocytes and basophils) in the circulation.
The most likely cause for this picture is a bacterial infection of the lower respiratory tract.

Answer 1.26

➥ case on page 125

It is not uncommon (though not particularly good practice), especially in puzzling clinical cases, to request a host of blood tests. Tumour markers for intra-abdominal pathology are sometimes used in this manner. However, due to the non-specific nature of these results, abnormal results can sometimes add to the diagnostic conundrum. The abnormal marker in this case is CA-125. This is most closely associated with ovarian malignancy. The clinical history is certainly in keeping with this, as the distended abdomen may reflect both tumour bulk and/or the presence of malignant ascites.

Answer 1.27

➥ case on page 125

His ascites white cell count shows a neutrophilia, with more than 250 cells/mm^3.

The albumin content is less than 25 g/l indicating a transudate.

The SAAG is 13 g/l (29 g/l - 16 g/l). This is in keeping with portal hypertension.

Gram staining shows the most typical finding in SBP - Gram-negative bacilli. In time, one might expect culture to yield *Escherichia coli* or *Klebsiella* species.

This man has spontaneous bacterial peritonitis, on a background of hepatic cirrhosis caused by alcohol. His clinical features are typical with general abdominal discomfort, often accompanied by pyrexia. This infection has also made him mildly encephalopathic, hence the confusion.

In a patient with a history of alcohol dependency, abdominal distension and pain, pancreatitis is a further differential diagnosis. However, this would cause an exudate, and one would expect the amylase level to be raised significantly.

Answer 1.28

➥ case on page 126

The PT and APTT are raised suggesting a tendency to bleed. The fibrinogen level is low indicating that fibrinogen has been used up. The D-dimer level is markedly raised indicating that the body's fibrinolytic system is working hard to disperse clots.

This pattern of abnormalities is typical of DIC, a not uncommon complication in patients with critical illness. Blood product support will be required, and the advice of a haematologist would be helpful.

Answer 1.29

➥ case on page 126

D-dimer is an extremely helpful blood test when sent in the correct circumstances. In a patient with a reasonable chance of having a blood clot, an elevated D-dimer would support the diagnosis. All too often, however, D-dimer is measured in patients with no clinical suggestion of thromboembolic disease. There are many causes for a raised D-dimer other than clot (eg commonly found in acutely unwell patients, malignancy, and following surgery or trauma), so, unless the patient has signs or symptoms in keeping with thromboembolism, the test should generally not be ordered. No investigations for thromboembolic disease are required in this woman in whom we are given no reason to suspect a blood clot.

Answer 1.30

➥ case on page 126

1. This elderly man has Paget's disease of the bone. He has an isolated ALP rise, in the absence of any liver disease. An ALP rise can occur for various reasons, including primary sclerosing cholangitis and bony metastases. However, in the context of this patient's symptoms, with deafness, Paget's disease is certainly possible.
2. The repeat bone profile demonstrates lowering of the ALP after successful treatment. He is likely to have received intravenous bisphosphonate therapy. Note that the majority of patients with Paget's disease are asymptomatic and the disease is often diagnosed incidentally when tests are requested for other reasons.

Answer 1.31

➥ case on page 174

1. The bilirubin and aminotransferases are raised. The CRP is highly elevated. He requires an ultrasound scan of the abdomen to investigate for an infective cause for his symptoms.
2. Viral hepatitis, a liver abscess and cholangitis are all potential causes.

Answer 1.32

→ case on page 128

1. The abnormalities seen include:
   - a raised MCV, with a slightly low platelet count
   - low values for urea, potassium, magnesium and, in particular, phosphate
   - a raised GGT
   - a low albumin.
2. The findings on these simple blood tests are classic for an individual who has consumed large quantities of alcohol for a significant time period. He may well have liver disease with portal hypertension, explaining the low platelet count. Poor nutrition may be responsible for some of the other abnormalities, and poor liver synthetic function could account for the albumin.

Answer 1.33

→ case on page 129

The course of primary biliary cirrhosis is variable. Patients may live with stable LFTs for a number of years. Decompensation may occur at any time with deterioration in the liver's synthetic function.

The chart shows LFTs over a period of 20 months. Initially only a moderately elevated ALP is seen in April 2004. Over the ensuing months the ALP continues to rise, and with this the albumin falls reaching a low of 28 g/l in December 2005.

The prothrombin time should also be checked. One would expect it to be raised indicating impaired production of clotting factors by the failing liver.

Answer 1.34

→ case on page 129

The blood tests show very mild elevations in AST and ALT. These are very minor and non-specific findings and could be caused by a variety of conditions, including viral hepatitis and drug-induced hepatitis. The only condition that meaningfully links a psychiatric disorder with these abnormal liver function tests is, however, Wilson's disease - a condition associated with copper overload. Tests that could be performed to investigate further include: serum copper level, serum ceruloplasmin level, slit-lamp examination of the eyes to look for copper deposition, 24-hour urinary collection for copper measurement and liver biopsy.

Answer 1.35

➥ case on page 130

1. There are a number of abnormalities on this set of results:
    - The haemoglobin is slightly low
    - The platelet count is slightly below normal
    - The WCC is low
    - The ESR is raised, with a normal CRP
    - Protein is noted in the urine.
2. The CRP is normal. This would go against an infectious cause for a raised ESR and be more suggestive of inflammation of some description. There are only a few conditions in which the ESR is elevated but the CRP remains normal. One such condition is systemic lupus erythematosus (SLE) which this patient's clinical features and test abnormalities are in keeping with.

Answer 1.36

➥ case on page 130

Some of the most rewarding data to interpret are those collated over a period of time when trends can be observed. This scenario illustrates the value of CRP in both supporting a clinical diagnosis and monitoring its response to treatment. On admission this patient's CRP is significantly raised, as one may expect in the presence of an abscess. With the commencement of antibiotics, one might hope for the CRP to improve as the abscess is treated. The worsening of her clinical state and the rising CRP suggest that either the antibiotics are ineffective against the causative organism or they are unable to penetrate the abscess. Day 4 sees a change in treatment, no doubt to an alternative antimicrobial. However, the CRP remains stubbornly high. It is only in the days following surgical intervention that the CRP begins to decrease, reflecting the successful treatment of the abscess.

Answer 1.37

➥ case on page 131

The key findings on this patient's blood tests are a microcytic anaemia and a raised CEA. Given his symptoms, these results should arouse a great deal of suspicion of colorectal carcinoma. Although proctoscopy was normal this visualises only a very small percentage of the large bowel and further imaging is required. In this case the tumour marker merely adds weight to a clinical suspicion.

Answer 1.38

➥ case on page 131

This patient may have liver cirrhosis secondary to hepatitis C. Her regular attendance at an outpatient clinic is at least in part for surveillance for hepatocellular carcinoma. Her α-FP level is within normal limits, indicating a low likelihood of this tumour being present. Regular surveillance ultrasound scans of the liver will be used in conjunction with α-FP measurements to seek out a hepatocellular carcinoma. A significant percentage of tumour markers are performed for monitoring so you should expect to interpret some normal results.

Answer 1.39

➥ case on page 132

α-Fetoprotein is one of the few tumour markers with a good specificity for two different tumours - hepatocellular carcinoma and testicular teratoma. Similarly testicular teratoma is unique in characteristically causing high levels of two tumour markers - α-FP and β-hCG. Both tumour markers are significantly elevated here indicating a high probability of testicular malignancy. Following treatment, these markers should be checked again and should have decreased.

Answer 1.40

➥ case on page 132

Time (h)	Plasma osmolality (mosmol/kg)	Urine osmolality (mosmol/kg)
0	297	115
1	300	117
2	305	115
3	309	115
4	316	114
5	324	113
6	326	115
7	332	116
8	336	115
Following desmopressin injection		750

Increasing plasma osmolality with time

No change in urine osmolality with time

Increase in urine osmolality following desmopressin injection

1. The random blood glucose level is normal. The patient therefore probably does not have diabetes mellitus. It is important to exclude this diagnosis, since it can also present with polydipsia and polyuria.

2. The diagnosis is cranial diabetes insipidus. The patient has a problem producing ADH. When deprived of water, he is unable to concentrate the urine. The plasma rapidly becomes more concentrated. Following an injection of synthetic ADH (desmopressin), the urine osmolality increases. This shows that the kidney is still sensitive to the effects of ADH, and excludes nephrogenic diabetes insipidus as the diagnosis.

Answer 1.41

➥ case on page 133

The urinary metanephrine levels are normal. This excludes phaeochromocytoma as a cause of the hypertension with some certainty.

The second test shows the results of an overnight dexamethasone suppression test. The morning cortisol level is greater than 50 nmol/l, suggesting a diagnosis of Cushing syndrome. The precise cut-off may vary from lab to lab.

Answer 1.42

➥ case on page 133

1. The two diagnoses that can be made from this one test are: diabetes mellitus and acromegaly.

   The glucose level before the start of the test is elevated in keeping with the label of impaired fasting glucose. However, the abnormally high glucose level 2 h after the glucose load confirms the diagnosis of diabetes mellitus.

   The growth hormone level is greater than 2.0 μg/l at all stages of the test, allowing the diagnosis of acromegaly to be made.

2. The most common cause of acromegaly is a pituitary tumour. This commonly extends in an upward direction and can compress the optic chiasma, causing a bitemporal hemianopia. Loss of temporal visual fields is the probable reason for presentation at the eye A&E.

Answer 1.43

➥ case on page 134

Pleural effusions can develop in acute pancreatitis. It is most typical for them to be unilateral; however, bilateral effusions are recognised. The key to diagnosis is the amylase level within the aspirated fluid.

Answer 1.44

➥ case on page 134

Pleural effusion is an uncommon but well-documented finding in rheumatoid disease. This is a systemic disease and a number of manifestations occur in the chest. Among these are: pleural effusion, pulmonary nodules, interstitial fibrosis, pleural thickening and bronchiolitis obliterans. This patient has a number of autoimmune diseases so it would not be unreasonable for her to be diagnosed with rheumatoid disease. The pleural effusion is an exudate. The rheumatoid factor level is hugely elevated at 556 IU/ml. In addition the glucose is low at 2.2 mmol/l in the effusion, further supporting the diagnosis.

Answer 1.45

➥ case on page 135

The WCC is not significantly raised.

The albumin level is greater than 25 g/l, indicating an exudate.

The SAAG is 1 g/l (29 g/l - 28 g/l), indicating a low probability of portal hypertension.

The diagnosis is seen on cytology.

This patient has an advanced intraperitoneal malignancy. The specific primary origin is unknown. The cells present may originate from a primary intraperitoneal malignancy or be due to intraperitoneal metastatic disease. A large volume of ascites in an elderly patient without known liver disease should always arouse the suspicion of malignancy. The CT findings are in keeping with a primary pelvic malignancy of likely ovarian origin.

Answer 1.46

➥ case on page 135

The ascites is an exudate, and there is no evidence of infection.

The SAAG is 3 g/l (32 g/l - 29 g/l), indicating a low probability of portal hypertension.

The amylase is elevated at 894 U/l, in keeping with acute pancreatitis.

Every effort should be made to persuade this man of the need to stay in hospital for further investigation and treatment of his pancreatitis.

Answer 1.47

➥ case on page 136

- Both males and females are affected
- Male-to-male inheritance is possible
- One of the parents of all affected cases is also affected.
- If one parent is affected, there appears to be approximately a 50% chance that a child will also be affected.

The inheritance pattern is therefore autosomal dominant.

Answer 1.48

➥ case on page 136

The finding of a normal N-terminal pro-BNP level in this man makes the diagnosis of cardiac failure extremely unlikely. Another cause for his breathlessness and crepitations should be found. A chest radiograph would seem like a useful first test.

Answer 1.49

➥ case on page 136

1. Oxygenation is abnormal. The patient has type 1 respiratory failure, with a low PaO_2 and normal $PaCO_2$.

   The pH is normal, as is the HCO_3^-.

2. This man's clinical history when taken in conjunction with his clinical signs and ABG is highly suggestive of pulmonary fibrosis. The fact that he worked in a shipyard may suggest exposure to asbestos, which is a potential cause of pulmonary fibrosis - especially at the lung bases as the CT scan suggests. Other causes for type 1 respiratory failure are listed in the box on page 21.
3. Long-term oxygen therapy (LTOT) could be considered. However, there are strict guidelines that must be met before LTOT is commenced.

Answer 1.50

➥ case on page 137

1. Oxygenation is abnormal, ie the PaO_2 is lower than normal for a patient breathing room air.

   The pH is high, indicating an alkalosis. The $PaCO_2$ is normal, and the

HCO_3^- is high. Using Fig 1.5 on page 24, you can work out that this represents an uncompensated metabolic alkalosis.

2. Poor oxygenation could reflect any disease process affecting the lungs. Common causes would be pulmonary oedema or pneumonia. The causes of a metabolic alkalosis are listed in the box on page 27. The patient in this case had a lower respiratory tract infection and vomiting.

Answer 1.51

➥ case on page 137

This patient has a significantly elevated troponin T indicating a significant amount of cardiac damage. The clinical information is consistent with myocardial infarction. The patient is at significant risk of cardiac arrhythmias and should be managed in a coronary care unit.

Answer 1.52

➥ case on page 138

1. Oxygenation is normal given that the FiO_2 is 35%.

   The pH is high indicating an alkalosis. The $PaCO_2$ and HCO_3^- are both low. Using Fig 1.5 on page 24, you can see that this pattern could be due to either a respiratory alkalosis with metabolic compensation or a predominant respiratory alkalosis with coexistent metabolic acidosis.

2. The likely cause for this ABG given the clinical history is hyperventilation. Thus the acid-base disturbance is a respiratory alkalosis with metabolic compensation. One of the most common causes is anxiety, but it may occur as a result of organic pathology such as a stroke or subarachnoid haemorrhage affecting the respiratory centre.

   A full history and examination would be essential to help rule out a serious cause of this acid-base disturbance.

3. Reassurance would be a key aspect of treatment in the case of anxiety. Re-breathing one's own exhaled air, using a paper bag, may also be beneficial.

Answer 1.53

➥ case on page 138

It is difficult to be sure whether or not the patient has had a myocardial infarction (MI) based on the information given. The chest pain was short-lived, and the ECG normal which points away from MI. Although the troponin T level is quite markedly raised over normal, there is an alternative explanation for this other than MI, namely renal failure. A reasonable course of action in this case would be to repeat an ECG and repeat the troponin T level after several more hours. If the patient has really had an MI, one would expect the ECG to change and/or the troponin level to change.

Answer 1.54

↪ case on page 139

1. There are several trends present:
   - The haemoglobin concentration falls after the operation, reflecting blood loss during surgery. It remains stable postoperatively, suggesting that the blood loss has stopped.
   - The elevated white cell count (WCC) probably reflects a response to the trauma of surgery, but infection should be borne in mind.
   - The sodium concentration is falling steadily.
   - There is a slow, minor elevation in urea and creatinine, perhaps suggesting a degree of dehydration.
2. The patient should be assessed for evidence of cerebral oedema, which would mandate urgent treatment of the hyponatraemia. He should also have an assessment of his hydration status. Useful first-line investigations would include serum osmolality, urinary electrolytes and urinary osmolality.
3. A low urinary sodium suggests low effective circulating volume. This can occur in heart/liver failure, but there is no reason to suspect those conditions in this case. More commonly, low urinary sodium is seen together with dehydration (healthy kidneys trying to hold on to salt and water). Treatment will involve cautious rehydration, ensuring that the sodium concentration is increased at an appropriate rate.

Answer 1.55

↪ case on page 139

He is not anaemic, but his red blood cells are larger than normal (high MCV). This is not due to vitamin B_{12} or folate deficiency. Other possibilities for this finding include thyroid disease and alcohol consumption. There are a range of causes for thrombocytopenia as detailed on page 80. The most likely unifying diagnosis in this case is alcoholic liver disease causing liver cirrhosis and portal hypertension. Portal hypertension can result in hypersplenism which is the cause of the low platelet count. Patients often understate the amount of alcohol that they consume, and it is relatively easy to exceed the recommended maximum limits set out by the government. It is always a good idea to try to quantify the amount of alcohol (ideally with units consumed) that a patient is taking - do not accept passive statements that convey little information.

Answer 1.56

➥ case on page 140

Yes. The creatinine concentration in the ascitic fluid would approximate more closely to that in blood than that in urine. Serum creatinine levels are reported in µmol/l, whereas urine concentrations are much higher and are therefore reported in mmol/l. The result here appears to be from urine, suggesting that the catheter has been sited correctly.

Answer 1.57

➥ case on page 140

1. The male hormone profile is in keeping with primary hypogonadism (low testosterone with high LH and FSH concentrations). It is more tricky to interpret the female hormone profile, because precise hormone levels depend on timing in the menstrual cycle. With that in mind, however, it is clear that the patient is producing oestradiol and therefore does not have ovarian failure. The progesterone is high, suggesting that recent ovulation has occurred. Although the prolactin concentration is high, this is due to the presence of macro-prolactin, because the mono-prolactin concentration (which represents biologically active hormone) is completely normal. The female results are therefore all satisfactory.
2. Primary hypogonadism in a male (ie testicular failure) has a variety of causes, eg Klinefelter syndrome, testicular trauma, mumps orchitis or undescended testes.

Answer 1.58

➥ case on page 141

1 The fluid meets Lights' criteria and is an exudate. Comparison of the cholesterol and triglyceride results with those of the serum reveals that this is a chylothorax. See page 40 for further detail on interpreting these results.

2. The most likely cause of a chylothorax here is damage to the thoracic duct during surgery.

Typical chylothorax fluid is shown in the following photograph:

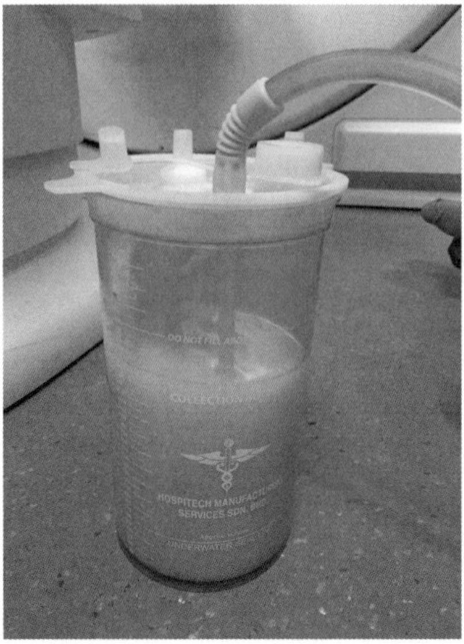

Answer 1.59

➥ case on page 141

This patient has hypocalcaemia and hypomagnesaemia. The magnesium abnormality is not severe enough to account for her presentation. The spasms are most probably due to hypocalcaemia. Hypocalcaemia is fairly uncommon. Vitamin D deficiency is probably the most common cause, but, in vitamin D deficiency, the serum phosphate is usually low. This patient's presentation is most probably due to hypoparathyroidism. It is possible that her parathyroid glands were damaged or removed at the time of her thyroidectomy.

Answer 1.60

➥ case on page 142

1. This patient has Cushing's disease, ie Cushing syndrome caused by an ACTH-secreting pituitary tumour. The 24-hour urine collection shows an abnormal quantity of free cortisol – this is suggestive, but not diagnostic, of Cushing syndrome. The administration of low-dose dexamethasone should normally result in negative feedback on the adrenal axis, but, in Cushing syndrome, autonomous cortisol secretion is unaffected by this and there is a failure to suppress cortisol release. In the high-dose test, significant suppression of cortisol is seen – this is typical of Cushing's disease (ie Cushing syndrome due to pituitary secretion of ACTH). In the CRH test, cortisol secretion is seen to increase, thus confirming Cushing's disease.

2. Inferior petrosal venous sampling with measurement of cortisol can be helpful in clinching the diagnosis. MRI of the brain would also be helpful in imaging the pituitary gland and planning surgical intervention.

Answer 1.61

➥ case on page 143

1. Three abnormalities can be seen in the first set of results:

    - Low sodium (hyponatraemia)
    - Low potassium (hypokalaemia)
    - High urea (uraemia).

    The low sodium and low potassium are a consequence of a prolonged period of vomiting combined with very limited oral intake. There has been a substantial loss of electrolytes without any means of replacement until admission to hospital. The patient is clinically dehydrated and the raised urea is a reflection of this.

Na^+	149 mmol/l	Marked rise from original sample
K^+	5.7 mmol/l	Marked rise from original sample
Urea	9.6 mmol/l	
Creatinine	69 µmol/l	
Cl^-	96 mmol/l	
HCO_3^-	25 mmol/l	

Na^+	133 mmol/l	More in keeping with original blood test
K^+	3.8 mmol/l	More in keeping with original blood test
Urea	8.9 mmol/l	
Creatinine	71 µmol/l	
Cl^-	94 mmol/l	
HCO_3^-	24 mmol/l	

2. Looking at the first repeat blood test, the sodium and potassium levels have both risen from the time of admission a few hours previously. There has been a dramatic change in electrolyte levels. The second repeat sample is very different again.

    The explanation for these findings is that the first repeat blood sample has been taken from the arm into which fluid is being infused. This is an erroneous sample.

    The second repeat sample comes from a 'non-drip' arm, and shows the true state of affairs, ie slowly improving electrolytes from the time of admission.

Answer 1.62

➥ case on page 144

Hb	82 g/l	Low
MCV	109.4 fl	High
Platelets	169 x 10^9/l	
WCC	6.2 x 10^9/l	
Iron	23 μmol/l	
Ferritin	49 μg/l	
TIBC	62 μmol/l	
Vitamin B_{12}	31 ng/l	Low
Folate	>10 μg/l	
Anti-parietal cell antibody	Titre < 1:120	
Anti-intrinsic factor antibody	Negative	

Schilling test

Without oral intrinsic factor: 0.03 μg radioactive vitamin B_{12} in 24-h urine sample (3% of oral dose) — Less than 10% of oral dose excreted in urine

With oral intrinsic factor: 0.03 μg radioactive vitamin B_{12} in 24-h urine sample (3% of oral dose) — Less than 10% of oral dose excreted in urine

Hydrogen breath test

Early peak in hydrogen excretion — Abnormal result

1. This patient has a macrocytic anaemia. Vitamin B_{12} is the only deficient haematinic, but the autoantibodies for pernicious anaemia are negative. The history states that the diet is balanced and no surgery has taken place on the bowel to interfere with the absorption of vitamin B_{12}. The Schilling test is abnormal. Normally, at least 10% of the oral dose of radiolabelled vitamin B_{12} is excreted in the urine. In this case, the excreted dose is low, and supplementation with intrinsic factor makes no difference. The likely pathology is therefore in the ileum.

2. The abnormal hydrogen breath test result points to the cause of anaemia - small bowel bacterial overgrowth. Patients with systemic sclerosis are prone to developing this condition. Definitive testing for bacterial overgrowth involves culturing small bowel contents. One would expect a normal Schilling test after an adequate course of appropriate antibiotics.

Answer 1.63

➥ case on page 145

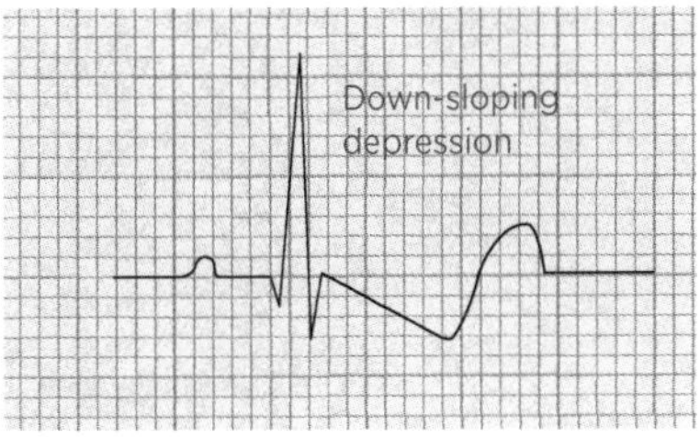

This patient has been prescribed digoxin for atrial fibrillation, and has digoxin toxicity. Digoxin is a drug with a narrow therapeutic ratio and a normal therapeutic range of 0.8–2.0 μg/l. A level as high as 2.9 nmol/l is enough for the symptoms described in this elderly patient. Digoxin levels can accumulate rapidly in patients with renal impairment. It is likely that this woman has become dehydrated following a bout of gastroenteritis. Renal impairment has caused the rise in plasma digoxin resulting in toxicity. Hypokalaemia is also present. This can exacerbate the symptoms of digoxin toxicity.

This iatrogenic problem is simply treated. Fluid resuscitation with the replacement of potassium intravenously and the exclusion of digoxin is appropriate in this case. The ECG shows down-sloping ST-segment depression ('reverse tick') often seen in patients on digoxin, and would have been a clue here that the patient was taking this drug. Sometimes an antidote (Digibind®) is required in the treatment of digoxin toxicity.

Answer 1.64

➥ case on page 146

This man has a normocytic anaemia. He is deficient in iron, vitamin B_{12} and folate. The red cell distribution width (RDW) is raised, indicating a wide variation in the size of circulating red cells. The patient is likely to have a dimorphic blood picture, with small red cells resulting from iron deficiency, and large cells resulting from deficiencies of vitamin B_{12} and folate. Crohn's disease is an inflammatory bowel disease involving the whole gastrointestinal tract so has the potential to cause deficiencies in all three haematinics. In this case, multiple operations have left him with a very short small bowel ('short gut syndrome').

Answer 1.65

➥ case on page 146

Creatinine clearance can be calculated using the following equation:

$$CL_{Cr} = \frac{U_{Cr} \times V \times 0.694}{B_{Cr}}$$

where U_{Cr} is the concentration of creatinine in urine (in mmol/l), V is the 24-h urine volume (in ml) and B_{Cr} is plasma creatinine in µmol/l

In this case:

$$CL_{Cr} = \frac{8 \times 1543 \times 0.694}{690} = 12.4 \text{ ml/min}$$

The creatinine clearance is 12.4 ml/min. Bearing in mind that the normal creatinine clearance is approximately 100 ml/min, it is clear that this man has significant renal impairment.

Answer 1.66

➥ case on page 147

1. The additional test is for parathyroid hormone (PTH).
2. These findings are in keeping with primary hyperparathyroidism.

The excess PTH, most likely from a parathyroid adenoma, is causing excess bone resorption resulting in a high calcium and ALP. Constitutional symptoms include bony aches, low mood and constipation, which can arise due to the hypercalcaemia. Hence the patient with hyperparathyroidism can have problems with 'bones, stones, moans and abdominal groans'.

Note that in primary hyperparathyroidism PTH is generally raised. However, a normal PTH level is also abnormal in a patient with hypercalcaemia and may be indicative of hyperparathyroidism. This is because PTH should normally be suppressed by negative feedback in the setting of hypercalcaemia.

Answer 1.67

➥ case on page 147

The most important pieces of information to ascertain from a paracetamol overdose patient are:

- **How much has been taken?**
- **When was it taken?**

Further questions to ascertain the psychiatric state and suicide risk are also clearly important.

In this case:

- **How much?**

16 tablets. Paracetamol tablets are normally 500 mg. Thus total dose = 16 x 500 mg = 8000 mg = 8 g.

- **Timing?**

4 h post-ingestion.

The 4 h level in this patient is 155 mg/l.

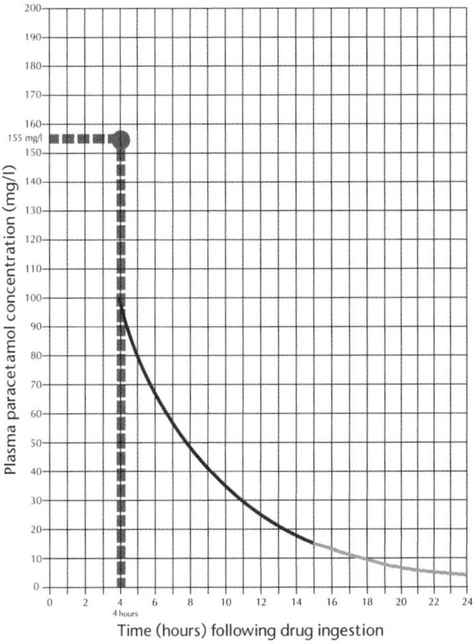

Using the graph illustrated earlier, one can interpret a paracetamol level of 155 mg/l at 4 h as high enough to warrant treatment.

Answer 1.68

→ case on page 148

- Both males and females are affected
- There are no instances of male-to-male transmission
- Male-to-female transmission is possible, with all daughters of an affected male having the condition.

The likely diagnosis is vitamin D-resistant rickets, with the inheritance pattern being X-linked dominant.

Answer 1.69

→ case on page 148

This man's U+E reveals an elevated urea. His creatinine is normal and his clinical history does not suggest dehydration. His full blood picture reveals information that helps in interpreting the significance of the elevated urea. His haemoglobin, MCV, white cell count and platelets are all abnormal. The raised MCV most likely represents chronic alcohol use.

During gastrointestinal bleeding, an increase in urea may occur. This is because urea is a breakdown product of digested blood. Similarly, during an active bleed, a rise in the white cell count and platelet count may occur.

The combination of the following is suggestive of gastrointestinal bleeding:

- Raised urea (with normal creatinine)
- Low haemoglobin
- Raised white cell count (in the absence of infection)
- Raised platelets.

Answer 1.70

→ case on page 149

This overdose case is more difficult, although perhaps more typical. The patient is only admitting to taking 'tablets', although the quantity, type and timing are more uncertain. At the time of presentation to hospital it is over 7 h since ingestion. This patient has taken alcohol with the tablets, has a raised paracetamol level and a mildly raised salicylate level. The patient also has mild impairment of her liver function tests.

When the paracetamol result is transferred to the nomogram, one can see that a level of 80 mg/l is well above the treatment line. Instigation of an infusion of *N*-acetylcysteine must commence immediately.

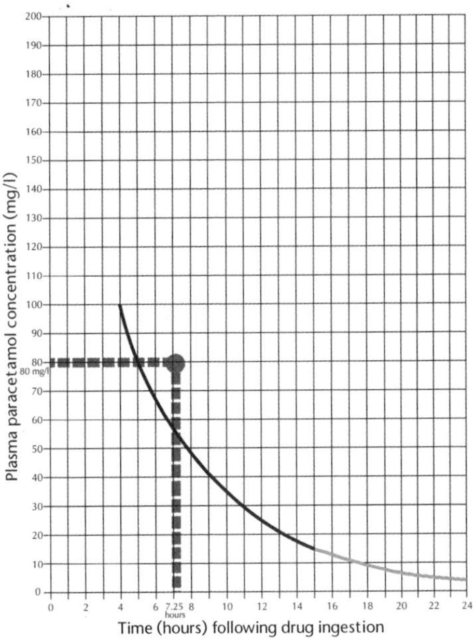

Answer 1.71

➥ case on page 150

1. The only abnormality on the liver biochemistry is a raised ALP. ALP may be raised in bone as well as liver disease (see page 12). An isolated ALP rise may be seen in both primary sclerosing cholangitis (PSC) and early primary biliary cirrhosis (PBC). The normal albumin suggests that the synthetic function of the liver remains intact. The immunological tests are the diagnostic key in this case. A substantially raised anti-mitochondrial antibody (AMA) is observed. Ninety-five per cent of patients with PBC will have a positive antibody for AMA-M2. In PSC the presence of autoantibodies is uncommon.

2. The most useful investigation to confirm and assess the extent of disease would be a liver biopsy.

Answer 1.72

➥ case on page 150

One must be particularly mindful in patients with psychiatric disease of the accuracy of information conveyed and compliance with medication. Lithium is a commonly used drug in bipolar affective disorder, but has one major drawback - overdose. It has a narrow therapeutic ratio. Patients on long-term lithium can become unwell due to toxicity even without deliberate overdose. Lithium toxicity can be fatal. The normal range is 0.4–1.5 mmol/l with levels above 2.0 mmol/l requiring treatment that may include haemodialysis. Levels between 1.5 and 2.0 mmol/l, as in this case, may require only fluid resuscitation and supportive treatment, along with temporary discontinuation of the drug.

Answer 1.73

➥ case on page 151

On 1 July, the patient developed thrombocytopenia. This has worsened steadily and significantly since. An extremely rare adverse drug reaction, 'heparin-induced thrombocytopenia (HIT)', can occur in patients receiving unfractionated or low-molecular-weight heparin. It is likely that this patient was receiving low-molecular-weight heparin in an attempt to prevent thromboembolic disease.

Answer 1.74

➥ case on page 151

These findings are in keeping with a diagnosis of osteomalacia. Osteomalacia is a metabolic bone disease in which there is a lack of calcium or phosphate (or both) for mineralisation of newly formed osteoid. As a result, bone is 'soft' and unable to withstand the stresses and forces of normal bone. Parathyroid hormone would need to be checked if there were any diagnostic doubt.

It is likely that this patient's coeliac disease is contributing to the development of osteomalacia through malabsorption of calcium. A vitamin D level should be checked here.

Answer 1.75

→ case on page 152

Date	14/02	15/02	16/02	17/02	
Na^+ (mmol/l)	135	135	134	136	
K^+ (mmol/l)	3.3	3.4	3.4	3.7	Slow increase
Urea (mmol/l)	2.1	2.2	2.2	2.3	Slow increase
Creatinine (μmol/l)	44	49	47	45	
Cl^- (mmol/l)	94	94	93	93	
HCO_3^- (mmol/l)	23	22	23	23	
Mg^{2+} (mmol/l)	0.39	0.37	0.38	0.51	Slow increase
PO_4^{3-} (mmol/l)	0.70	0.61	0.41	0.40	Dangerous drop in first 3 days
Adjusted Ca^{2+} (mmol/l)	2.32	2.05	2.12	2.22	Drop on day 2
Albumin (g/l)	33	32	33	32	

This scenario illustrates the issue of refeeding in those patients who have been nutritionally depleted for some time. When feeding is commenced, a rapid and precipitous drop often occurs, in particular, in phosphate levels.

Answer 1.76

→ case on page 152

This patient has a microcytic anaemia. The striking abnormality on her FBP is that the MCV is extremely low, whereas the haemoglobin concentration is only slightly below the reference range. She originates from the Maldives - an area where thalassaemia is common. It is probable that this woman has thalassaemia (most likely to be β-thalassaemia trait). Haemoglobin electrophoresis will confirm the diagnosis. Concomitant iron deficiency is possible, so sending blood for iron studies would also seem sensible.

Answer 1.77

→ case on page 153

1. Oxygenation is normal.

   The pH is low indicating an acidosis. The $PaCO_2$ and HCO_3^- are both low. Using Fig 1.5 on page 24 you can see that this indicates either a metabolic acidosis with respiratory compensation or a predominant metabolic acidosis with coexistent respiratory alkalosis.

   Remember to calculate the anion gap with any case of metabolic acidosis. In this case the anion gap is calculated as follows: (131 + 4.5) - (96.1 + 12.6) = 26.8. Thus this is a raised anion gap metabolic acidosis.

2. Bearing in mind the causes of a raised anion gap metabolic acidosis shown in the box on page 27, the following tests would be helpful: urinalysis for ketones, plasma lactate levels and salicylate levels.

3. This pattern can be seen when salicylates (eg aspirin), methanol or ethylene glycol is taken in excess.

Answer 1.78

➥ case on page 154

1. Oxygenation is abnormal. The patient has type 2 respiratory failure, with low PaO_2 and high $PaCO_2$.

   The pH is low, indicating an acidosis. The $PaCO_2$ is high, as is the HCO_3^-. Using Fig 1.5 on page 24 you can see that this pattern could represent either respiratory acidosis with metabolic compensation, or a predominant respiratory acidosis with a coexistent metabolic alkalosis.

2. The most likely diagnosis is an acute exacerbation of chronic obstructive pulmonary disease (COPD). This would be in keeping with the clinical findings. The acid–base disturbance would therefore represent respiratory acidosis with metabolic compensation. Note that the compensation is only partial, since the patient remains acidotic. An acute exacerbation of COPD is the most common cause of a respiratory acidosis with a raised HCO_3^-.

   Many patients with COPD have high resting CO_2 levels, causing a respiratory acidosis. However, with time, the kidneys compensate for this acidosis by retaining HCO_3^-. Thus, in the 'normal' state, many patients with COPD have a normal pH, with a raised $PaCO_2$ and a raised HCO_3^-, such as that shown in the ABG below:

pH	7.38
PaO_2	9.1 kPa
$PaCO_2$	6.8 kPa
HCO_3^-	36.0 mmol/l
BE	5 mmol/l

   During an acute exacerbation, however, the $PaCO_2$ levels increase, giving rise to a respiratory acidosis.

3. Patients may often benefit from non-invasive ventilation (NIV) using bilevel positive airway pressure (BiPAP). If deterioration occurs, intubation and ventilation may be required.

Answer 1.79

→ case on page 154

The patient has a metabolic acidosis, with a high anion gap. She also has a significant osmolar gap, because the calculated osmolality (294.5 mosmol/l) is much lower than the measured osmolality.

A normal osmolar gap is around 2 mosmol/l, so the gap here (352 – 294.5 = 57.5 mosmol/l) is clearly very high. This means that there is a significant quantity of an unmeasured, osmotically active substance in the patient's blood. This abnormality is often due to the presence of ethanol or a toxic alcohol, most commonly ethylene glycol (antifreeze), in the patient's blood. From the results, it can be seen that the ethanol result does not fully explain the gap. (Please note that the ethanol result is given in mmol/l to aid your comprehension - this is not the normal unit for reporting ethanol concentration.) One should be suspicious of ethylene glycol poisoning in this case, and a level should be requested. Treatment of ethylene glycol poisoning often includes utilising dialysis to clear ethylene glycol from the blood and the administration of an antidote (most commonly fomepizole).

Answer 1.80

→ case on page 155

1. The abnormalities shown in the FBP and U+E are:

   - Normocytic anaemia
   - High chloride
   - Hypokalaemia
   - Low HCO_3^-.

   The hypokalaemia is severe and could cause cardiac arrhythmias at this level.

2. The pH is low, as is the $PaCO_2$ and HCO_3^-. This patient has a metabolic acidosis with partial respiratory compensation. The anion gap is 136 – (110 + 14) = 12 mmol/l, which is normal. This is a normal anion gap metabolic acidosis.

3. There are a limited number of causes of this acid-base disturbance (see page 27). The coexistence of hypokalaemia and metabolic acidosis is an uncommon finding (hyperkalaemia usually accompanies acidosis), and should raise suspicions of an underlying diagnosis of renal tubular acidosis (RTA). RTA can involve disease of the proximal or distal renal tubules and can in itself have a wide variety of causes. The clue to the unifying diagnosis in this case comes from the patient's symptom of ocular grittiness. The diagnosis here is RTA secondary to Sjögren syndrome. Immunological testing will confirm this (see page 98 for details).

Answer 1.81

➥ case on page 156

The abnormality on the FBP is the high WCC. A differential WCC result is not given, so it is difficult to speculate as to the cause based on these blood results alone. The key to making the diagnosis is the correct interpretation of the blood film. The diagonal arrow highlights a smear cell, whereas the vertical arrow highlights a chronic lymphocytic leukaemia (CLL) cell. The diagnosis is CLL, a condition that is not uncommonly detected in seemingly well individuals who have blood tested for other reasons.

Answer 1.82

➥ case on page 157

1. This man presents with neuromuscular irritability. This is commonly a feature of hypocalcaemia. Although his serum calcium concentration is low, when corrected for the hypoalbuminaemia it is actually normal. Hypocalcaemia is therefore not to blame for his symptoms. Hypomagnesaemia can also present in this way, and is the cause of the presentation in this case.
2. The most likely cause for the hypomagnesaemia, based on the information provided, is the use of a proton pump inhibitor. The mechanism of action may relate to impaired magnesium absorption in the gut.

Answer 1.83

➥ case on page 157

1. This man has severe hyponatraemia, a low HCO_3^- level (suggesting possible metabolic acidosis), renal impairment (which might be chronic kidney disease or acute kidney injury; the current results would need to be compared with historical results to differentiate the two) and a normal serum osmolality. His urine is reasonably concentrated.

   The normal serum osmolality raises the possibility that the hyponatraemia is actually pseudohyponatraemia (ie the true sodium level might well be normal). Possible causes are high concentrations of protein in the serum (as seen in multiple myeloma) and hypertriglyceridaemia (as seen in genetic disorders of lipid metabolism).
2. Putting all these findings in the context of the patient's presenting complaint, the most likely cause is acute pancreatitis secondary to hypertriglyceridaemia. To get the correct diagnosis, you would need a good understanding of his test results and knowledge of common causes of acute pancreatitis.

Answer 1.84

→ case on page 158

1. The patient is clinically 'euthyroid', ie there is no sign of hypo- or hyperthyroidism. The set of results that fits with this picture is most likely to be correct. The second set of results (normal values) is correct.
2. The first set of results suggests secondary hyperthyroidism, but this is not replicated on the second run. It is possible that there was a sample mix-up, and that the set of results obtained first time around belongs to another patient. These two sets of results have been obtained from separate laboratories, which are probably using different methods to analyse the blood samples. Another explanation for the difference in results is that the patient has a substance or substances in his blood (commonly antibodies) that affect the method used by the first laboratory, but not that used in the second laboratory.

This case illustrates an important point – always interpret data with the patient in mind. If the data do not appear to fit the case, something unusual might be going on. Always ask for help in such a scenario as, in this case, there may be an unusual but completely innocent explanation for the findings.

Answer 1.85

→ case on page 158

1. The results show an acidosis, which is most probably a metabolic acidosis because the HCO_3^- is low. A complete blood gas analysis would be helpful to confirm this with certainty. The anion gap is high.
2. Considering the potential causes of a high anion gap metabolic acidosis, there is nothing in the history to suggest poisoning, and the patient is not taking paracetamol or salicylates. Renal function is satisfactory. A district nurse is administering parenteral nutrition, so starvation ketosis is unlikely. The blood glucose is normal, so diabetic ketoacidosis is unlikely. 'Lactate' is normal. A regular lactate assay gives a result for L-lactate, not D-lactate. D-lactic acidosis is the diagnosis here, and a lactate level would be required to confirm this perceived diagnosis. D-lactic acidosis most commonly occurs in patients with abnormal bowel anatomy, when the abnormal bacteria in the bowel lumen metabolise carbohydrate. The patient's episodes of drowsiness are probably due to periodic worsening of the acidosis, although the codeine might also have a part to play.

Answer 1.86

➥ case on page 159

This question is tricky. The key to finding the answer is to remember that the total WCC is equal to the sum of the component parts of the differential white cell count.

DON'T FORGET

Total white cell count = neutrophil count + lympocyte count + eosinophil count + monocyte count + basophil count

In this case, the neutrophil count and lymphocyte count together cannot account for the total white cell count [$(7.4 \times 10^9/l) + (2.5 \times 10^9/l) < 13.2 \times 10^9/l$]. There must be a further type of white blood cell in elevated numbers. It is impossible to tell for certain what this cell type might be. However, the likely diagnosis here is helmintic (worm) infection. A full differential white cell count would reveal a raised level of eosinophils.

Answer 1.87

➥ case on page 159

1. Care should be taken when interpreting these results. Note that the TOTAL T_4 level is given, not the FREE T_4 level. It is the free level that is important physiologically. It is impossible to make any further comments on these tests other than to say that the total T_4 level is raised, and the TSH is normal.
2. First, the free T_4 level should be measured. In this case it was normal (result not shown), indicating normal thyroid function. The patient therefore has an elevated total T_4 level with a normal free T_4 level. The reason for this is increased levels of TBG. The most likely reason for this is a high oestrogen state (eg pregnancy or use of the oral contraceptive pill). Since the question states that the patient is not on any medication, the most likely diagnosis here is pregnancy. The second test that should be performed is therefore a pregnancy test.

Answer 1.88

➥ case on page 160

The key to even thinking about the rare disease in this case starts with the basics in interpreting the patient's FBP. The neutrophil and lymphocyte counts do not account for the elevated total WCC. The missing piece of information in the question is the eosinophil count which is highly abnormal in this case. The diagnosis here is Churg–Strauss syndrome, a rare vasculitic disease associated with a peripheral eosinophilia.

Answer 1.89

➥ case on page 160

- Both males and females are affected
- Male-to-male and male-to-female transmission do not occur
- Affected females pass the condition on to all offspring.

The inheritance pattern is mitochondrial.

Answer 1.90

➥ case on page 161

This situation is a common cause for concern. The details omitted from the history above are that the patient has chronic renal failure, and receives haemodialysis three times per week via his indwelling central venous catheter. The raised urea and creatinine are a reflection of the chronic renal failure in this case. This would be apparent if these results were compared with the old results.

The cause of the deranged coagulation is most likely because blood has been drawn from the central venous catheter, which is often flushed with a heparin solution. The next step should be to repeat the coagulation profile using blood taken from a peripheral vein.

2

INTERPRETING MEDICAL IMAGING

9

INTERPRETING CHEST AND ABDOMINAL RADIOGRAPHS

Introduction to medical imaging

The interpretation of imaging investigations is a comprehensive topic that forms a specialty in its own right. Its influence and remit in contemporary medicine are vast, forming huge amounts of 'digital data' for interpretation.

X-ray images are technically known as 'radiographs', and it is essential that medical students and trainee doctors have a sound basic understanding of these, in particular chest and abdominal films. Likewise an appreciation and insight into the more advanced imaging investigations at their disposal are increasingly important, in particular the ever popular and influential computed tomography (CT) imaging. A good professional relationship with the radiology department, including thoughtful and selective referral, can hugely aid patient care.

This chapter and the following chapter do not aim to be a concise undergraduate textbook on radiology, nor an exhaustive description of characteristic radiological findings in common diseases. They act as a guide to approaching the interpretation of common radiographs and the core cross-sectional imaging modalities. In the clinical cases featured, the emphasis will be on inpatient films, ie radiographs that one might be expected to interpret during work on general medical and surgical wards or in an emergency department. No film will be viewed in isolation without clinical information. As with all the data interpretation considered in this book, investigations should be assessed in the light of the clinical scenario and laboratory results. This should also be the gold standard to aspire to in clinical practice.

DON'T FORGET

Always interpret X-ray findings in their clinical context.

Compare images with old ones if possible.

Interpreting a chest X-ray

The chest X-ray (CXR) is the single most requested imaging investigation and is also the most likely film to feature in daily practice or an undergraduate exam. It provides a perfect prompt for questioning other aspects of a patient's condition and for exploring management strategies. To be able to comment confidently on the film's findings, and have an understanding of how to approach interpretation, an appreciation of normality is required. Don't forget that a CXR is a two-dimensional representation of a three-dimensional structure.

One may think of a CXR as a picture that contains five 'shades' on a black-and-white scale. Four shades represent natural 'tissues' and one represents artefacts.

The shades seen are:

1. Bone is WHITE
2. Gas is BLACK.
3. Soft tissue is GREY
4. Fat is DARKER GREY.
5. Most man-made things on the film are BRIGHT WHITE.

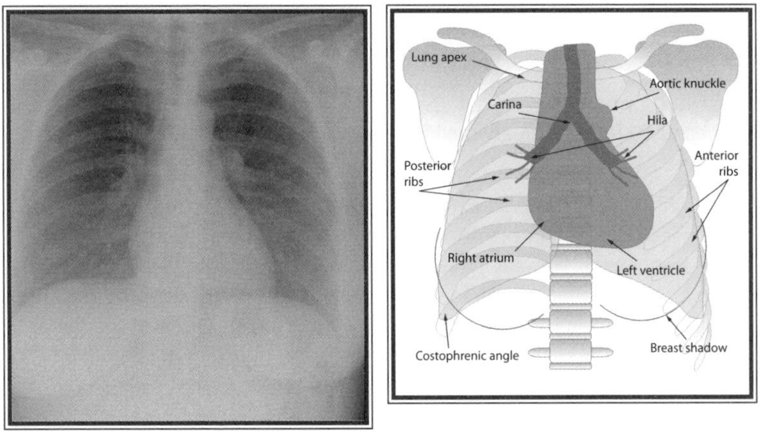

Fig 9.1: CXR.

Film specifics and technical factors

Before proceeding to interpret a CXR, always comment on film specifics and technical factors as shown in the boxes below.

FILM SPECIFICS (DETAILS)
Name of patient
Age and date of birth
Location of patient
Date taken
Film number (if applicable)

FILM TECHNICAL FACTORS
Type of projection (see box below)
Markings regarding any special techniques used (eg taken in expiration)
Rotation
Inspiration
Penetration

TYPES OF PROJECTION
Posteroanterior (PA): the X-ray tube is behind the patient and film against the chest. The GOLD standard projection
Anteroposterior (AP): the X-ray tube is in front of the patient and film against the back
Supine: the patient is lying on his or her back
Erect: the patient is upright
Semi-erect: the patient is partially upright
Mobile: the X-ray has been taken with a mobile X-ray unit. This should be used for very sick patients only (on the ITU/HDU/CCU usually)

These descriptions may be combined. For example, an acutely unwell patient who has a CXR taken on an intensive therapy unit (ITU) may have a mobile, semi-erect AP film.

You might think of this part of the interpretation like the safety announcement on an airplane: necessary to acknowledge, but tedious and of little consequence. However, this could not be further from the truth. Changes in these parameters can give the impression of abnormalities in the structures visualised. For example, a widened mediastinum, on an AP chest X-ray may provoke the impression of a thoracic aortic dissection, or a pneumothorax may be overlooked if one does not appreciate that the chest X-ray is supine rather than erect.

Assess the film in detail

Just as one would approach a clinical system examination in a methodical manner, a structured systematic approach is needed for thorough interpretation.

It is good practice to mention a clear-cut abnormality at the outset. A reasonable way to say this would be, 'The technical quality of the film is satisfactory. The most striking abnormality on initial assessment is ...'.

In the context of an assessment, the examiner will then expect the candidate to demonstrate an organised approach to looking at the rest of the film. Do not stop when one abnormality has been noted - there may be more to see.

DON'T FORGET

Keep looking - multiple findings may give the definitive diagnosis.

Structures to assess

1. Heart and major vessels

Assess:

- Size of the heart overall
- Size of individual chambers of the heart
- Size of pulmonary vessels
- Evidence of stents, clips, wires, valves and pacemakers
- Outline of the aorta, inferio and superior vena cava.

DON'T FORGET

Do not comment on heart size on an AP chest X-ray because it appears magnified.

2. Lungs

Assess:

- Size
- Intrapulmonary pathology
- Bronchovascular lung markings.

3. Pleura

Assess:

- Thickness or calcification
- Fluid or air in the pleural space.

4. Mediastinum (including hila)

Assess:

- Width of the mediastinum
- Contour of the mediastinum
- Size and density of the hila
- Level and symmetry of the hila.

5. Bones and soft tissues

Assess:

- Diffuse or focal bony abnormalities
- Surgical emphysema
- Breast presence/absence and symmetry.

6. Review areas

Be particularly careful not to miss the following REVIEW areas. They should be specifically checked, as abnormalities in these areas may be easily overlooked.

- Costophrenic angles (A)
- Lung apices (B)
- Behind the heart (C)
- Below the diaphragm (D)
- Breast shadows (in females) (E).

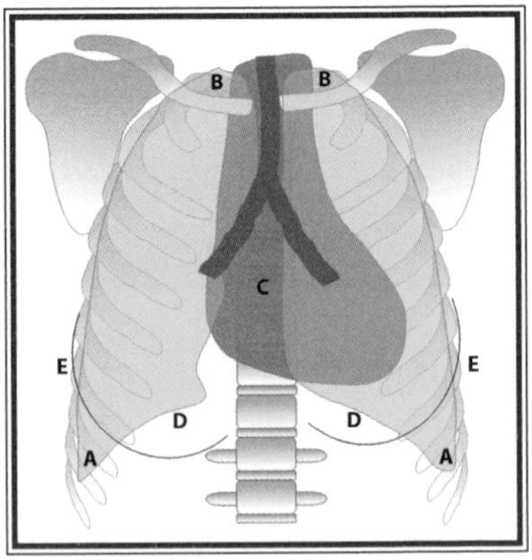

Fig 9.3: Review areas on a chest X-ray assessment.

Interpreting an abdominal X-ray

The abdominal X-ray (AXR) has a more limited value in diagnosis than a CXR. Its chief use is in the diagnosis of bowel obstruction and renal tract calculi, although other pathology may be identified. Even in these cases, the abdominal X-ray is often just a 'stepping stone' to further imaging with ultrasonography or CT. Indiscriminate requests for the abdominal X-ray are discouraged.

The radiation exposure of an AXR is also considerably higher compared with a CXR. One AXR is equivalent to 35 CXRs.

As with a CXR, an appreciation of normality is vital.

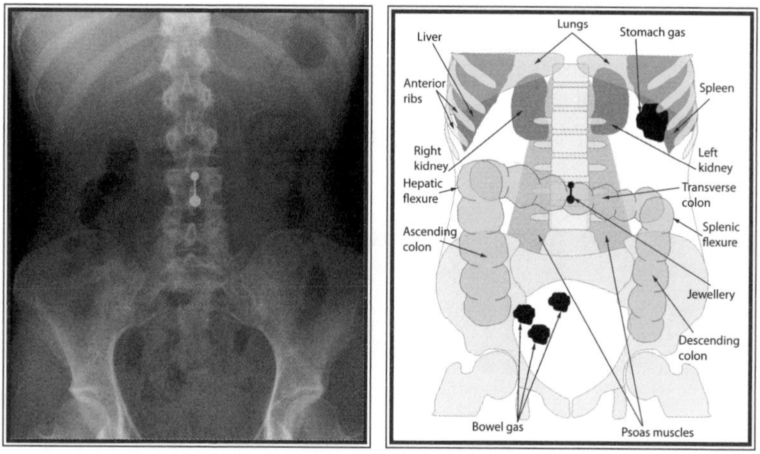

Fig 9.4: An almost normal AXR (this person has jewellery in the umbilicus).

Film specifics and technical factors

The initial assessment of an AXR is similar to a CXR.

FILM SPECIFICS	FILM TECHNICAL FACTORS
Name of patient Age of patient Location of patient Date taken Film number (if applicable)	Type of projection (supine is standard) Markings of any special techniques used Adequate anatomical coverage

Assess the film in detail

A simple guide to interpretation is shown below. Working through these headings, one covers 'black bits', 'white bits', 'grey bits' and 'bright white bits' in turn. Alternatively one may take an anatomical approach to interpretation.

Structures to assess

'Black bits' (gas)

Intraluminal gas

Intraluminal gas can be normal. However, its presence can be abnormal if it is in the wrong place or if too much is seen.

The maximum normal diameter of the large bowel is 5.5 cm. Small bowel should be no more than 3.5 cm in diameter. The natural presence of gas within the bowel allows assessment of calibre, although the amount varies between individuals. The caecum is not considered to be dilated unless wider than 8.0 cm in diameter.

Large and small bowel may be distinguished in adults by looking at bowel wall markings.

> **DON'T FORGET**
>
> The haustra of the large bowel extend only a third of the way across the diameter of the large bowel from each side. The valvulae conniventes of the small bowel traverse the whole diameter.

It is usual to see small volumes of gas throughout the gastrointestinal tract and the absence in one region may in itself represent pathology. For example, if gas is seen to the level of the splenic flexure and nothing is apparent distal to this, a site of obstruction - a 'cut-off' point - is assumed.

Similarly, displaced bowel loops may suggest an intra-abdominal mass or collection.

Extraluminal gas

When a bowel loop or any other gas-containing structure perforates, its contained gas becomes extraluminal. Extraluminal gas is never normal, but it may be seen following intra-abdominal surgery or laparoscopy, when strictly speaking it is not pathological.

CAUSES OF EXTRALUMINAL GAS
Post-abdominal surgery/laparoscopy
Perforation of viscus (eg bowel, stomach)
Abscess/collection

DON'T FORGET

An erect CXR (not AXR) is the best projection to diagnose a pneumoperitoneum (gas in the peritoneal cavity), as it is more sensitive.

'White bits'

Calcification

Calcified structures are often seen on an AXR. The main question to ask is: 'Does their presence have any important implications?' Calcification can be broadly divided into three types:

1. Calcification that is an abnormal structure, eg gallstones, renal calculi, calcified splenic artery aneurysm.
2. Calcification that is within a normal structure, but represents pathology, eg pancreatic ductal calcification.
3. Calcification that is within a normal structure, but is not clinically significant, eg lymph node calcification or a calcified pelvic phlebolith.

Bones are normal 'white' structures. On the AXR they comprise mainly those of the thoracolumbar spine and pelvis. Findings are often incidental.

'Grey bits'

Soft tissues

Soft tissues represent most of the contents of the abdomen and feature prominently in the AXR. However, these tissues are poorly visualised and delineated when compared with other imaging techniques such as ultrasound, CT or MRI.

The outlines of the kidneys, spleen, liver and bladder (if filled) can be seen in addition to psoas muscle shadows. An AXR should not, however, be requested to specifically look at these structures.

'Bright white bits'

Foreign bodies

Foreign bodies represent an interesting final observation. Objects may have been deliberately placed, for example, an aortic stent, an inferior vena cava filter or abdominal drain. Sterilisation clips and intrauterine devices are common findings in women. Other objects that may be seen include ingested and rectal foreign bodies, as well as items in the path of the X-ray beam, such as belt buckles, dress buttons and umbilical jewellery.

Other imaging modalities

A range of other imaging modalities is in regular use - the majority of which do not feature significantly in undergraduate exams. Knowledge of their importance in diagnosis should be sufficient, in particular which investigation should be requested for different common clinical scenarios.

IONISING RADIATION TECHNIQUES
Contrast/fluoroscopic studies (mostly use barium)
Computed tomography (CT)
Positron emission tomography (PET)
Nuclear (radionuclide) imaging

NON-IONISING RADIATION TECHNIQUES
Ultrasound
Magnetic resonance imaging (MRI)

INTERPRETING CHEST AND ABDOMINAL RADIOGRAPHS - WHAT YOU NEED TO KNOW

How to present imaging investigations in an exam - structured guidance

- Be methodical in your approach
- Check and present the patient demographic parameters first in all instances
- State what investigation has been offered and if required the specifics (the type of view, if with contrast)
- Go through the investigation by a review of either anatomical structures or systems
- Take time to describe any abnormal finding in detail
- Include the relevant negatives, if you are able to appreciate what these are
- Summarise your findings
- To complete give your radiological impression or differential
- You may wish to recommend or suggest other investigations, if relevant.

10

CROSS-SECTIONAL IMAGING

The medical community has become ever more dependent on 24/7 imaging when delivering patient care. As practices evolve so do the demands and expectations of medical imaging, with a progressive 'chase to the top'. Imaging with CT is now routine, even out of hours, with MRI playing a more restricted role in cross-sectional imaging.

With the exception of CT of the head, clinicians rarely view cross-sectional images without the direct involvement of a radiologist. However, an understanding and appreciation of such images are useful skills to have. With this in mind, together with examination expectations, a reasonably detailed guide to interpreting head CT is provided here, along with an overview of normal anatomy as visualised on other cross-sectional imaging modalities. The aim of this material is not only to aid learning and assist in examinations, but also to be of practical use in everyday working practice.

A detailed review of how to approach each of these different investigations and the diverse range of potential pathologies can be found in specific clinical radiology texts. Suffice to say that the approach for all of these cross-sectional studies is standard and similar to that for plain films (see Chapter 9).

PRACTICAL POINTS

- Large-bore secure peripheral venous access is always ideal for CT studies
- CT angiographic studies require 14-G or 16-G cannulas in the antecubital fossa to ensure optimal contrast opacification
- IV contrast is not required for all studies, but is vital in body trauma
- Renal function - ideally estimated glomerular filtration rate (eGFR) - is needed before IV contrast studies
- Consider the pros and cons of the clinical scenario when giving contrast to those with renal impairment
- More is not always better - target the scan or the sequences to the chief clinical concern
- Appreciate that CT and MRI are not always the best studies for a clinical query. More does not always equate with better

Review and presentation of cross-sectional imaging

- Be methodical in your approach
- In all instances check and present the patient demographic parameters first
- State what investigation has been offered and, if required, the specifics (eg the type of view; if contrast has been used)
- Go through the investigation by reviewing either anatomical structures or systems
- Take time to describe any abnormal finding in detail
- Include the relevant negatives, if you can appreciate what these are
- Recognise, but don't dwell on, incidental findings (which are common)
- Summarise your findings
- To complete, give your radiological impression or differential diagnosis
- You may wish to recommend or suggest other investigations, if relevant.

CT Head

The most commonly requested CT scan is the CT head. Quick and inexpensive to acquire, and fast to report, an ever-growing number of clinicians view CT head independently. For this reason an introduction to CT head is included and key pathologies are featured in the clinical cases.

Specific National Institute for Health and Care Excellence (NICE) guidelines have been written with respect to the indications for CT head following trauma. These include:

- Glasgow Coma Scale (GCS) <13 when first assessed or GCS <15 2 hours after injury
- Suspected open or depressed skull fracture
- Signs of base-of-skull fracture
- Post-traumatic seizure
- Focal neurological deficit
- More than one episode of vomiting. Scottish Intercollegiate Guidelines Network (SIGN) guidance suggests two distinct episodes of vomiting.
- Coagulopathy + any amnesia or loss of consciousness since injury
- More than 30 minutes of amnesia of events before impact.

Normal anatomy

The normal appearances of key structures in the supra- and infratentorial brain are shown in Figs 10.1–10.5.

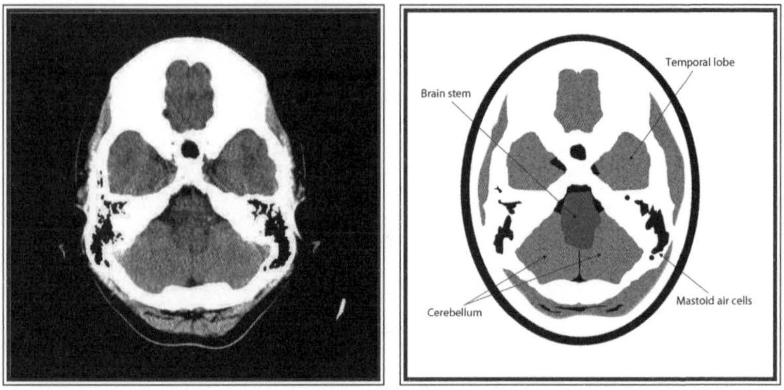

Fig 10.1: Normal CT head anatomy (a).

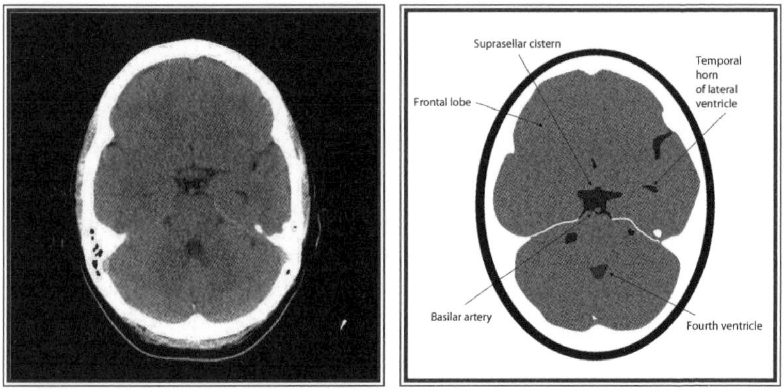

Fig 10.2: Normal CT head anatomy (b).

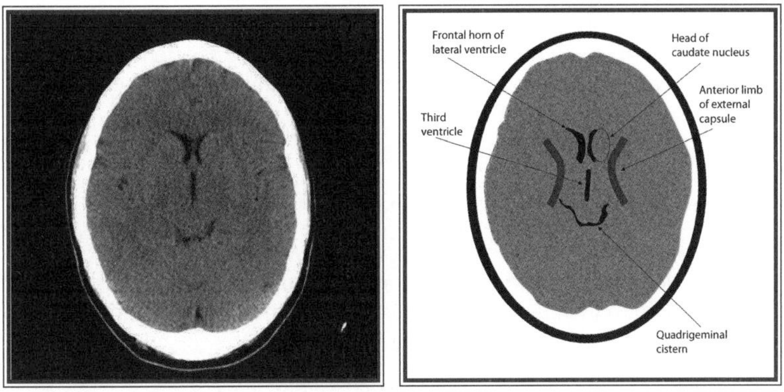

Fig 10.3: Normal CT head anatomy (c).

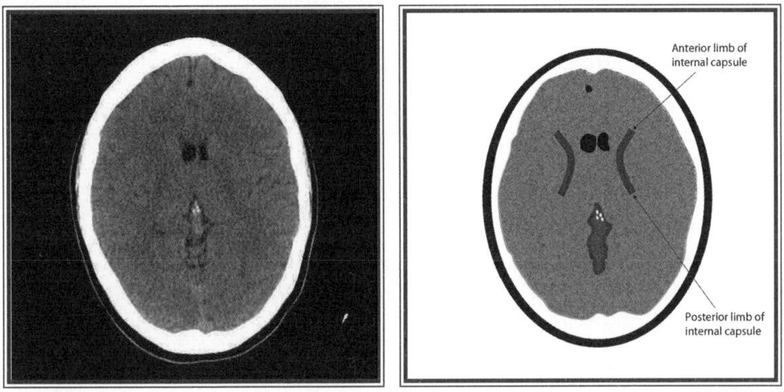

Fig 10.4: Normal CT head anatomy (d).

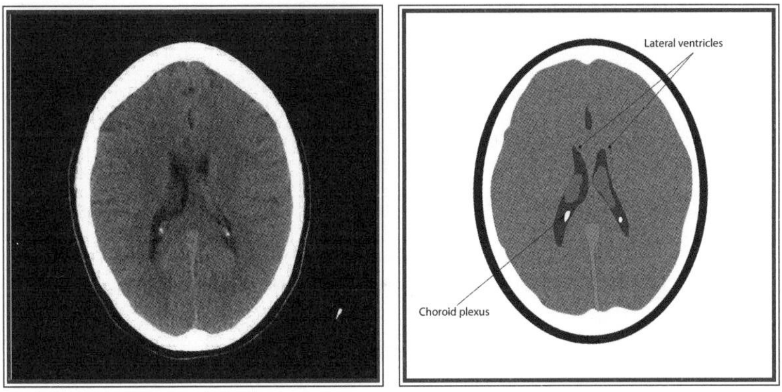

Fig 10.5: Normal CT head anatomy (e).

Key basic facts

CT demonstrates a wide-ranging grey scale, referred to as attenuation. In the brain this is often stated to be hypo-, iso- or hyperdense in relation to normal brain parenchyma. Bearing this in mind:

- CSF in the brain will appear black.
- The bone of the skull will appear white.
- Grey and white matter within the brain have different attenuations. The densely packed nerve cell bodies of the grey matter have a higher attenuation than the nerve axons of the white matter, meaning that surprisingly white matter is darker than grey matter on CT.
- Blood contains protein, making it dense, and areas of acute haemorrhage appear as high attenuation (white) on a CT scan.
- Areas of dead or damaged brain tissue (encephalomalacia or ischaemic brain) will become less dense, meaning that they will appear darker than the surrounding brain (low attenuation).
- Intravenous contrast on CT highlights blood vessels or vascular areas of the brain. It is also useful for identifying areas of high cell turnover, such as tumours and infection. Aneurysms, tumours and abscesses all become brighter after contrast administration.

DON'T FORGET

If there is concern over intracranial haemorrhage, the scan must be performed unenhanced. Acute blood and contrast look the same!

Assessment of images

Try to answer the following questions:

- Is the ventricular system the appropriate size?
- Is there any acute blood present? If so, is it intraparenchymal, subarachnoid or an extra-axial collection?
- Is there any evidence of ischaemia? If so is it focal or territorial in nature?
- Is there normal differentiation between the grey and white matter of the brain?
- Is there space around the cord at the level of the foramen magnum?
- Are the sulci effaced or the ventricles displaced, suggesting mass effect?
- Check the bony skull (on bone window settings) to look for a fracture or other bony abnormality.

Check the review areas to finish:

- Is there anything in the ventricular system, eg blood in the occipital horns?
- Are the visualised orbits normal?
- Is there any abnormality in the mastoid air cells or paranasal sinuses?

Normal anatomy as seen on other cross-sectional imaging modalities

1. CT of the neck

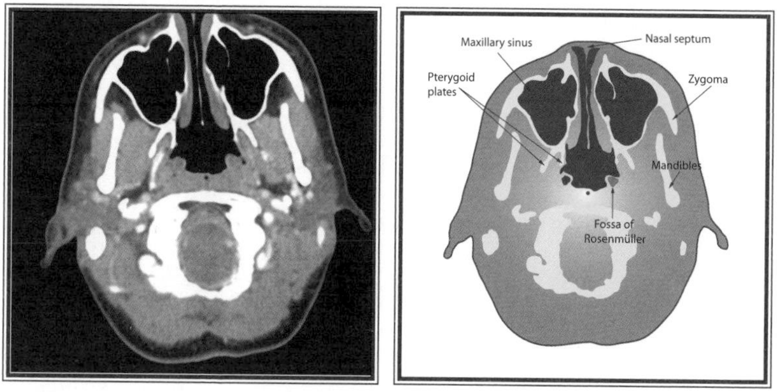

Fig 10.6: Axial CT of the neck (arterial phase): normal anatomy (a).

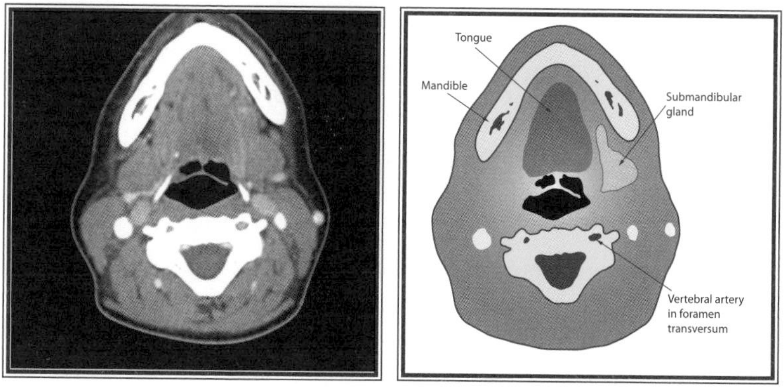

Fig 10.7: Axial CT of the neck (arterial phase): normal anatomy (b).

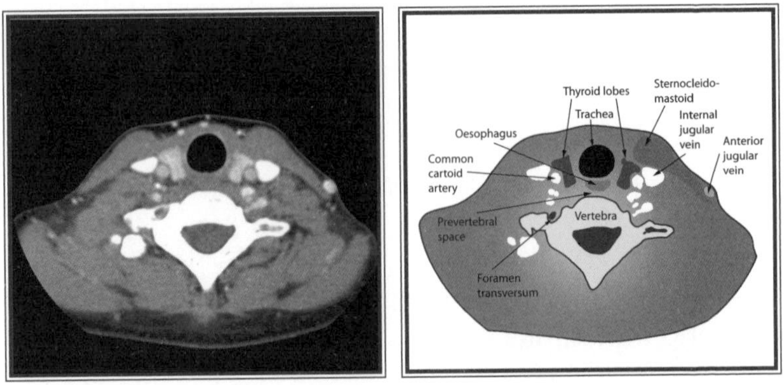

Fig 10.8: Axial CT of the neck (arterial phase): normal anatomy (c).

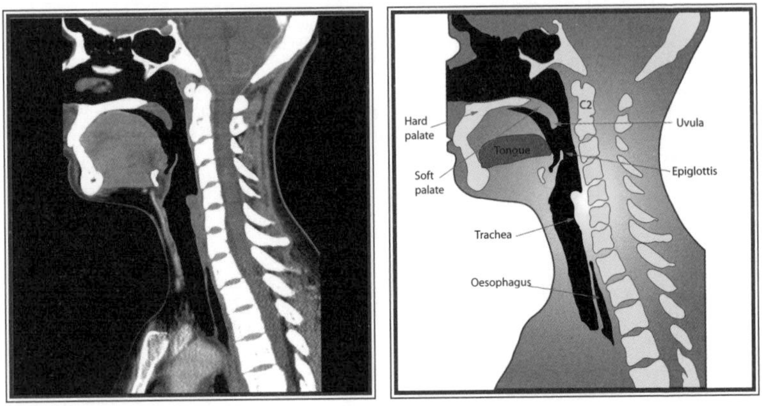

Fig 10.9: Sagittal CT of the neck (arterial phase): normal anatomy.

2. CT of the cervical spine

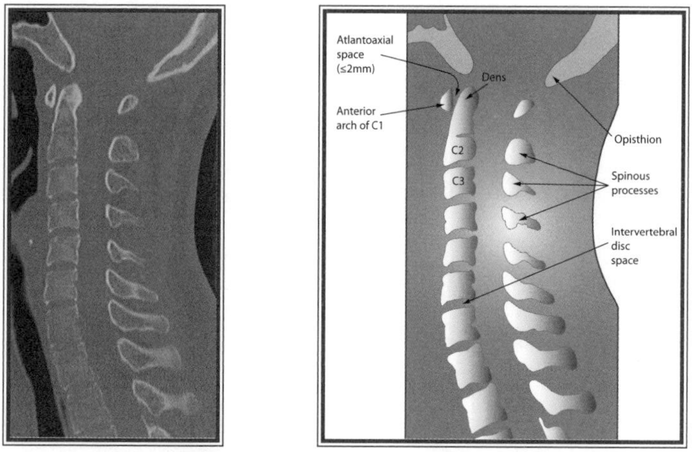

Fig 10.10: Sagittal CT of the cervical spine: normal anatomy.

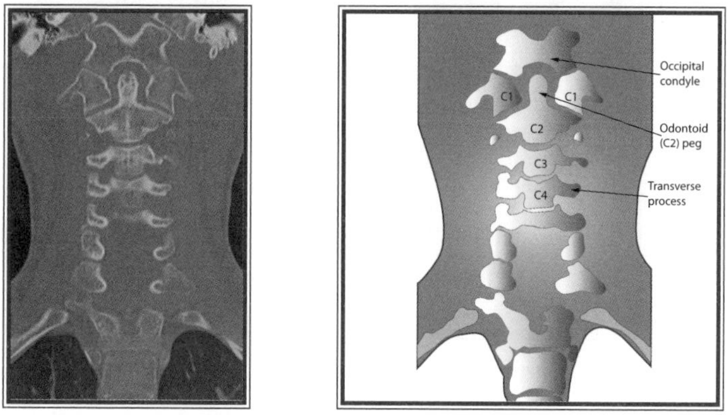

Fig 10.11: Coronal CT of the cervical spine: normal anatomy.

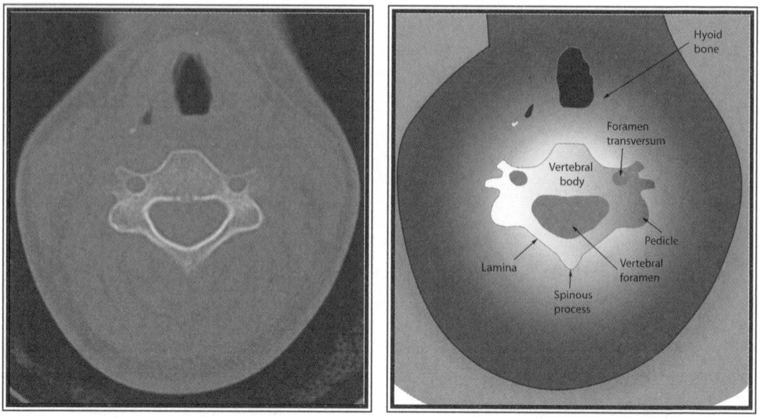

10.12: Axial CT of the cervical spine (bone window): normal anatomy.

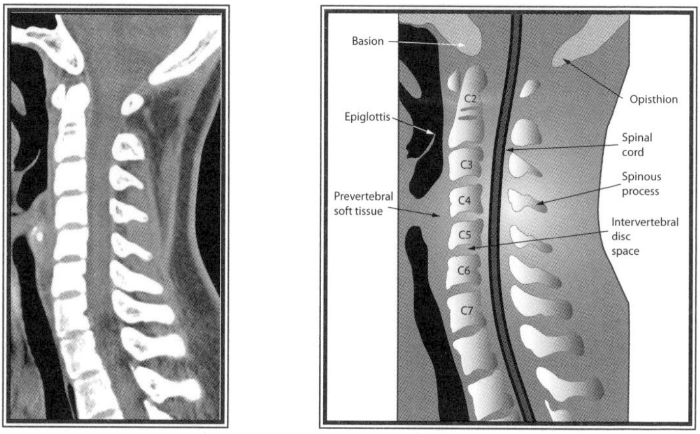

10.13: Sagittal CT of the cervical spine (soft tissue window): normal anatomy.

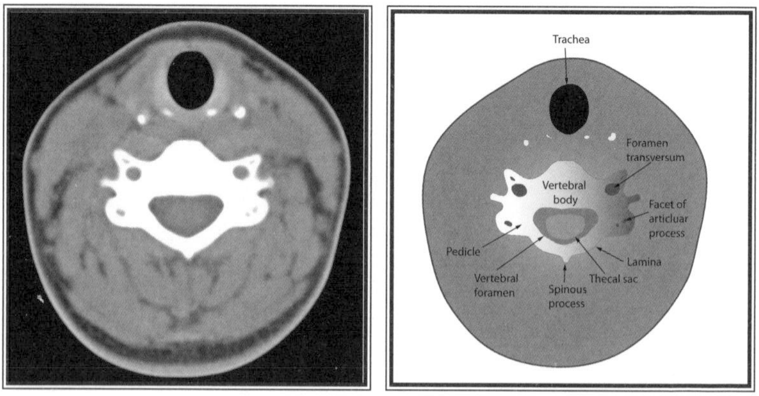

10.14: Axial CT of the cervical spine (soft tissue window): normal anatomy.

3. CT of the chest

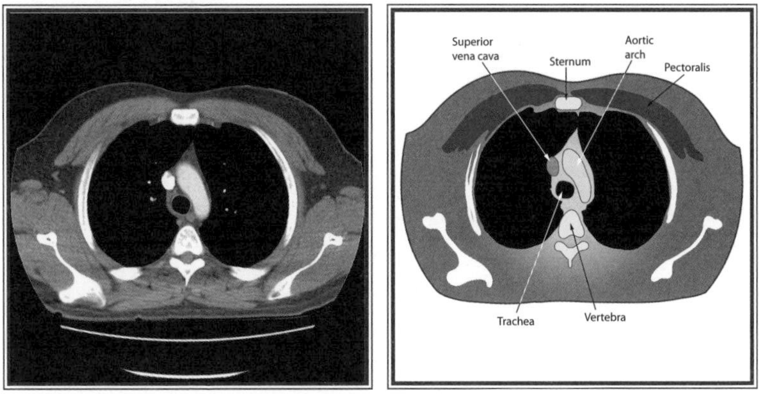

Fig 10.15: Axial CT of the chest (arterial phase): normal anatomy (a).

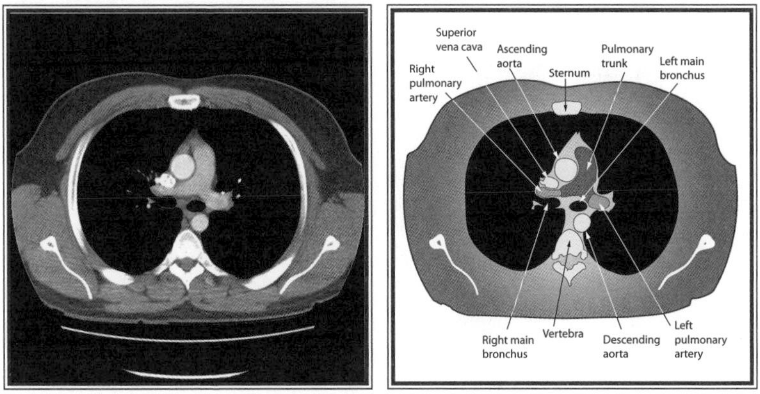

Fig 10.16: Axial CT of the chest (arterial phase): normal anatomy (b).

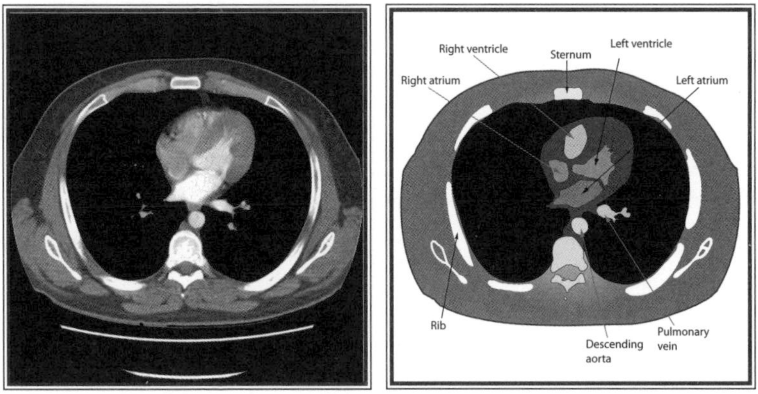

Fig 10.17: Axial CT of the chest (arterial phase): normal anatomy (c).

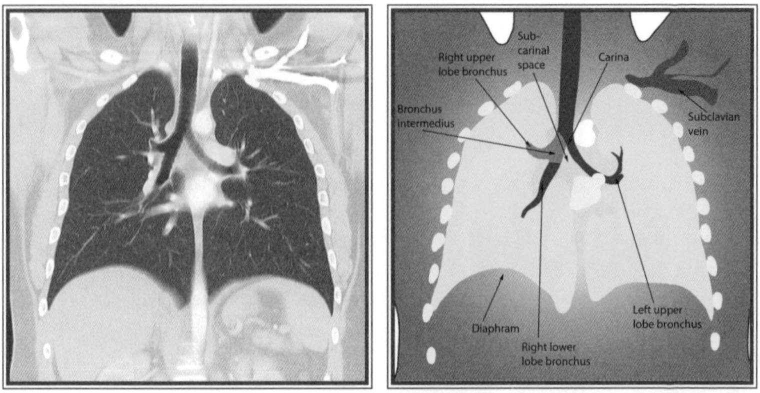

Fig 10.18: Coronal CT of the chest (lung windows): normal anatomy.

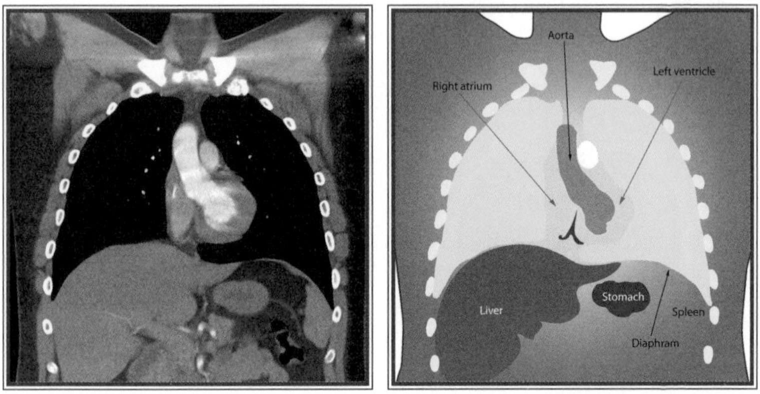

Fig 10.19: Coronal CT of the chest (mediastinal windows): normal anatomy.

4. CT of the abdomen

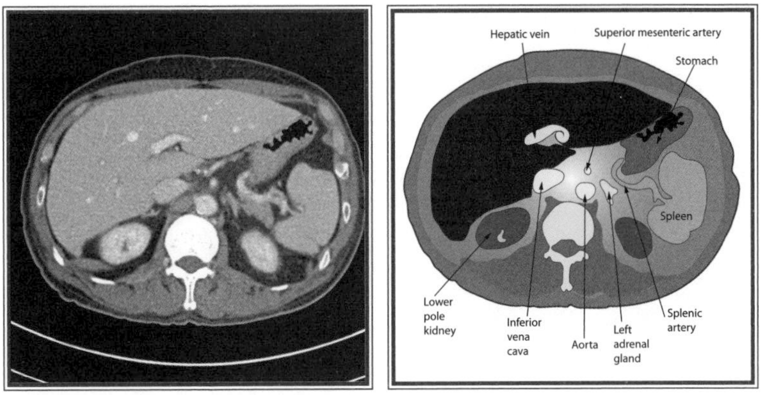

Fig 10.20: Axial CT of the abdomen (portal venous phase): normal anatomy (a).

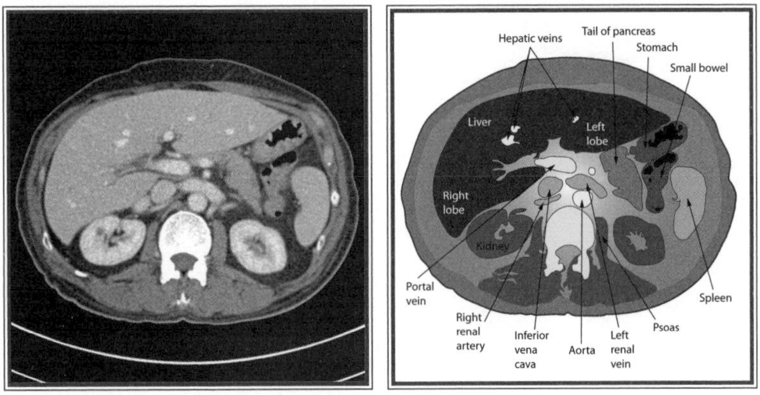

Fig 10.21: Axial CT of the abdomen (portal venous phase): normal anatomy (b).

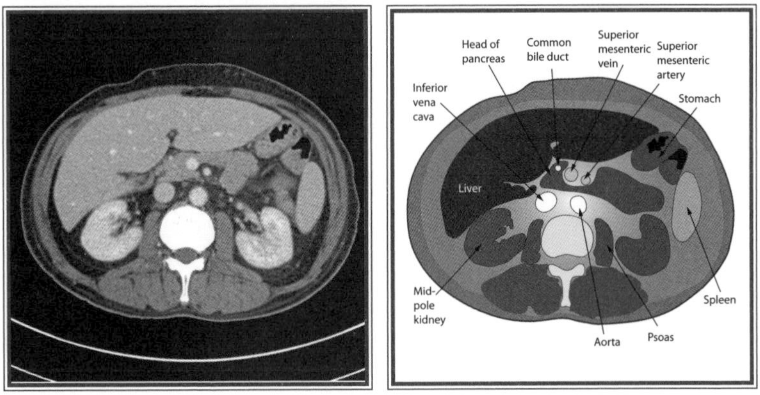

Fig 10.22: Axial CT of the abdomen (portal venous phase): normal anatomy (c).

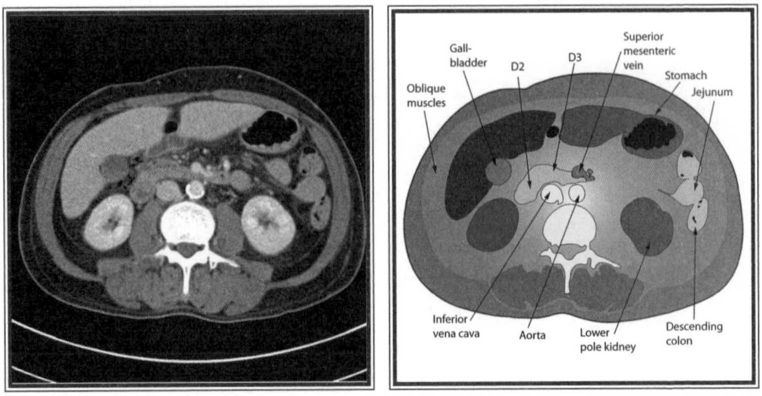

Fig 10.23: Axial CT of the abdomen (portal venous phase): normal anatomy (d).

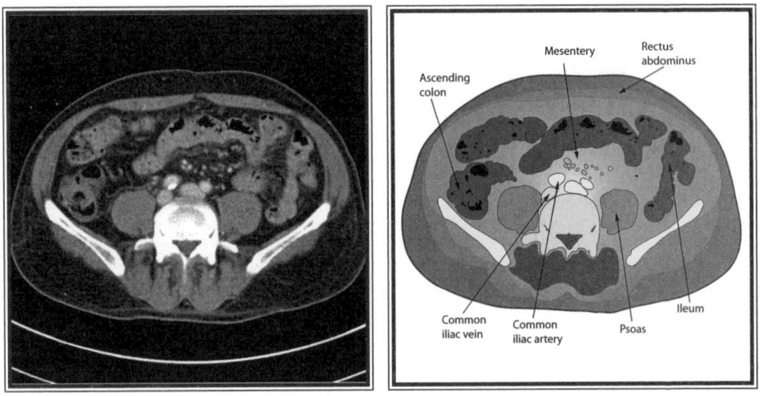

Fig 10.24: Axial CT of the abdomen (portal venous phase): normal anatomy (d).

5. MRI of the brain

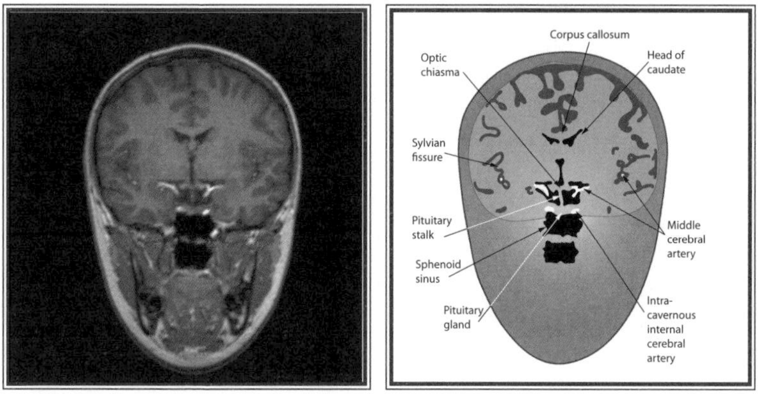

Fig 10.25: Coronal T1 MRI brain: normal anatomy.

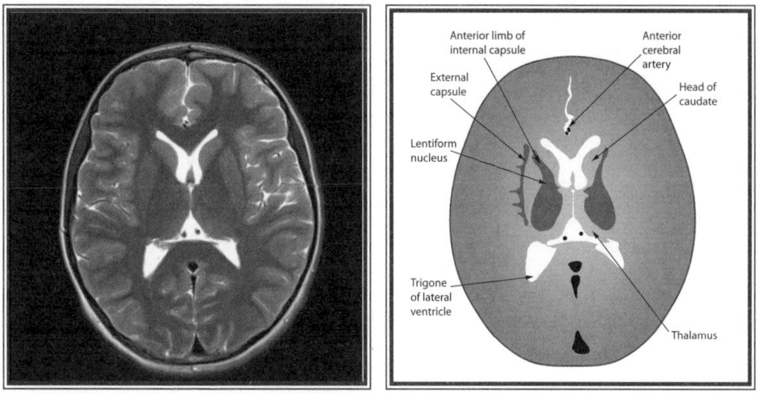

Fig 10.26: Axial T2 MRI brain: normal anatomy (a).

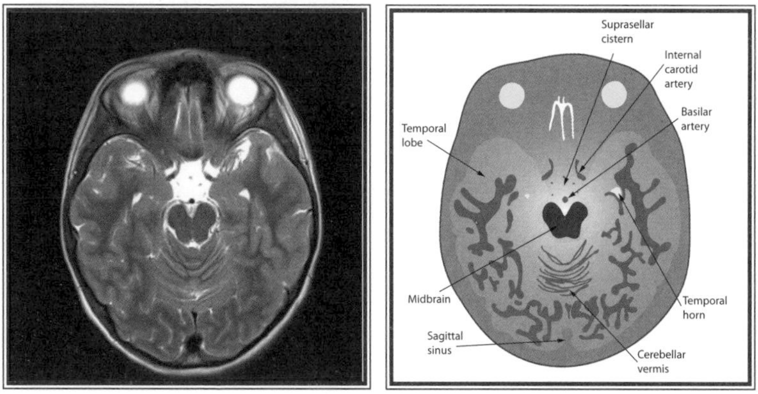

Fig 10.27: Axial T2 MRI brain: normal anatomy (b).

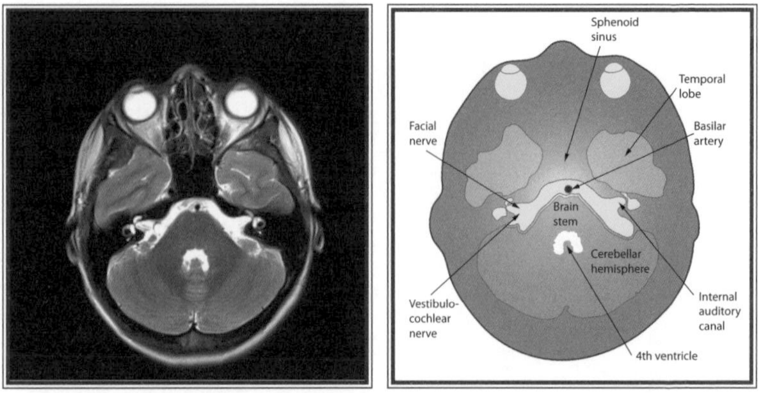

Fig 10.28: Axial T2 MRI brain: normal anatomy (c).

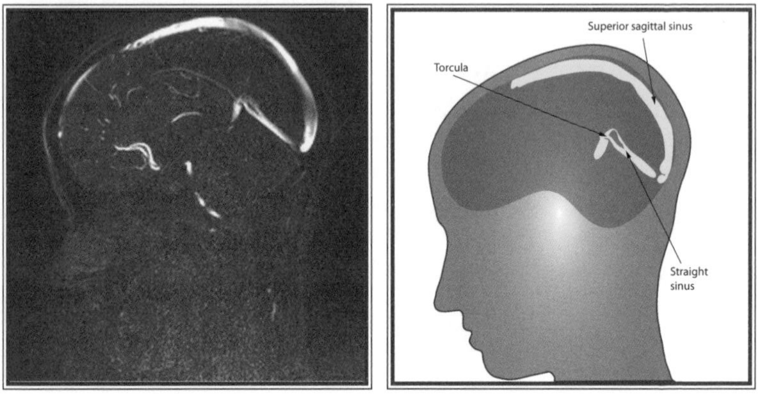

Fig 10.29: Sagittal MR venogram: normal anatomy.

6. MRI of the lumbar spine

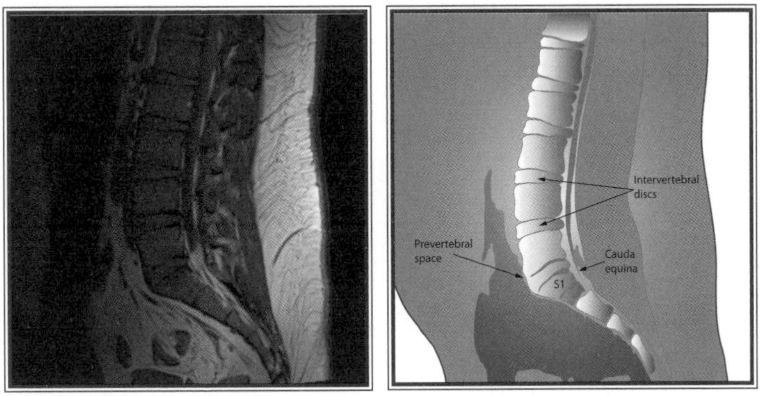

Fig 10.30: Sagittal T1 MRI lumbar spine: normal anatomy (a).

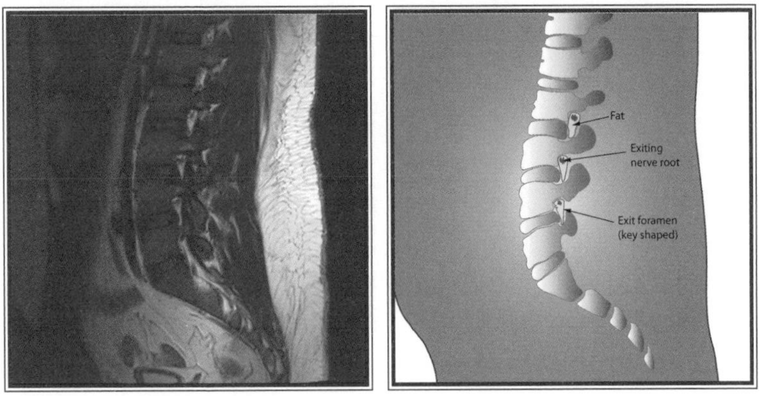

Fig 10.31: Sagittal T1 MRI lumbar spine: normal anatomy (b).

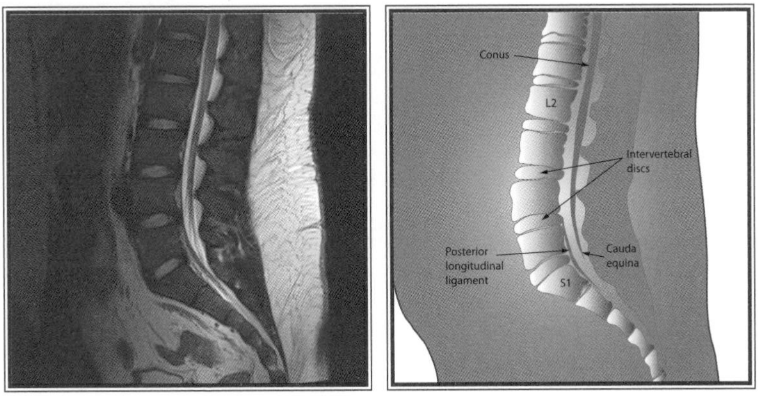

Fig 10.32: Sagittal T2 MRI lumbar spine: normal anatomy.

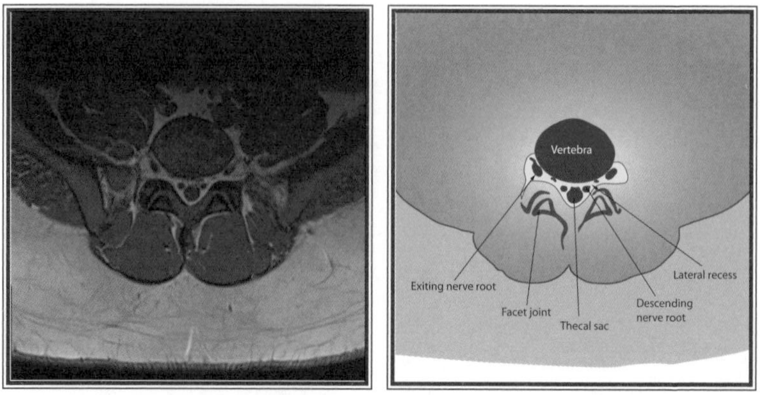

Fig 10.33: Axial T1 MRI lumbar spine: normal anatomy.

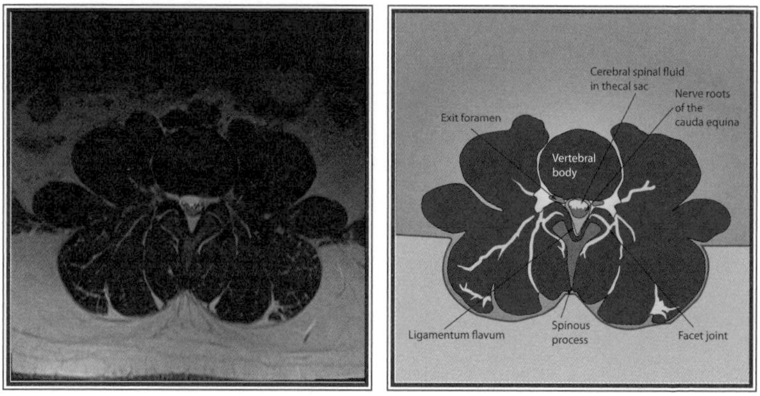

Fig 10.34: Axial T2 MRI lumbar spine: normal anatomy.

CROSS-SECTIONAL IMAGING – WHAT YOU NEED TO KNOW

- Ensure that the indication for your request is valid with a clinical question
- Be aware of the significant radiation doses involved with CT investigations
- Safety is the paramount concern with MRI requests given the dangers of the magnetic field
- Provide the clinical information and clinical query and the radiologists will do the most appropriate test (including whether contrast is required)
- Windowing enables most CT to be viewed in various ways to assess different structures from a single acquisition
- MRI requires multiple and variable numbers of sequences to enable complete interpretation
- Adequate renal function is a precursor to contrast administration in both CT and MRI
- Have a structure to approach cross-sectional imaging review just as with plain radiographs.

2 INTERPRETING MEDICAL IMAGING: CASES

These cases all share one theme, something that one should consider with all out-of-hours imaging requests:

> 'Will this study influence immediate patient management and clinical outcome?'

Case 2.1

This 23-year-old university student presents to A&E acutely short of breath.

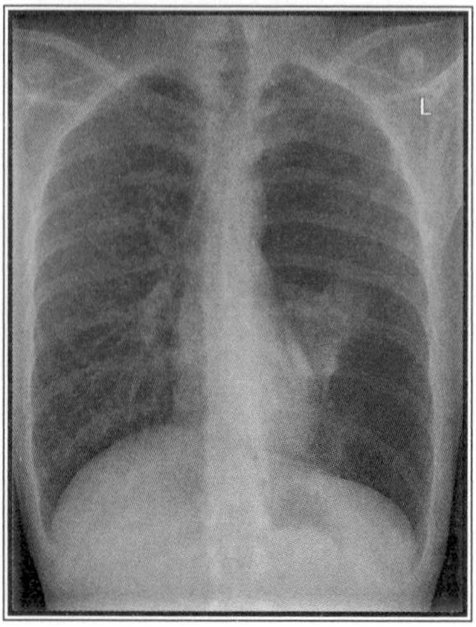

1. Describe the findings on the CXR.
2. List five conditions that predispose to this condition.

→ **answer on page 270**

Case 2.2

This 46-year-old retired hairdresser has become increasingly short of breath over the past 6 months. She complains of a dry cough. Pulmonary function tests and CXR were requested.

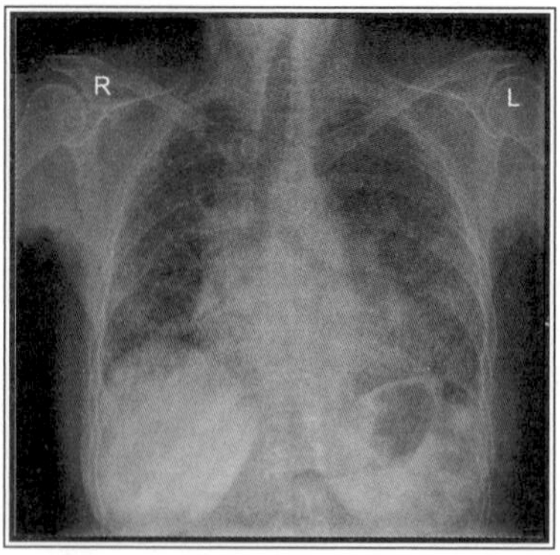

1. How would you describe the lungs on this CXR?
2. What are the possible causes for these findings?
3. What are her pulmonary function tests likely to demonstrate?

→ **answer on page 270**

Case 2.3

This 55-year-old man attended his local hospital feeling increasingly short of breath over the past week. He has lost 6 kg in weight recently. He is a smoker of 60 pack-years. His CXR is shown.

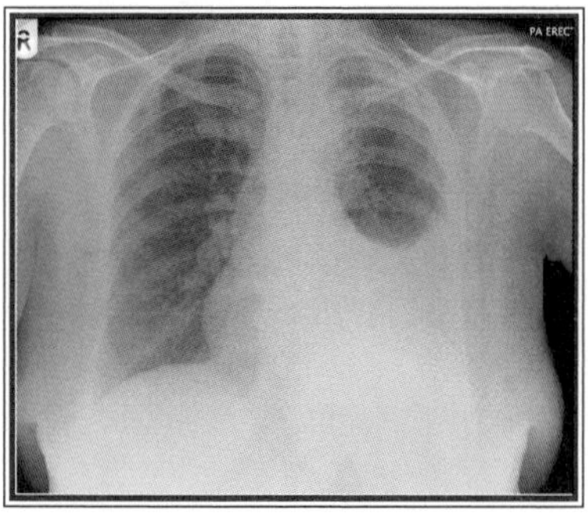

1. Describe the appearances on the CXR.
2. List the causes of this finding, and state the most likely cause in this patient.
3. What other simple test may assist in forming a diagnosis?

➥ **answer on page 271**

Case 2.4

This 45-year-old smoker of 30 pack-years attends his GP with increasing shortness of breath over the past 2 weeks.

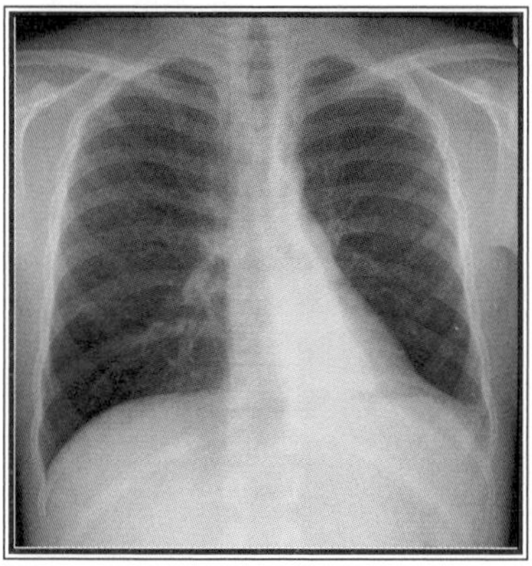

1. Describe the abnormality on this CXR.
2. What is your concern regarding these appearances and what would you recommend?

➥ **answer on page 272**

Case 2.5

This 21-year-old patient, well known to the local hospital, attends A&E with acute-on-chronic shortness of breath.

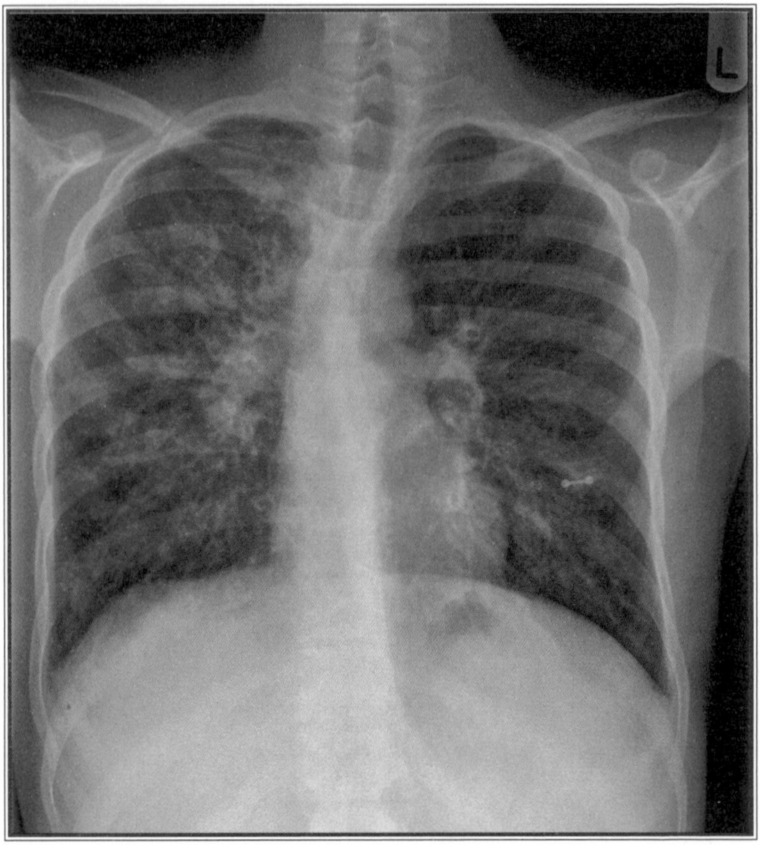

1. Describe the appearances on this CXR.
2. Give a short summary of the underlying condition.

➥ **answer on page 273**

Case 2.6

This 62-year-old patient presented to A&E with chest pain and shortness of breath.

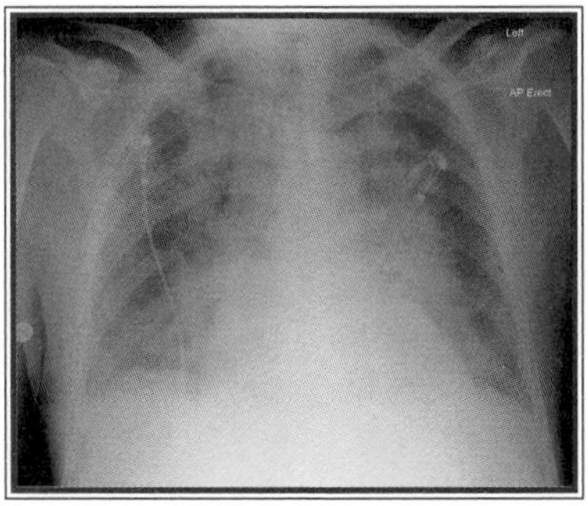

1. Describe the appearance on this CXR.
2. What conditions may cause these appearances with a normal-sized heart?

➥ **answer on page 273**

Case 2.7

This 34-year-old woman attends A&E with chest pain. She is known to the departmental staff from previous admissions.

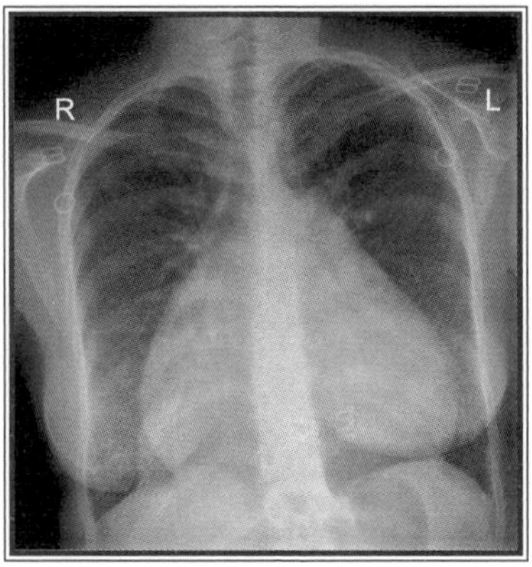

1. Describe the appearances on this CXR, especially the cardiac outline.
2. What else might you consider doing to establish the exact cause of these appearances?

➥ **answer on page 274**

Case 2.8

This 52-year-old man attends his GP complaining of non-intentional weight loss of 8 kg.

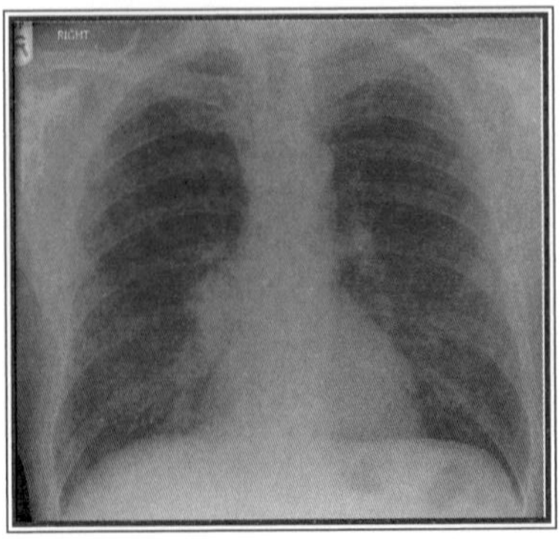

1. Describe the appearances on the CXR.
2. Provide a short differential diagnosis.

→ **answer on page 275**

Case 2.9

A 32-year-old man attends A&E complaining of shortness of breath and the development of a rash on his shins.

A CXR was requested.

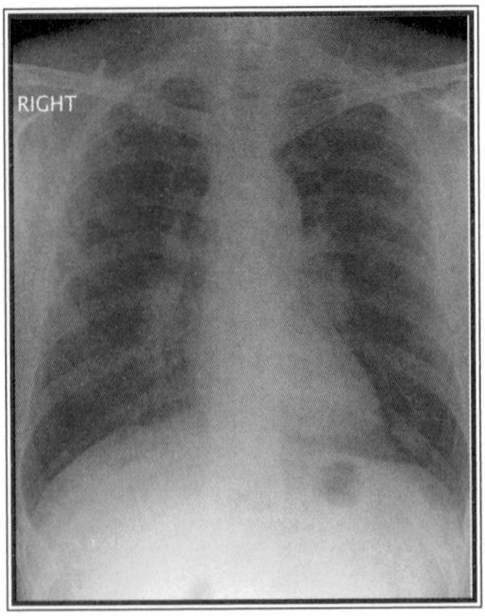

1. Outline any abnormal findings seen on this film.
2. Give a differential diagnosis for this appearance.

→ **answer on page 275**

Case 2.10

This 61-year-old woman complains of non-specific symptoms, including malaise and anorexia.

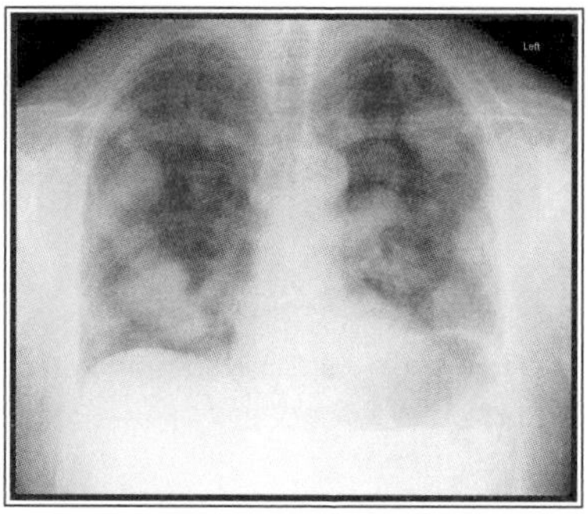

1. Succinctly describe the appearances on this film and the likely diagnosis.
2. Which primary tumour types are most likely to result in these appearances?

→ **answer on page 276**

Case 2.11

This 39-year-old woman attends A&E with a high fever, following a recent holiday overseas.

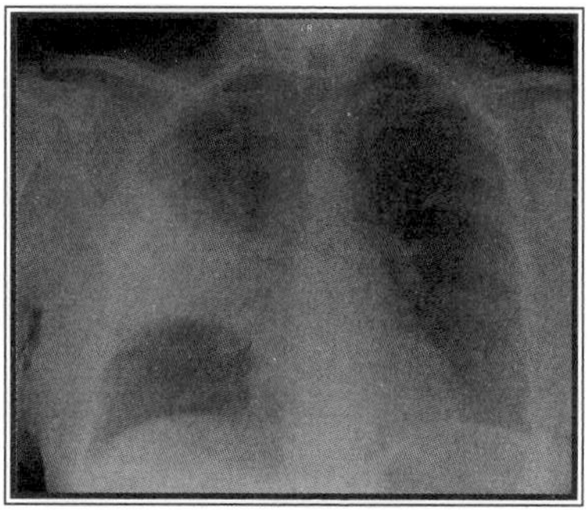

1. Describe the appearances on the CXR.
2. What follow-up imaging is necessary? How long after treatment should this be performed and why is it performed?

→ **answer on page 277**

Case 2.12

This 55-year-old retiree has a CXR as part of a medical insurance assessment.

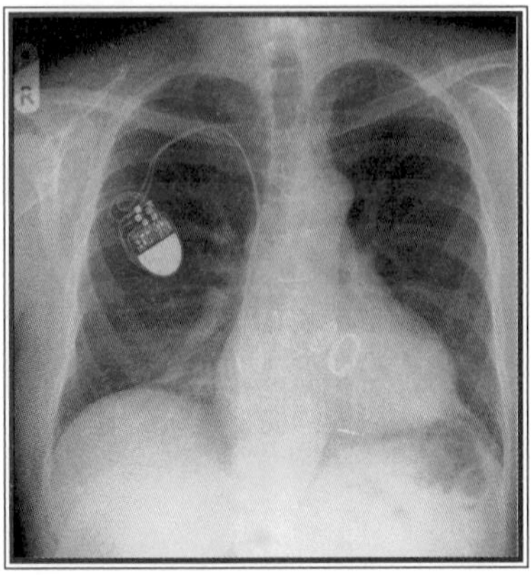

1. Report the CXR including what previous surgery has been performed.
2. List five indications for the surgery performed.

➥ **answer on page 277**

Case 2.13

This 57-year-old woman is attending a follow-up clinic after previous surgery.

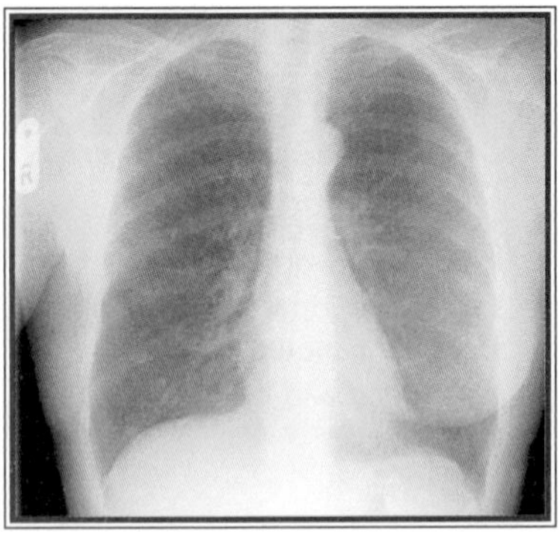

1. Describe the appearances on the CXR.
2. Name the other review areas when examining a CXR.

➥ **answer on page 278**

Case 2.14

This 63-year-old man attends A&E complaining of a short history of abdominal distension.

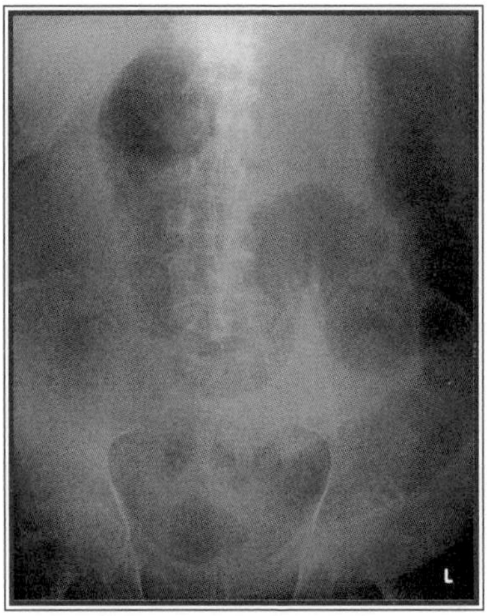

1. Describe the appearance on this AXR.
2. What investigation should be performed next and how will it be useful?

→ **answer on page 279**

Case 2.15

A 55-year-old man was admitted with acute abdominal pain and a CXR was performed.

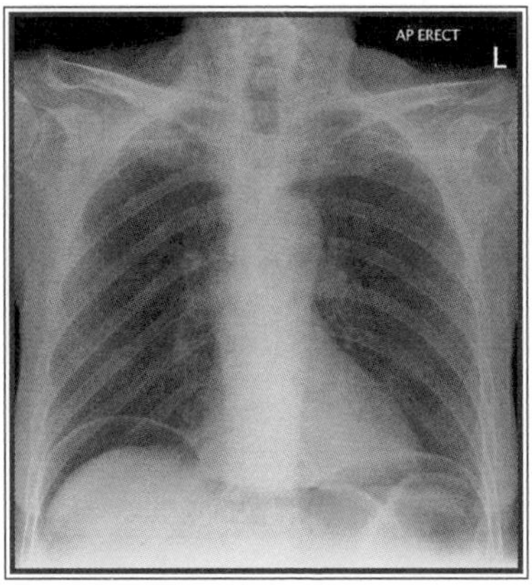

1. What abnormality is seen on this film?
2. What projection has been used?
3. List some causes of this finding.

→ **answer on page 279**

Case 2.16

This 69-year-old woman was admitted to the surgical ward with malodorous vomiting and a distended abdomen. An AXR was taken while she was in A&E.

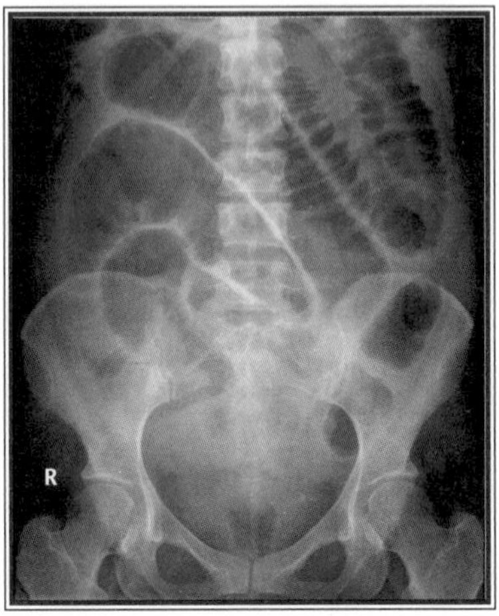

1. Describe the findings on the AXR.
2. What are the causes of this abnormality?

➥ **answer on page 280**

Case 2.17

This 77-year-old nursing home resident is brought to hospital because her carers are concerned about an enlarged abdomen over the last 24 hours.

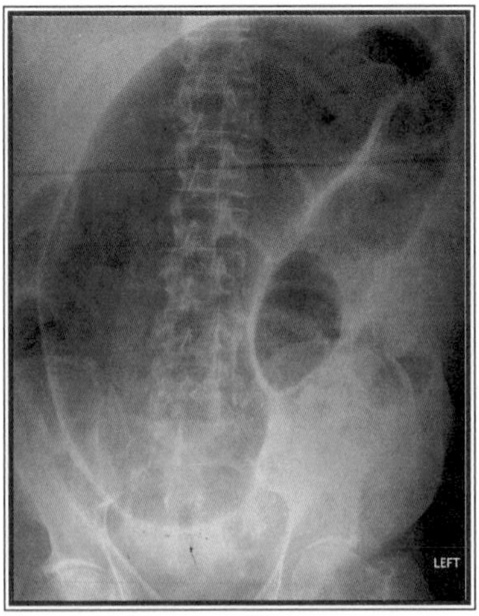

1. Describe the appearances on the AXR.
2. What are the treatment options for this condition?

➥ **answer on page 280**

Case 2.18

This 35-year-old man is a regular attendee at the hospital with severe upper abdominal pain.

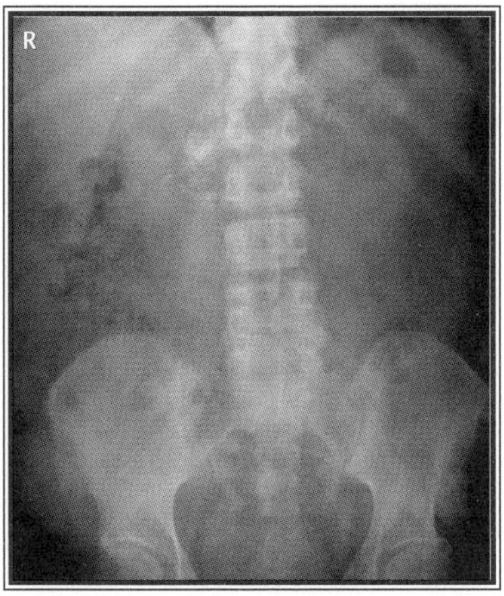

1. Give a brief report of your findings on this AXR.
2. List the potential complications after acute pancreatitis.

➥ **answer on page 281**

Case 2.19

This 75-year-old man complains of an ongoing aching pain in the centre of his abdomen.

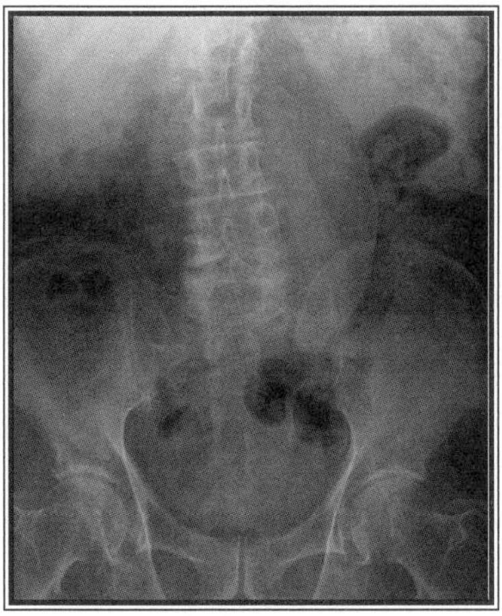

1. Describe the findings on this AXR.
2. What additional imaging investigation is recommended?

➥ **answer on page 282**

Case 2.20

This 43-year-old man complains of left-sided flank pain.

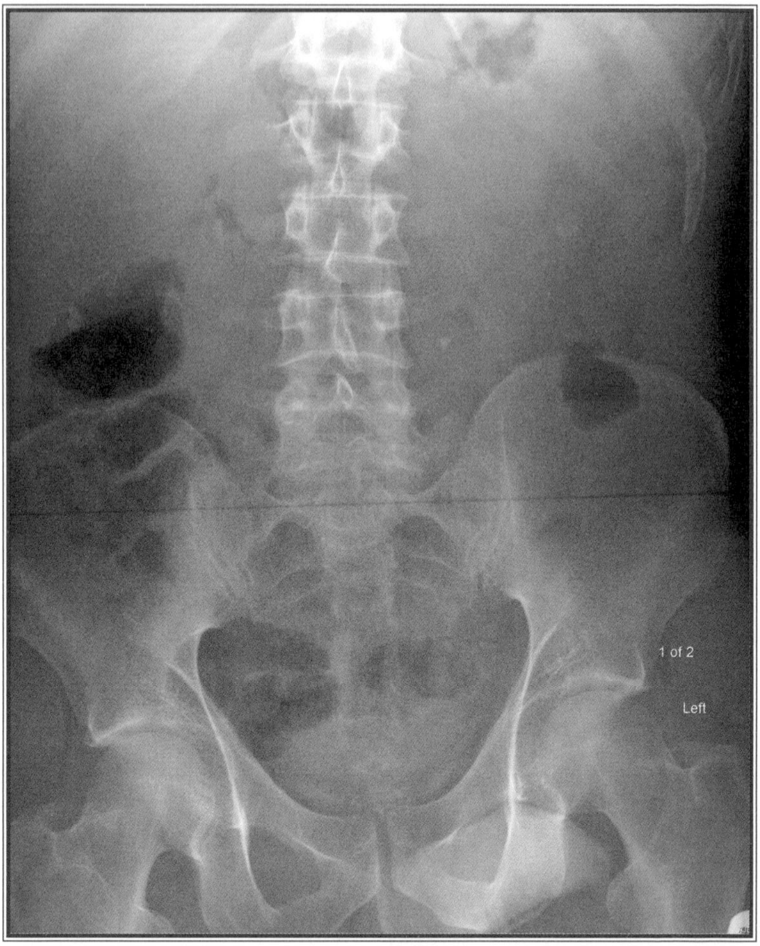

1. Describe any abnormalities present on this AXR.
2. Which imaging modality is best for imaging this pathology?

➥ **answer on page 282**

Case 2.21

This 37-year-old woman complains of lower abdominal pain and early bladder fullness.

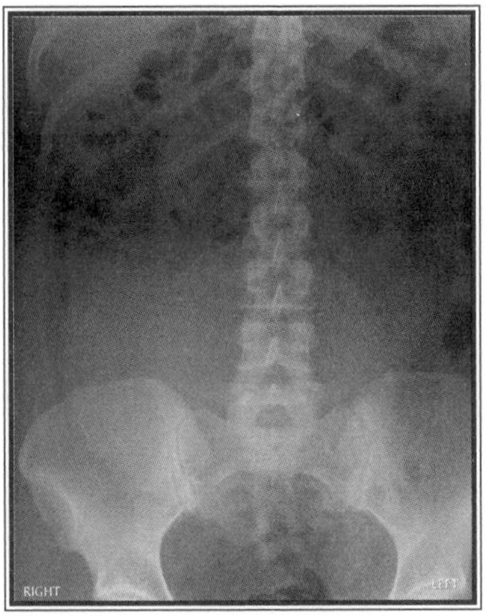

1. Describe the abnormality present on the AXR.
2. Give a differential diagnosis and suggest an additional imaging technique to assess further.

➥ **answer on page 283**

Case 2.22

This 37-year-old woman attended A&E complaining of a severe sudden headache.

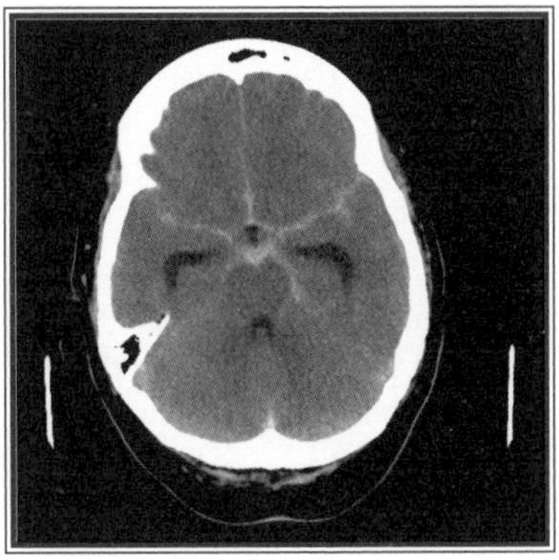

1. Describe the appearances on the CT head.
2. What other imaging investigation(s) would be helpful in the patient's management plan?

➥ **answer on page 283**

Case 2.23

This 39-year-old man was brought to A&E by his wife, because he had developed a progressively worsening headache over the past 2 weeks. This was particularly severe first thing in the morning.

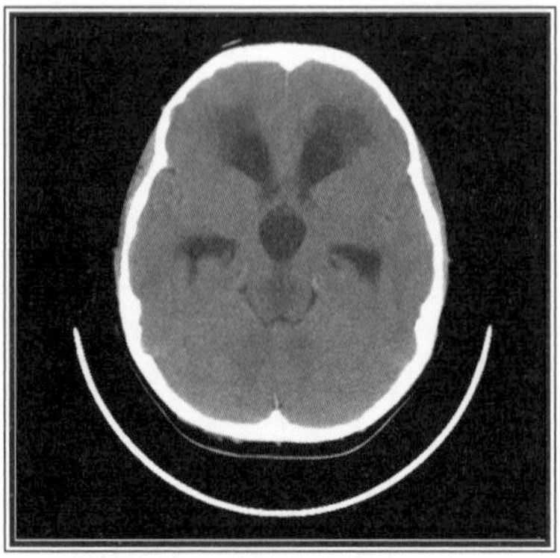

1. Describe the appearances seen.
2. List potential causes for these appearances.

➥ **answer on page 284**

Case 2.24

This 55-year-old woman was brought to A&E by her relatives who state that she has been confused over the past 24 hours. She had a mastectomy for breast cancer 2 years ago.

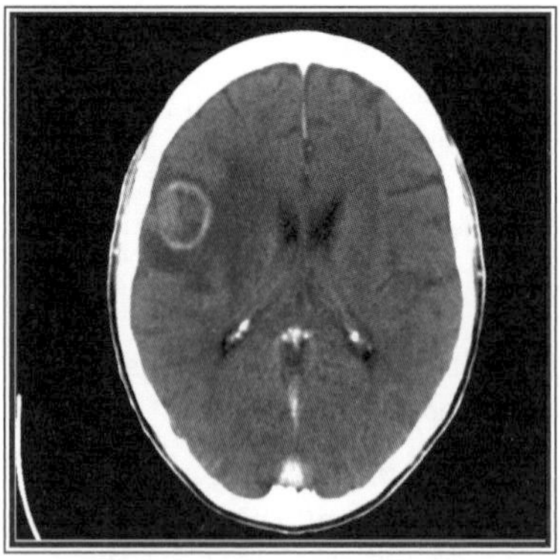

1. Describe the appearances on the CT head.
2. If this had been the patient's first presentation, what would the potential differential diagnosis have been?

➥ **answer on page 284**

Case 2.25

This 24-year-old intravenous drug user is accompanied to A&E by his friend who states that he has been confused over the last 3 days and has a fever.

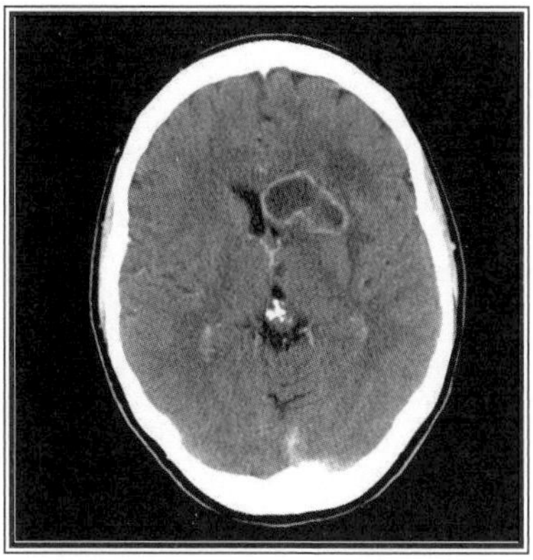

1. Describe the appearances seen.
2. Name some other complications that commonly occur in those using intravenous drugs.

➥ **answer on page 285**

Case 2.26

This 18 year old was involved in a skiing accident 2 hours previously. His GCS on arrival at A&E is 9/15.

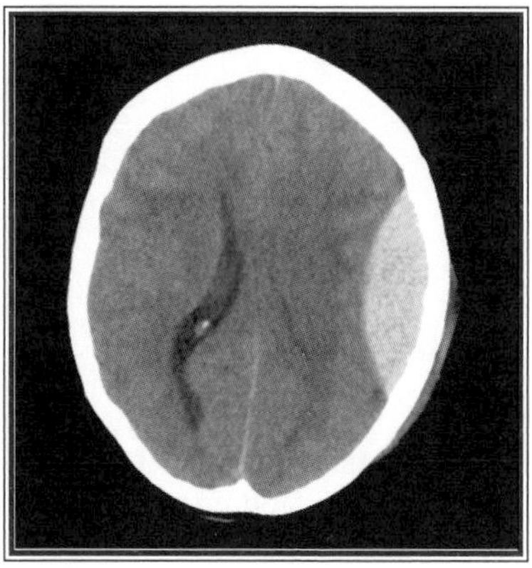

1. Describe the appearances seen.
2. What is normally associated with this finding on CT and which vessel is typically damaged?

➥ **answer on page 286**

Case 2.27

This 77-year-old widow is found at home by her neighbour. On arrival at A&E her GCS is 12/15.

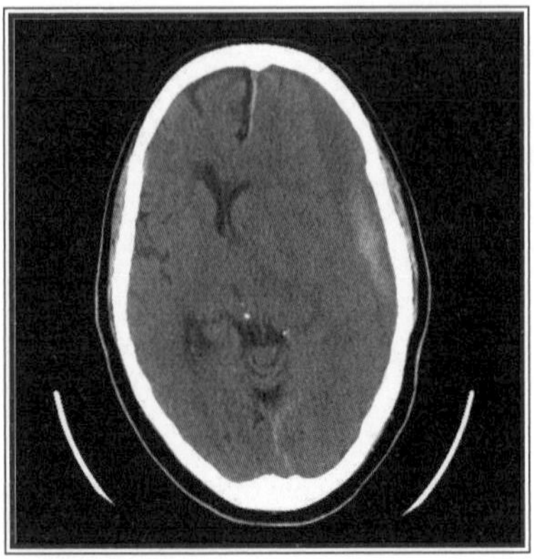

1. Describe the appearances seen.
2. There is no history of severe head trauma. How might this haematoma have arisen?

➥ **answer on page 286**

Case 2.28

This 66-year-old man gives a 3-hour history of right-sided weakness. Examination confirms a right hemiparesis.

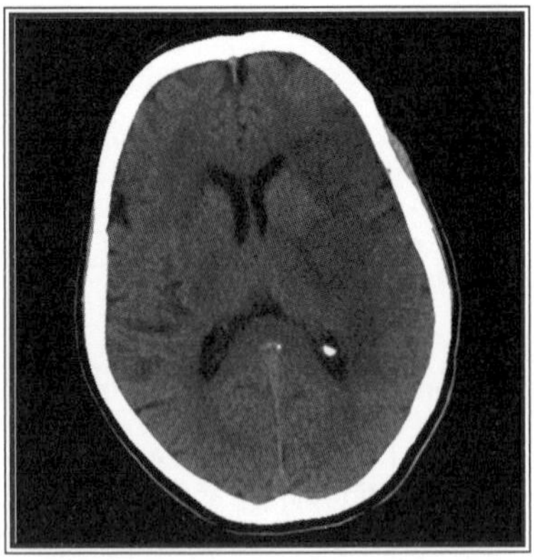

1. Describe the appearances seen.
2. Explain the concept of 'time is brain' in the modern management of this disease process.

➥ **answer on page 287**

Case 2.29

This 62-year-old man developed a left-sided visual deficit 3 months previously. On this occasion CT was performed after head trauma.

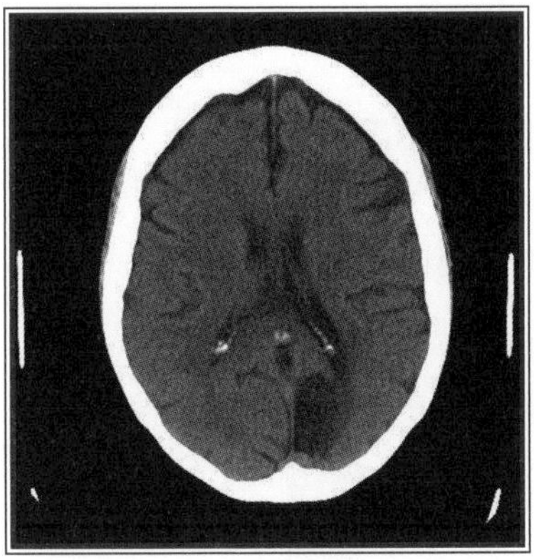

1. Describe the appearances seen.
2. List a few factors that predispose this condition.

→ answer on page 287

Case 2.30

This middle-aged woman was brought to the hospital by her son after being found slumped in a chair at home and with speech difficulties.

CT head was performed on admission. MRI of the head was performed later during routine working hours.

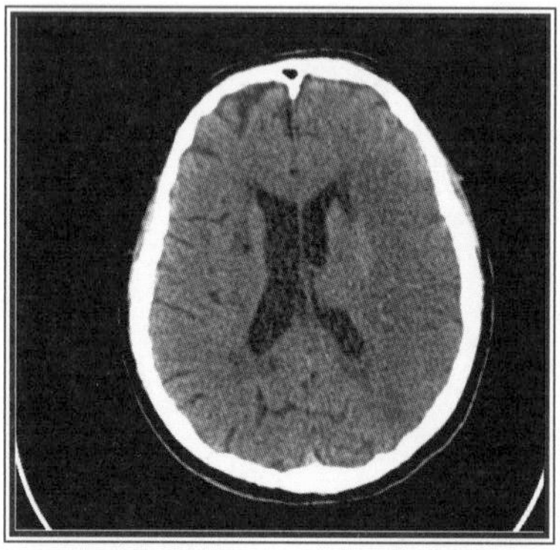

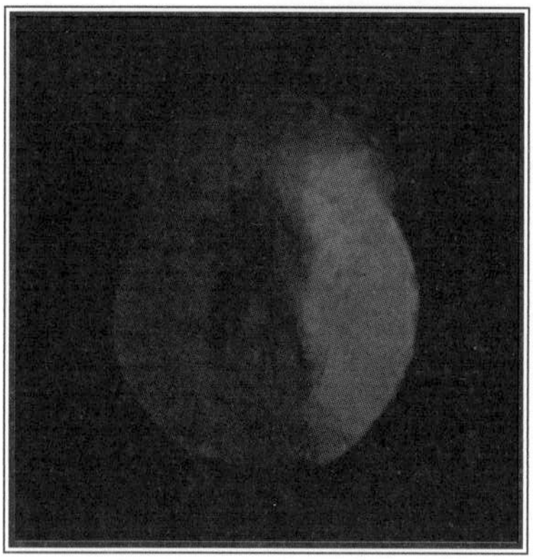

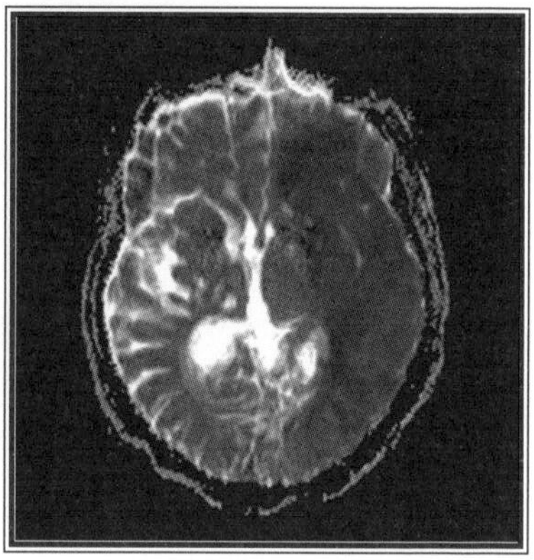

What do these investigations show?

➥ answer on page 288

Case 2.31

A previously well 60-year-old woman was admitted with a 3-day history of fever and altered mental status. Her relatives were concerned about her mental status. There had been no recent prior travel or medical history.

The admission CT was abnormal and it was recommended that an MRI of the brain be performed.

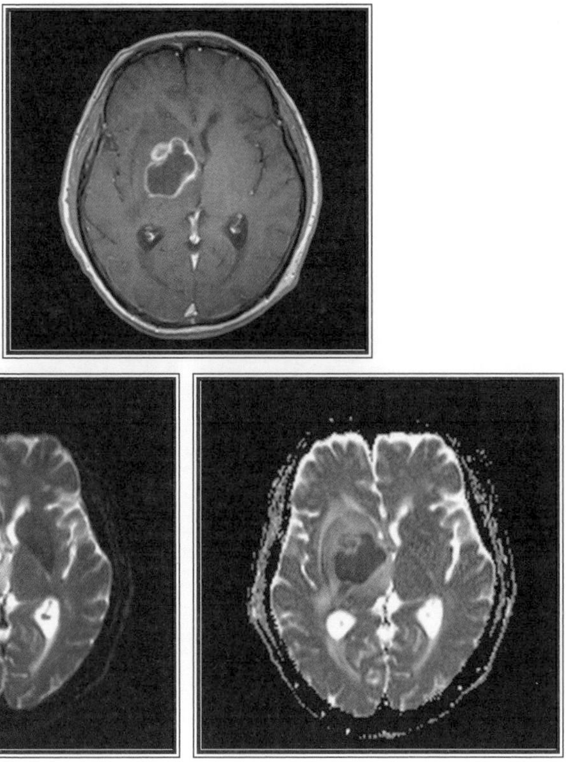

What does this show?

→ **answer on page 289**

Case 2.32 +

This 53-year-old woman arrives via ambulance after a collapse in a local shopping centre. She complains of chest pain and is clearly short of breath. Her respiratory rate is 40 breaths/min and her BP 90/44 mmHg.

A bedside echocardiogram suggests right heart strain. A CT pulmonary angiogram (CTPA) is performed.

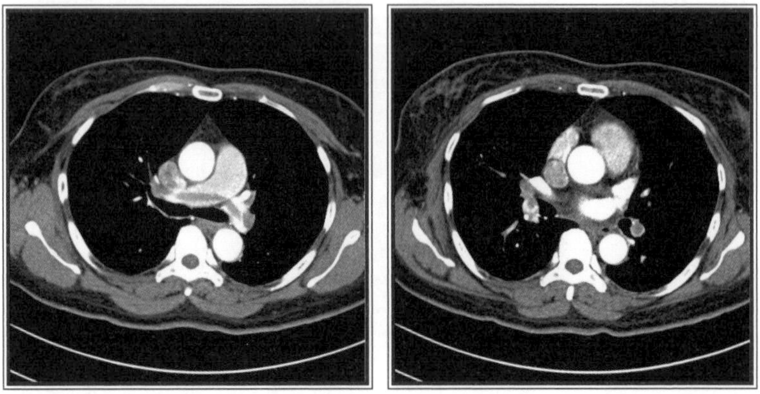

What does this show?

➥ **answer on page 289**

Case 2.33 +

This patient is admitted with severe right flank pain and fever.

A CT-KUB (CT of the kidneys, ureters and bladder) was performed given the clinical concerns about an obstructive uropathy. A nephrostomy was then performed.

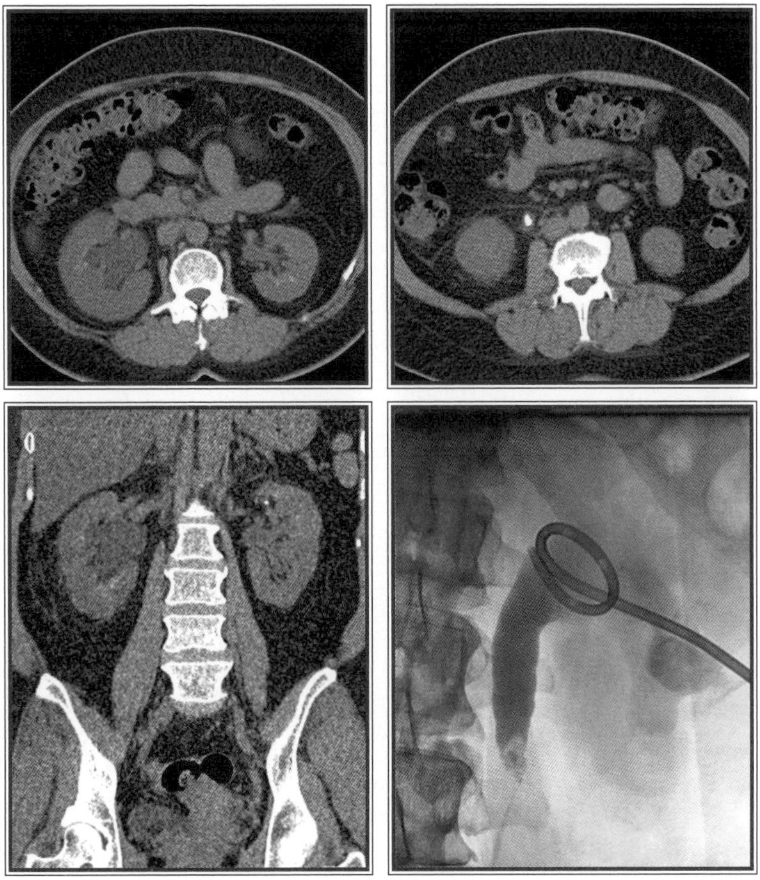

What does this show?

→ **answer on page 290**

Case 2.34

This 70-year-old man is admitted moribund to A&E with a BP of 70/20 mmHg. The patient flinches on palpation of the abdomen.

A CT of the abdomen was requested to identify the cause of his haemodynamic instability.

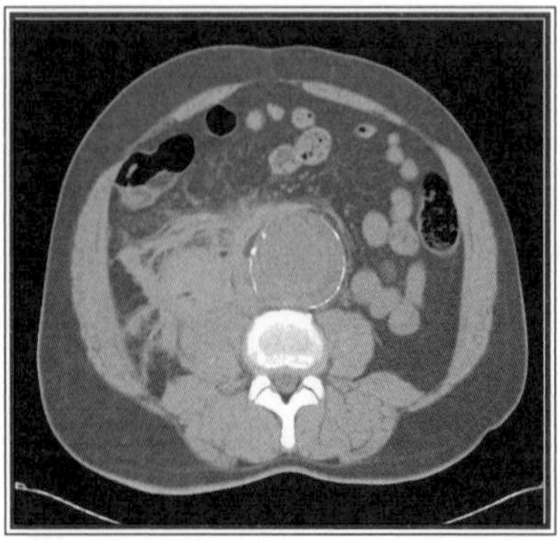

What does this show?

➥ **answer on page 291**

Case 2.35

This 33-year-old construction worker fell from 30 metres. He complains of severe back pain and tingling in both legs.

His bowel and bladder function normally. CT was performed on admission.

MRI of the lumbar spine was undertaken as a matter of urgency.

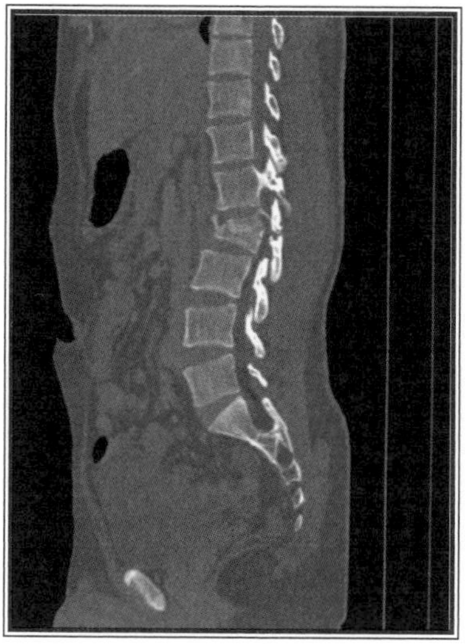

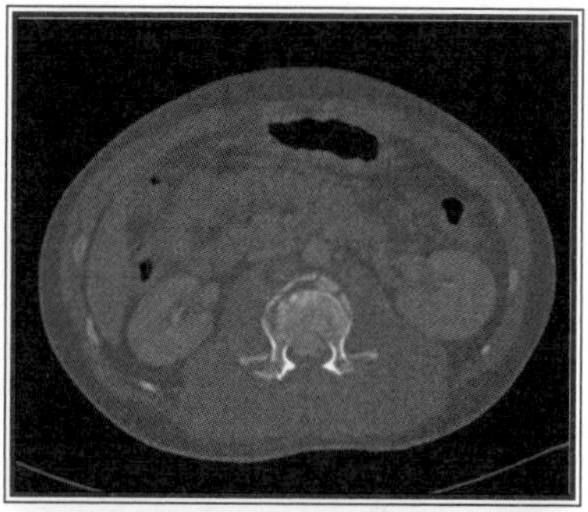

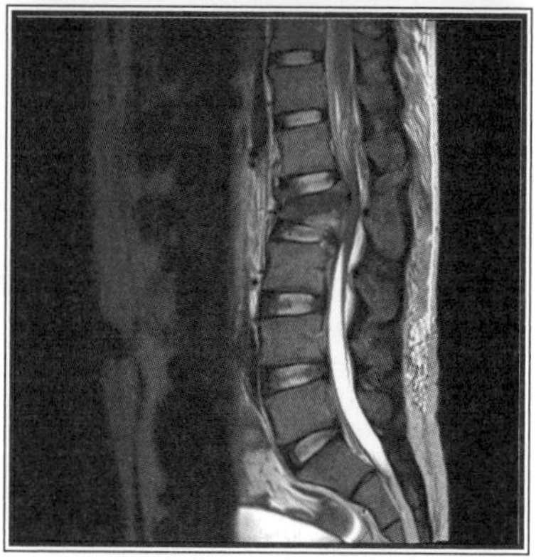

What does this show?

→ **answer on page 291**

Case 2.36 ++

This 80-year-old woman is brought to A&E by her daughter due to a short history of chest pain.

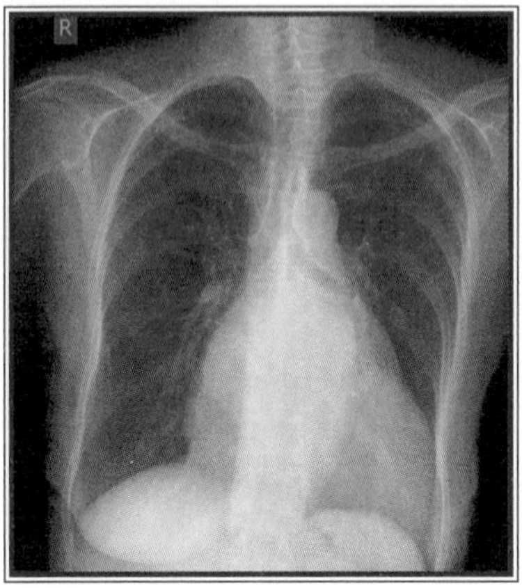

1. Outline the features on the CXR that suggest mitral valve disease.
2. If this patient presented with cardiac failure due to her underlying condition, what signs might be present?

→ **answer on page 292**

Case 2.37 ++

This 67-year-old woman was admitted with shortness of breath and weight loss. A large lung mass was seen on her CXR. Other investigations confirmed that the lesion was a bronchial carcinoma at the left lung apex.

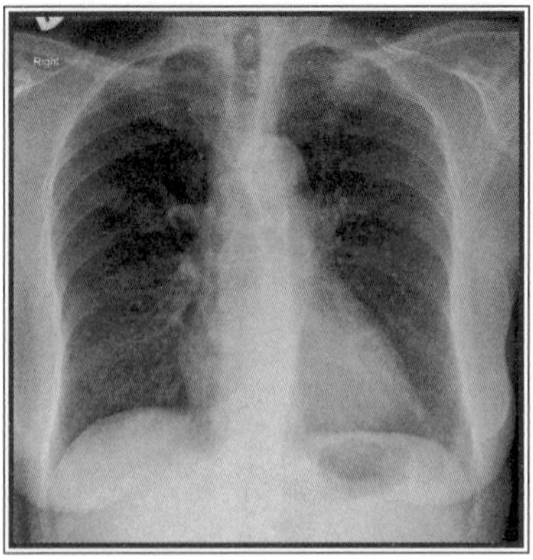

1. What other findings might be seen on a CXR in a patient with bronchial carcinoma?
2. What else could cause the appearance of a mass like this on a CXR?
3. What other imaging investigation would be helpful?

→ **answer on page 292**

Case 2.38 ++

This 34-year-old man is admitted with weight loss, shortness of breath and fever.

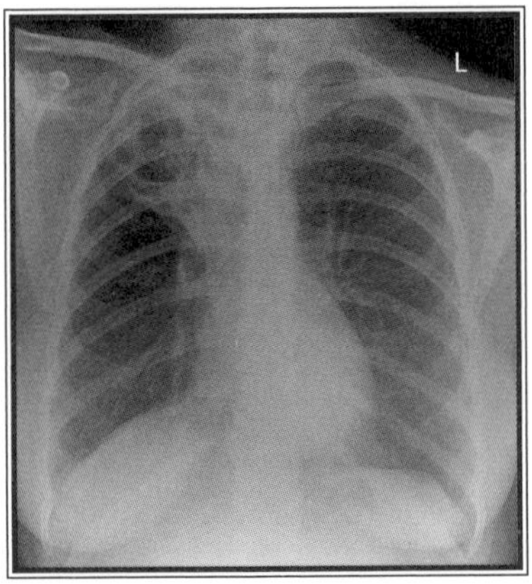

1. Describe the findings on this CXR.
2. What are the potential causes of such an appearance?

➥ **answer on page 293**

Case 2.39 ++

This 67-year-old ex-coalminer presents with a history of weight loss over the past month, now accompanied by shortness of breath.

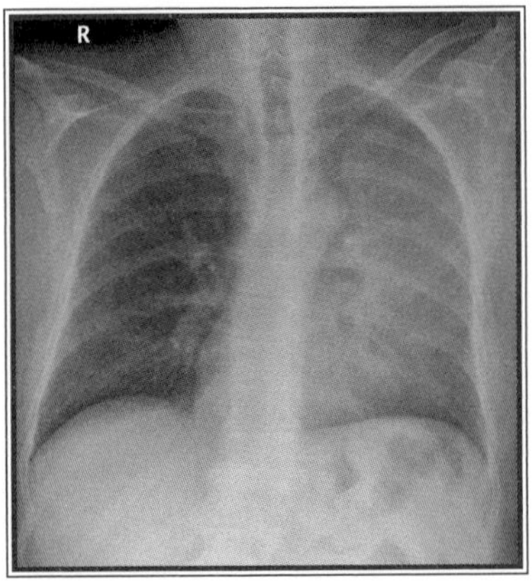

1. Describe the appearances on the CXR.
2. What further investigations are required and why?

➥ **answer on page 294**

Case 2.40 ++

This 30-year-old man presents with fatigue, for which a CXR is among numerous investigations.

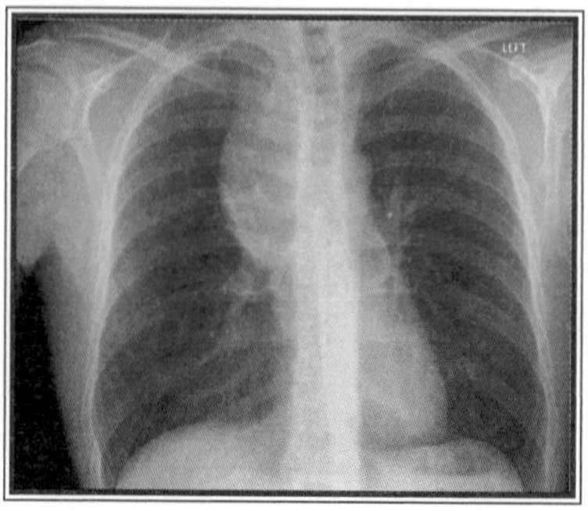

1. Describe the appearances on this CXR.
2. Give a short differential diagnosis and outline how you might establish the exact diagnosis.

➥ **answer on page 294**

Case 2.41 ++

This 38-year-old woman attends A&E with abdominal distension and discomfort lasting the previous 12 hours.

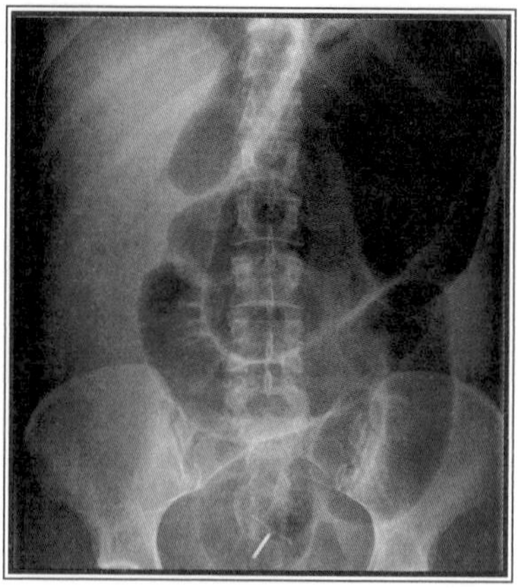

1. Describe the findings on the AXR and provide a diagnosis.
2. Which group of patients typically get this condition?

➥ **answer on page 295**

Case 2.42 ++

This 25-year-old man presented with upper abdominal discomfort. An AXR was performed because the admitting doctor was concerned about bowel obstruction.

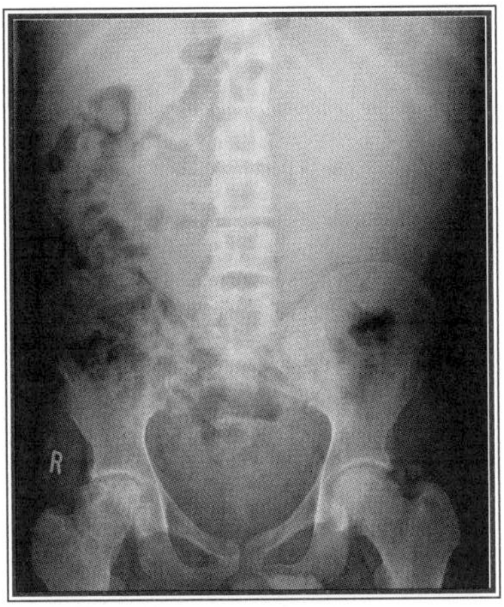

1. Describe the appearances on the abdominal radiograph.
2. List some potential causes, and the most likely cause here.

➥ **answer on page 295**

Case 2.43 ++

This 69-year-old man developed a severe headache while attending a local football match.

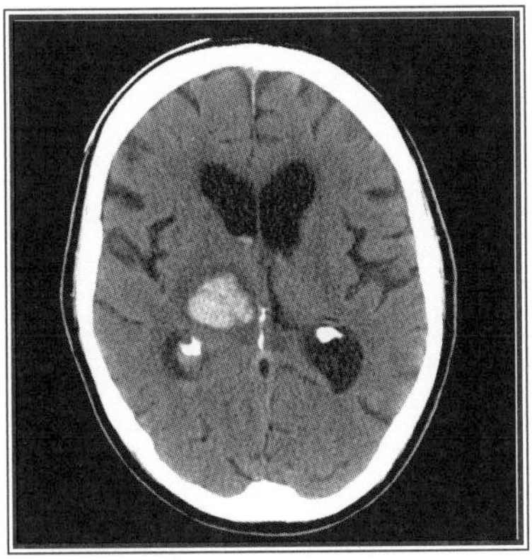

1. Describe the appearances on the CT.
2. What is the most likely cause for these appearances?

➥ **answer on page 296**

Case 2.44 ++

This 35 year old was found on the street late at night. She was intubated at the scene for a GCS of 3/15.

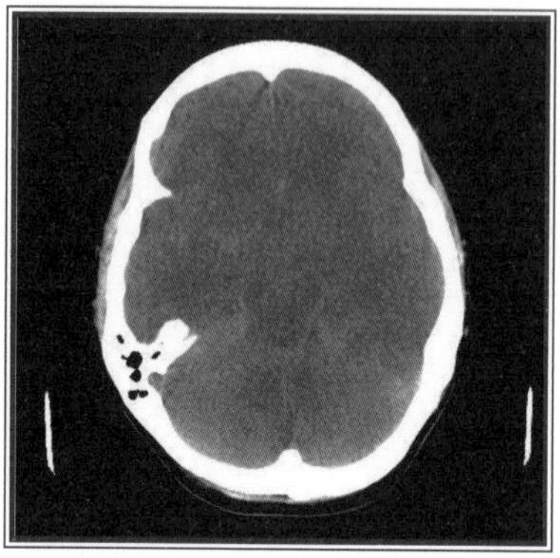

1. Describe the appearances on the image.
2. What is the likely cause?

↪ **answer on page 296**

Case 2.45 ++

This 78-year-old woman has developed progressive right-sided weakness in recent days.

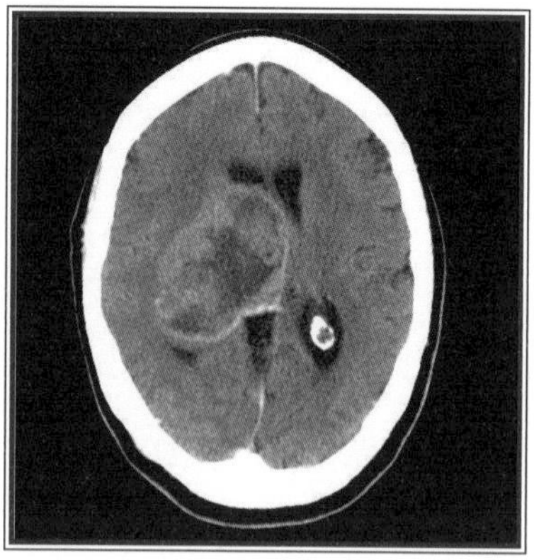

1. Describe the appearances on the image.
2. Name three types of this that occur in the supra- and infratentorial brain.

↪ **answer on page 297**

Case 2.46 ++

This 44-year-old patient with poorly controlled diabetes presents with progressive swallowing difficulties over the last 3 days. She is now pooling saliva in her mouth and her husband says that she is behaving 'out of sorts'.

A CT of the neck was requested after an ENT review. Endoscopy could not be safely performed.

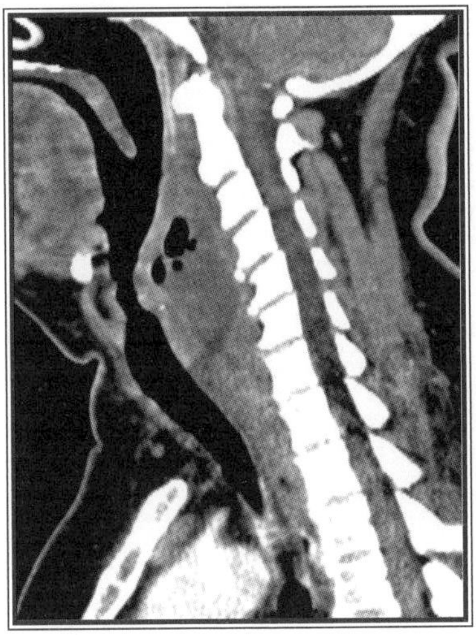

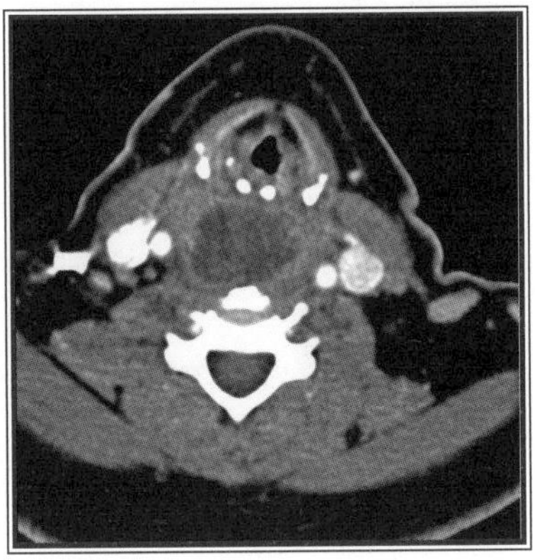

What does this show?

➥ **answer on page 297**

Case 2.47

This 29-year-old postgraduate student is admitted with acute intrascapular pain, which started while at the cinema. There is no history of trauma.

An ECG suggests that this is not cardiac in origin. A CT of the chest is undertaken.

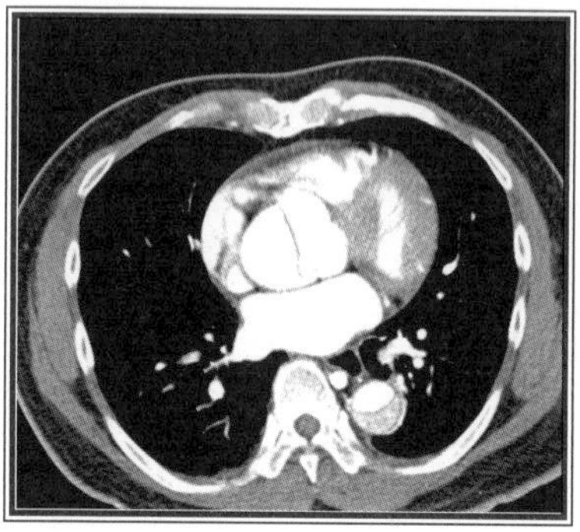

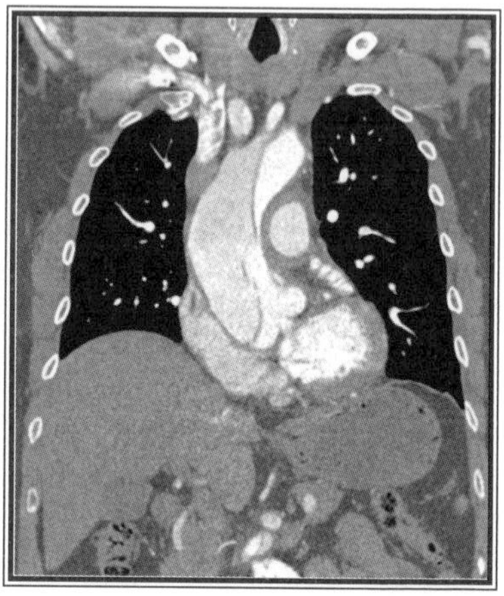

What does this show?

➥ **answer on page 298**

Case 2.48

This 55-year-old patient with long-standing poorly controlled diabetes was admitted with fever and hypotension. On examination the patient was tender to palpation in the right upper quadrant with a two-finger-breadth hepatomegaly.

A CT of the abdomen (portal venous phase) was performed.

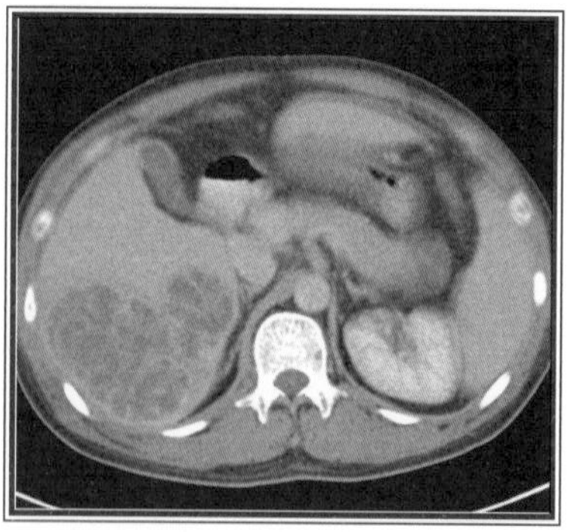

What does this show?

➥ **answer on page 298**

Case 2.49 ++

This 69 year old with no past medical history complains of a progressively distended abdomen over the past 2 days. Over the past 6 hours she has vomited repeatedly. On examination the abdomen is distended, but not peritonitic. The patient is apyrexic. A CT of the abdomen is performed.

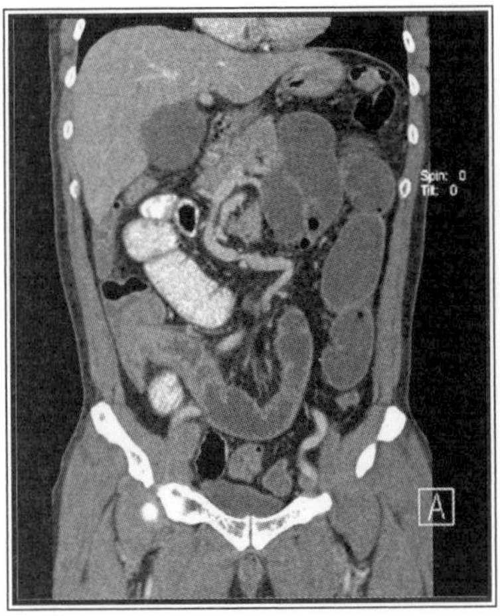

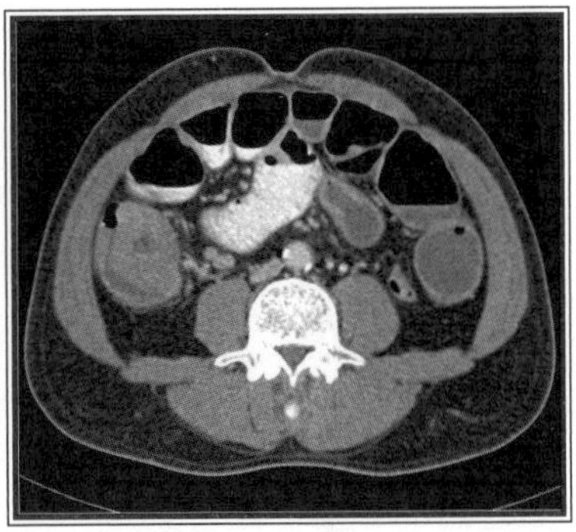

What does this show?

➥ **answer on page 299**

Case 2.50 ++

This 73 year old complains of a 2-day history of increasing abdominal distension. He has not passed any stools for 36 hours, although he admits to flatulence.

A CT of the abdomen was requested after the junior surgeon reviewed the patient and the abdominal radiograph.

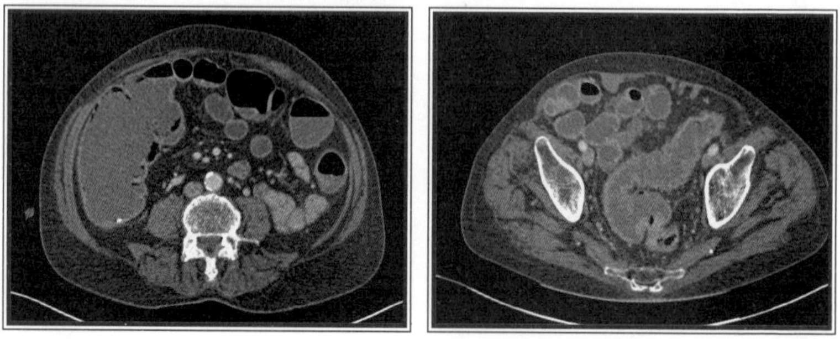

What does this show?

→ **answer on page 299**

Case 2.51 ++

This 77-year-old woman with a prior history of stroke and myocardial infarction was admitted with acute abdominal pain and dehydration.

Examination revealed a diffusely tender abdomen. She was haemodynamically unstable with a BP of 82/38 mmHg. Blood gas analysis demonstrated a high anion gap metabolic acidosis.

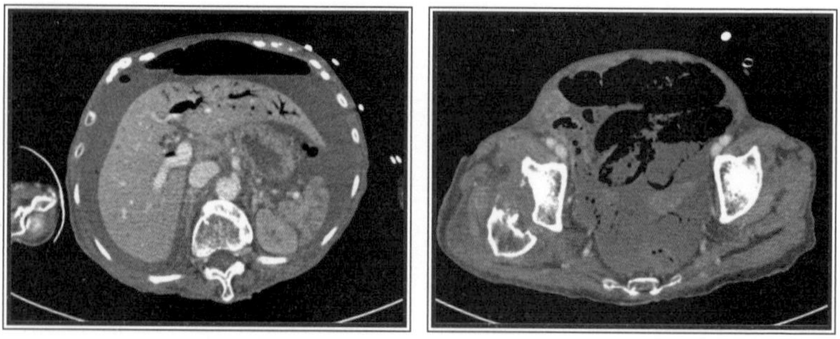

What does this show?

→ **answer on page 300**

Case 2.52 ++

This 30-year-old man complains of a week-long history of bilateral leg weakness, the findings of which are objectively reinforced on clinical examination. He has a mild pyrexia and an elevated white cell count.

MRI of the spine is performed.

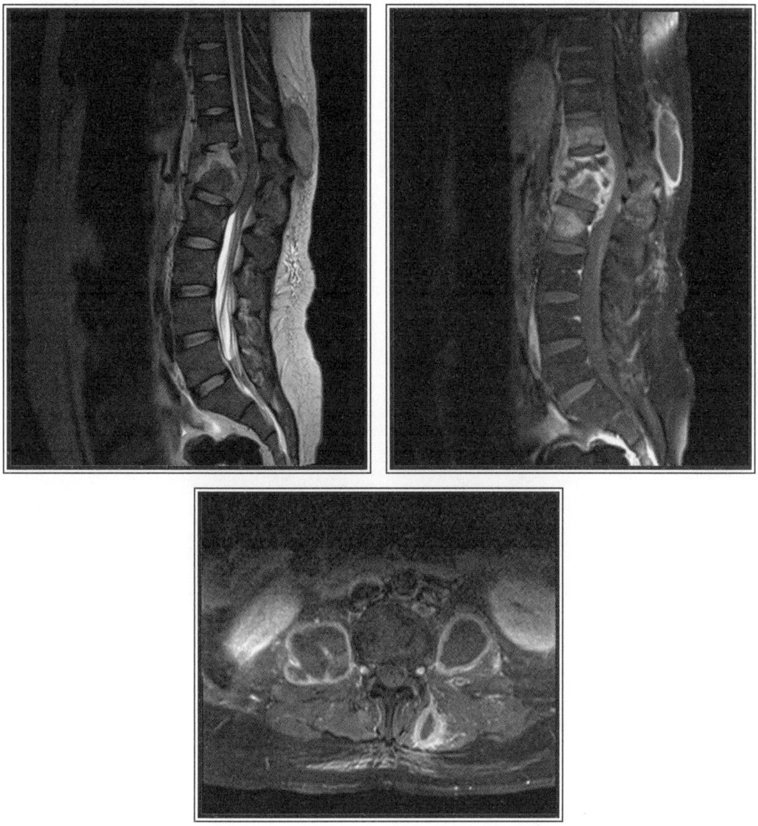

What does this show?

➥ **answer on page 300**

Case 2.53 ++

This patient complains of bilateral leg weakness after a fall. He has a known parotid malignancy.

MRI of the spine was performed due to concerns about cord compression.

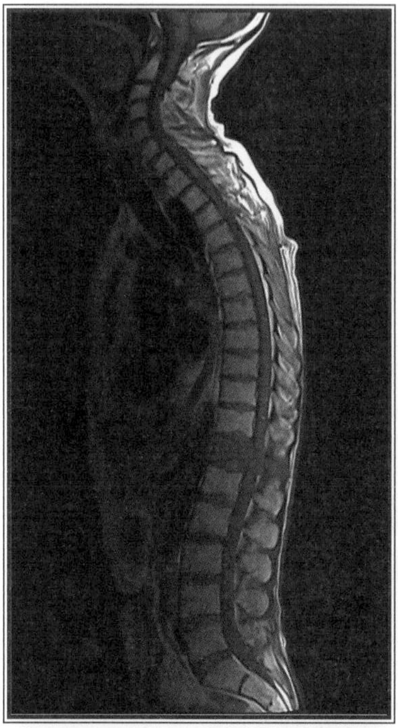

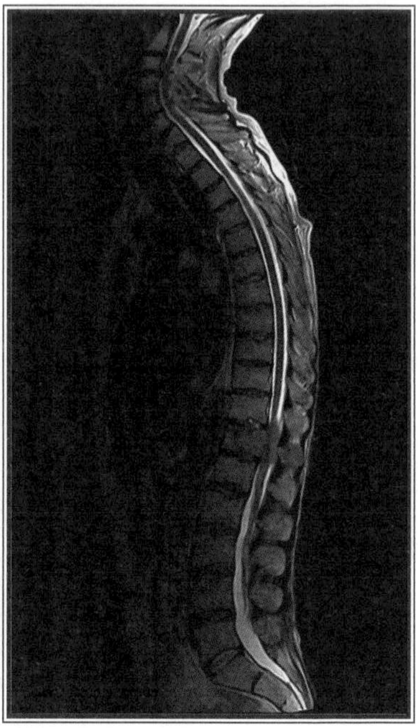

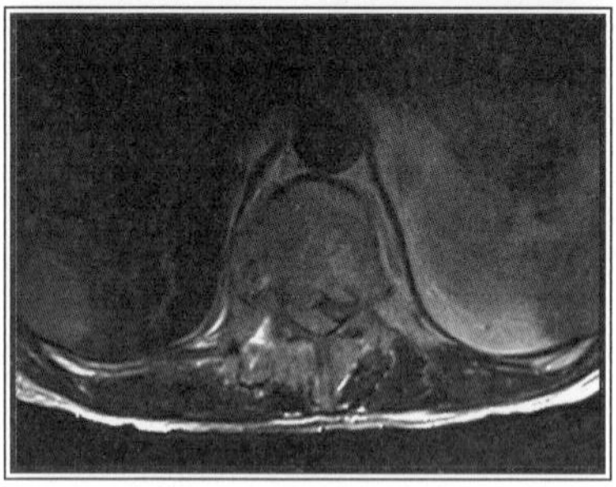

What does this show?

➥ **answer on page 301**

Case 2.54 +++

This 36-year-old woman complains of sudden-onset, right-sided weakness with a mild headache and discomfort in the neck. There is no history of trauma.

Clinical examination revealed a dense, right-sided hemiplegia. A CT of the brain was normal.

MRI of the brain and the carotid arteries as undertaken on the request of the neurologist.

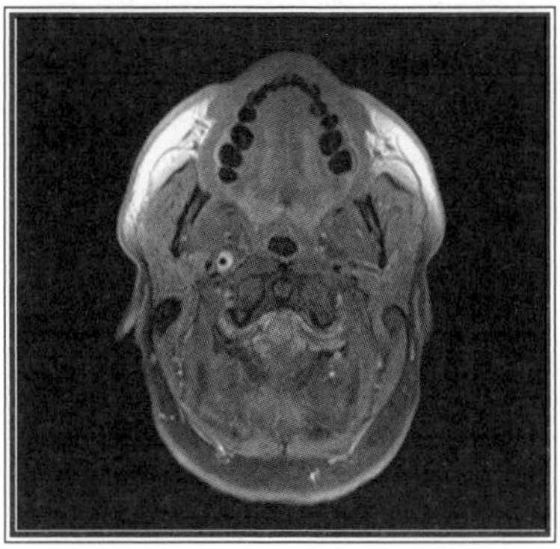

What does this show?

➥ **answer on page 301**

Case 2.55 +++

This 35-year-old woman gives a 3-day history of non-resolving headache. She has no prior medical history, and has not travelled recently. On examination no abnormal neurological signs are identified. A non-contrast CT was performed, and a subsequent MRI was undertaken.

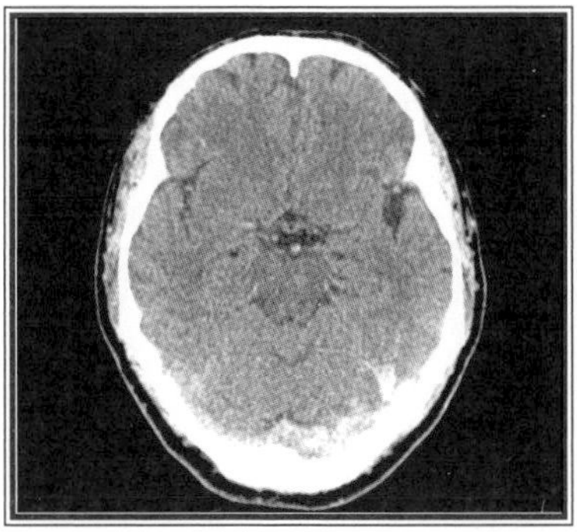

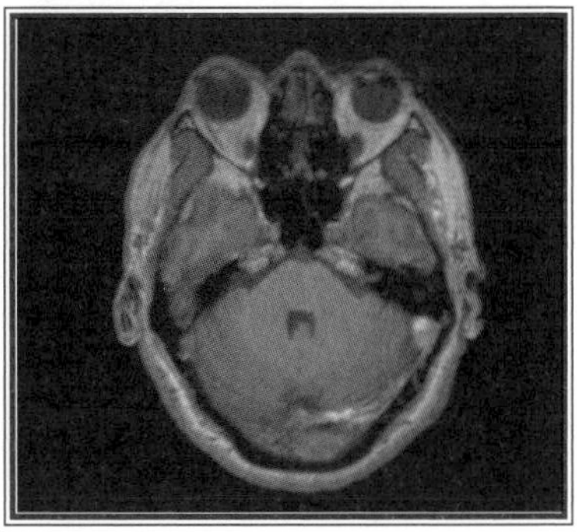

What does this show?

➥ **answer on page 302**

Case 2.56 +++

This 29 year old has a 3-day history of a swollen left eye, which she is now unable to open. She has no history of trauma. Her temperature is 38.1°C in triage.

After a clinical review a CT of the orbits and sinuses was requested.

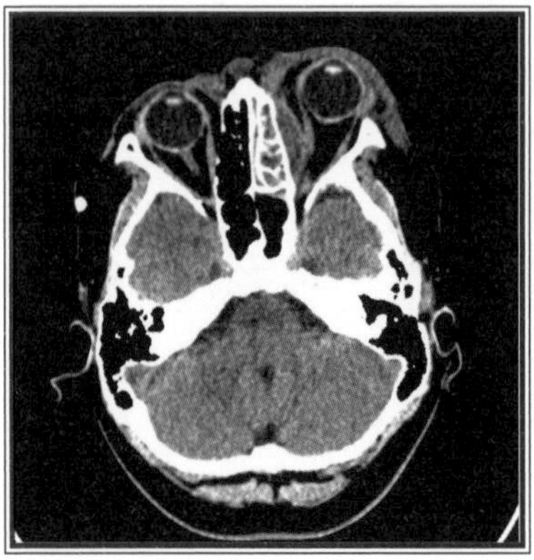

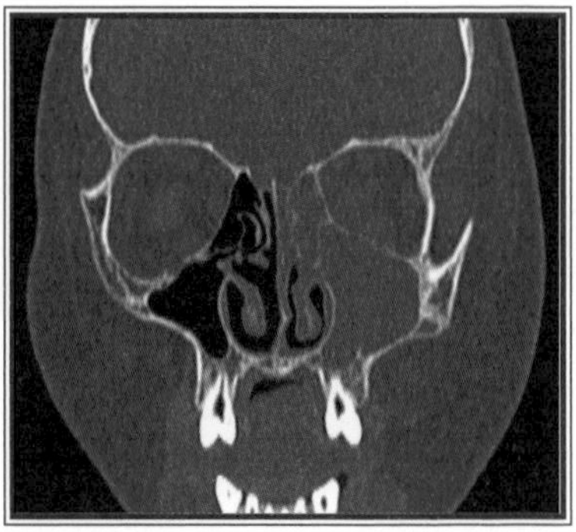

What does this show?

➥ **answer on page 302**

Case 2.57 +++

This 23-year-old man was involved in a high-speed road traffic accident. He is haemodynamically unstable on arrival in A&E. The trauma team are very concerned. A body CT is performed to assess for a source of bleeding.

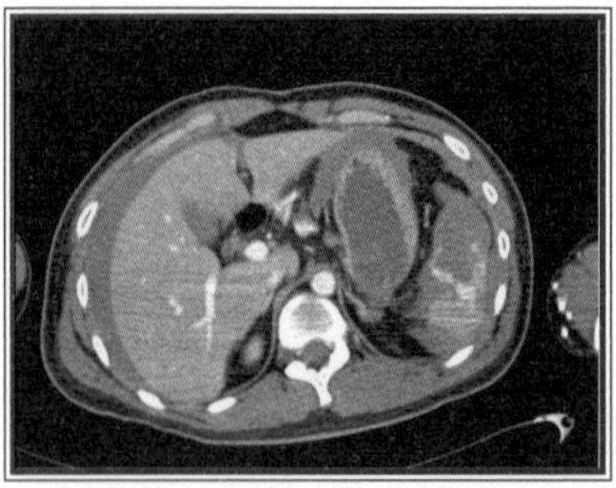

What does this show?

➥ **answer on page 303**

Case 2.58 +++

This 87-year-old, previously fit and well woman has a 6-hour history of lower abdominal pain. She has been passing motions before today.

On examination, she has left iliac fossa pain and peritonism.

A CT of the abdomen is performed.

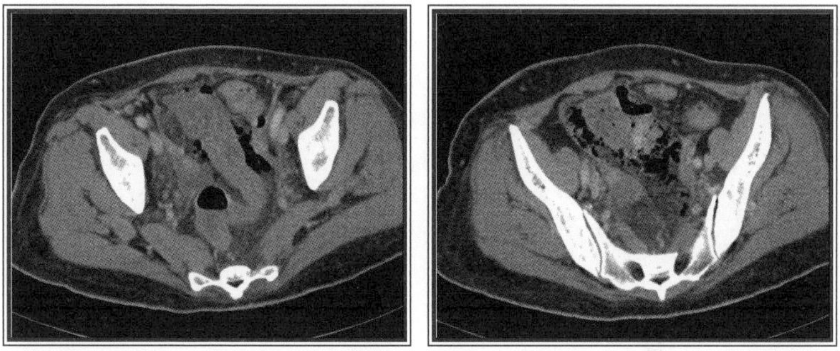

What does this show?

→ **answer on page 303**

Case 2.59 +++

This 25-year-old man was the passenger in a high-speed RTA. He was found unconscious at the scene, although the CT of his head was reported as normal.

After regaining consciousness in A&E he complains of neck pain.

Given the high-energy nature of the incident, a CT of the cervical spine was requested.

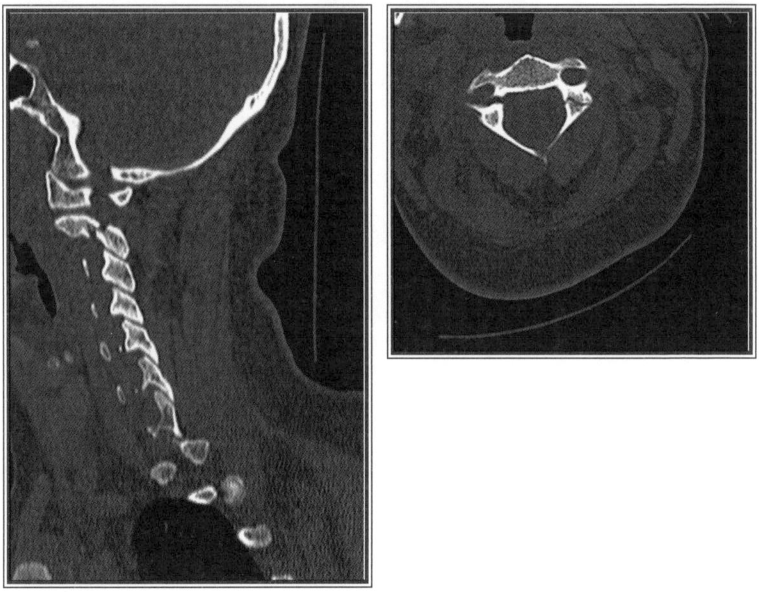

What does this show?

→ **answer on page 304**

INTERPRETING MEDICAL IMAGING: ANSWERS

2

Answer 2.1

➥ question on page 232

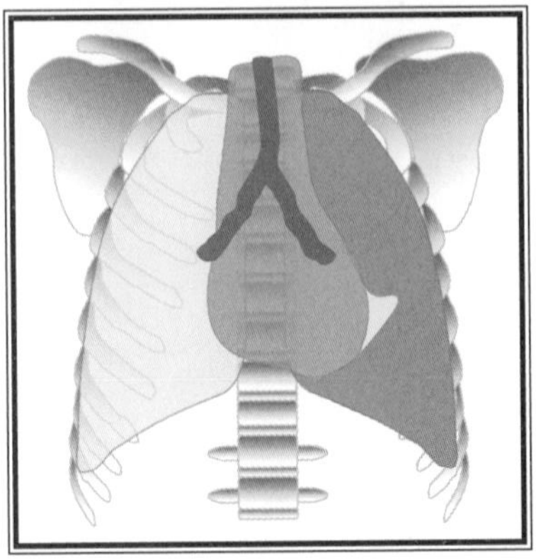

1. The left hemithorax is translucent with absent pulmonary markings. The collapsed left lung is apparent centrally. No evidence of mediastinal shift.

   The appearances are consistent with a large left-sided pneumothorax.

2. Numerous chronic pulmonary diseases predispose to pneumothoraces. These include: chronic obstructive pulmonary disease (COPD), asthma, pulmonary fibrosis and cystic fibrosis. Other important causes of pneumothorax include: trauma, congenital pulmonary blebs and iatrogenic reasons (eg central venous line insertion, mechanical ventilation).

Answer 2.2

➥ question on page 232

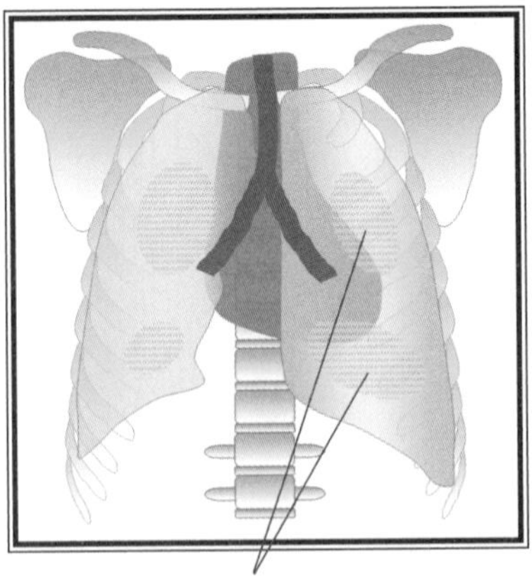

1. Diffuse reticulonodular ('lines and dots') shadowing is evident in both lungs. This has lower zone predominance.

   The appearances of this CXR are of pulmonary (interstitial) fibrosis.

2. The causes may be divided according to whether the fibrosis predominantly affects the upper or lower zones.

MEMORY AID

Upper lobe fibrosis (mnemonic = BREAST)	Lower lobe fibrosis
Berylliosis (uncommon)	Cryptogenic fibrosing alveolitis
Radiation fibrosis	Drug induced (eg amiodarone, methotrexate)
Extrinsic allergic alveolitis	Asbestosis
Ankylosing spondylitis	Connective tissue diseases (eg rheumatoid disease)
Sarcoidosis	
Tuberculosis	

3. Spirometry would demonstrate a restrictive pattern (see page 341 for further details).

Answer 2.3

➥ question on page 233

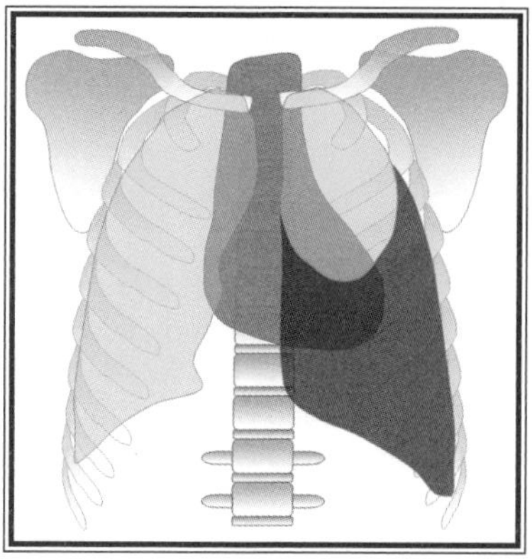

1. There is an area of increased radio-opacity in the lower left hemithorax. The edge can be seen to taper at the lateral aspect of the chest, forming a meniscus. There is no shift of mediastinal structures. This is a moderately sized, left-sided pleural effusion.
2. For unilateral pleural effusions, the causes are mostly exudates. These include:

- malignant tumours (both primary and metastatic disease)
- pneumonia
- pulmonary embolus or infarction
- rheumatoid disease.

A malignant effusion would be most likely in this patient because of his weight loss and smoking history.

3. A diagnostic pleural aspiration could be performed. This will help distinguish whether the effusion is an exudate or transudate based on the protein content (see page 40 for details).

In this case, malignant cells may be identified when the pleural fluid is examined cytologically.

Answer 2.4

➥ question on page 233

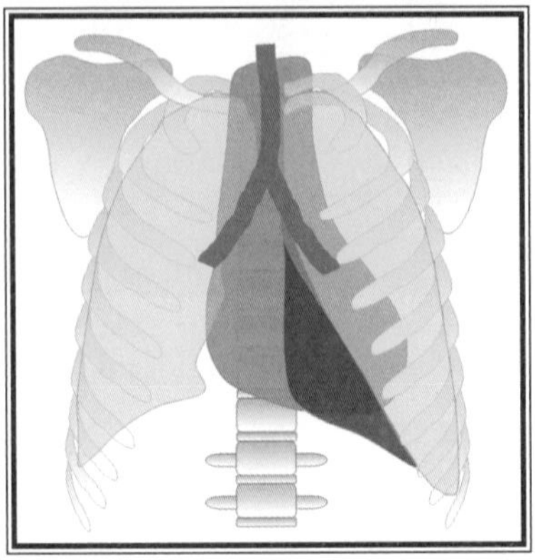

1. A triangular density is present in the left retrocardiac position, which is separate from the left heart border. The medial aspect is difficult to delineate, but the abnormality has a 'sail-like' appearance. The left hilum is inferiorly displaced and there is volume loss within the left hemithorax.

   The appearances are consistent with a 'tight' left lower lobe collapse.

2. The nature of further investigation depends on the clinical scenario. The three most common causes of a left lower lobe collapse are:

   (a) a central hilar or endobronchial mass

   (b) an endobronchial foreign body

   (c) an endobronchial mucus plug.

   In children, a foreign body is most likely and, in a postoperative or ITU patient, a mucus plug. Both can be dealt with by bronchoscopy. In adults, especially smokers, left lower lobe collapse must always be viewed with suspicion for an underlying tumour. Bronchoscopy and CT of the chest are indicated, after clinical assessment by a respiratory team.

Answer 2.5

➥ question on page 234

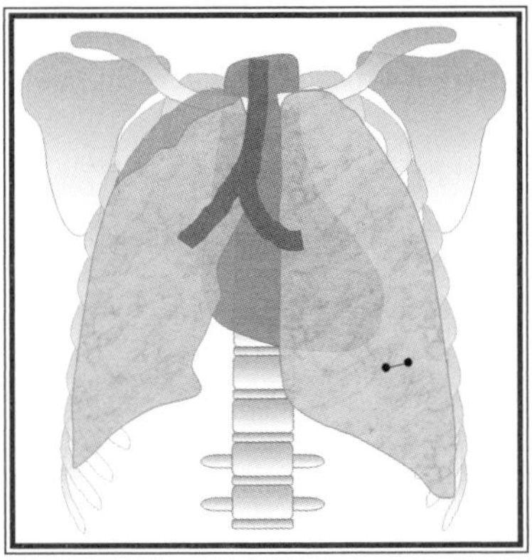

1. Throughout both lungs there are increased interstitial markings, most pronounced in the upper lobes, consistent with fibrosis. At the right lung apex, the lung edge is apparent with no lung markings peripheral to this, consistent with a small apical pneumothorax.

   Given the patient's young age this would be compatible with a pneumothorax on a background of cystic fibrosis.

2. Cystic fibrosis is the most common lethal inherited disease in white individuals. It is an autosomal recessive disorder, for which most carriers of the gene are asymptomatic. It is caused by defects in the *CFTR* gene, which encodes a protein that functions as a chloride channel, and also regulates the flow of other ions across the apical surface of epithelial cells. It is a disease of exocrine gland function that involves multiple organ systems, albeit most commonly associated with pulmonary manifestations. Pancreatic insufficiency is also a common element of the disease. The median survival is now 36 years of age.

Answer 2.6

➥ question on page 235

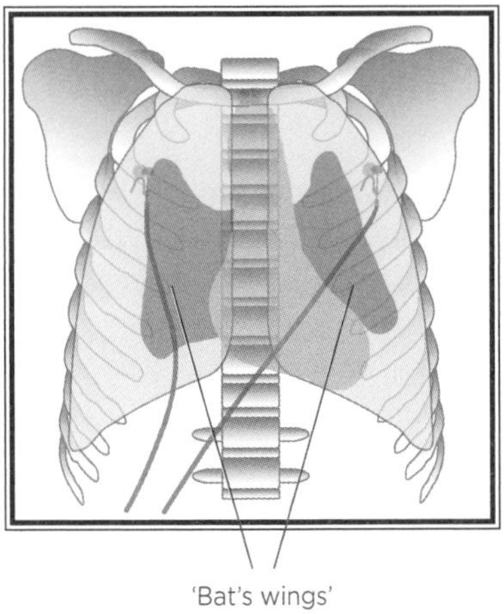

1. This AP erect film demonstrates evidence of bilateral perihilar consolidation ('bat's wings'). The remainders of both lungs are plethoric. The AP projection indicates an ill patient; however, it does limit the assessment of cardiac size.

   The appearances are in keeping with acute pulmonary oedema.

continued overleaf

2. The most common cause of pulmonary oedema is cardiac failure, which is typically associated with cardiomegaly. However, pulmonary oedema can occur in a number of situations where the heart is normal in size. These include:

   (a) in acute renal failure - so-called 'flash' pulmonary oedema

   (b) non-cardiogenic pulmonary oedema in adult respiratory distress syndrome (ARDS)

   (c) after aggressive fluid resuscitation

   (d) with a massive acute myocardial infarction/valve rupture

   (e) in association with a subarachnoid haemorrhage.

Answer 2.7

➥ question on page 235

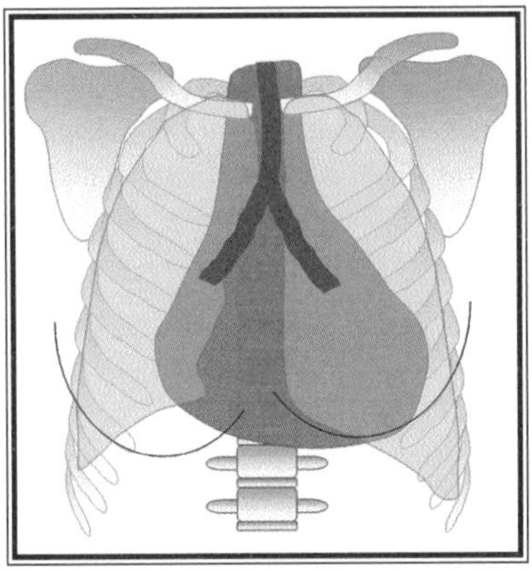

1. The heart is severely enlarged with a globular configuration, suggesting a diffuse cardiac abnormality rather than individual chamber enlargement. There is no evidence of cardiac failure.

   The differential diagnosis for these appearances includes congenital cardiac disease, cardiomyopathy and a pericardial effusion.

2. Important aspects that may help establish the exact cause include:

   (a) a full clinical history, including childhood illness and a family history of cardiac disease

   (b) a review of previous radiological investigations, eg old films may indicate that the cardiomegaly is longstanding and therefore unlikely to be due to a pericardial effusion

   (c) an echocardiogram.

Answer 2.8

➥ question on page 236

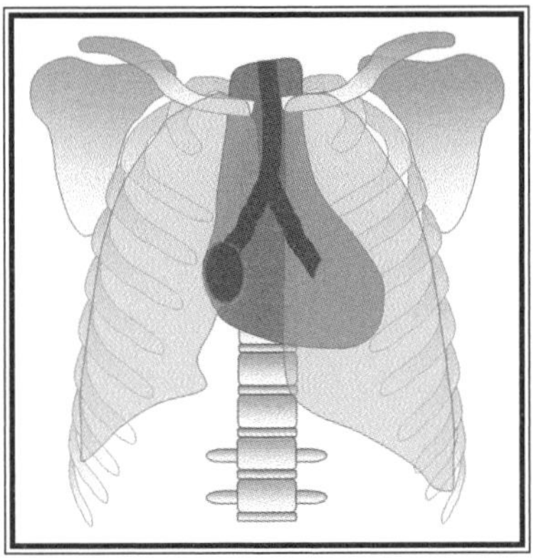

1. The inferior aspect of the right hilum is dense and enlarged. The left hilum and paratracheal regions are normal. The lungs are clear. Further investigation advised.
2. The differential diagnosis for unilateral hilar enlargement includes:
   (a) bronchial carcinoma
   (b) tuberculosis
   (c) lymphoma
   (d) metastatic mediastinal lymph node disease
   (e) atypical sarcoidosis
   (f) vascular anomaly.

Answer 2.9

➥ question on page 236

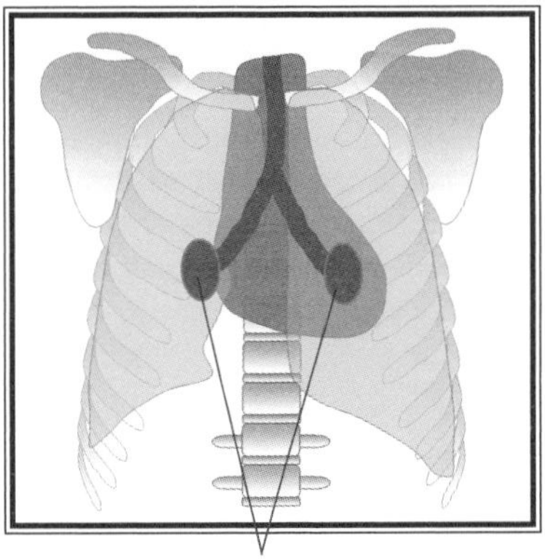

1. The mediastinal contour is abnormal. There is bilateral hilar enlargement. When bilateral hilar enlargement is observed the three important potential diagnoses are sarcoidosis, lymphoma (enlarged nodes) and pulmonary hypertension (enlarged pulmonary vessels). You should therefore pay special attention to the lungs to assess for the presence of other signs that might point to one of these diagnoses.

continued overleaf

DISEASE	SUPPORTING FEATURES
Sarcoidosis	Interstitial fibrotic change
Lymphoma	Enlargement of other nodes (paratracheal)
Pulmonary hypertension	Peripheral pruning Chronic lung disease (ie the cause of secondary pulmonary hypertension)

2. Causes of bilateral hilar enlargement include:
   - sarcoidosis
   - lymphoma
   - pulmonary hypertension (primary and secondary)
   - metastatic nodal disease.

Answer 2.10

➥ question on page 237

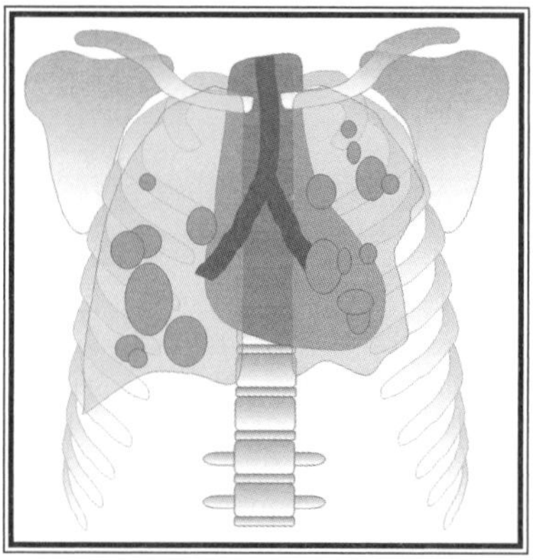

1. Multiple masses in both lungs of variable size, measuring up to 4 cm, consistent with pulmonary metastases. The appearances are those of 'cannon-ball' metastases and identification of the primary tumour is recommended, with CT of the chest, abdomen and pelvis.
2. The most likely primary tumour to cause cannon-ball metastases is renal cell carcinoma. Others include testicular malignancy and choriocarcinoma.

Answer 2.11

➥ question on page 237

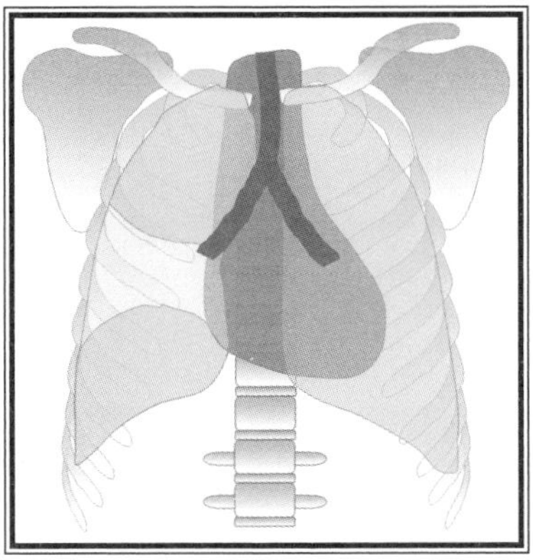

1. Dense consolidation is evident in the right upper and mid-zones, clearly delineated inferiorly by the horizontal fissure. This, combined with the right heart border remaining distinct, implies that the consolidation is in the right upper lobe The left hilum cannot be clearly visualised in its entirety. The left lung is clear.

   The appearances are in keeping with right upper lobe pneumonia.

2. A follow-up CXR is indicated with a dense lobar pneumonia, especially a case like this, where the hilum cannot be properly assessed.
   A lobar pneumonia may be the presentation of something more sinister underlying it, such as a central bronchial carcinoma, which has resulted in a distal 'obstructive' pneumonia. A follow-up film should be performed 6 weeks after antibiotic treatment. For every decade of life after 60 years of age, an additional week should be added. Radiological resolution may lag behind clinical resolution. The follow-up film enables assessment for resolution of the pneumonia for any underlying mass.

Answer 2.12

➥ question on page 238

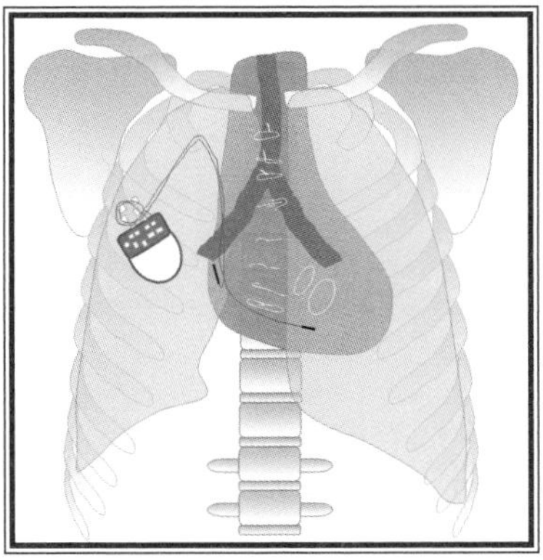

1. Dual lead pacemaker. Median sternotomy, aortic and mitral valve replacements. The heart is mildly enlarged, but there is no evidence of cardiac failure. The lungs are clear.

2. Cardiac valve replacement may be with a tissue or metallic valve. Only the latter will be visible on chest X-ray. Most commonly a single valve is replaced.

continued overleaf

The most common valve replacements are those of the 'left side of the heart' - the mitral and aortic valves. Indications for valve replacement include:

(a) endocarditis

(b) rheumatic heart disease (usually mitral valve)

(c) congenital valve disease (eg a biscupid aortic valve)

(d) severe acquired valve incompetence or stenosis

(e) acute valvular rupture.

Answer 2.13

➥ question on page 238

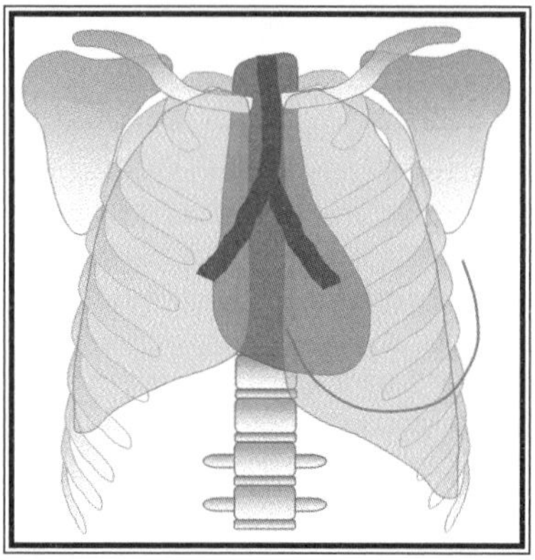

1. The right breast shadow is absent in keeping with a mastectomy. No evidence of recurrent disease in the lungs. Normal bony skeleton.
2. There are five key areas to review on a chest X-ray:

   (a) breast shadows (in females)

   (b) below the diaphragm

   (c) retrocardiac space

   (d) hila

   (e) lung apices

Answer 2.14

➥ question on page 239

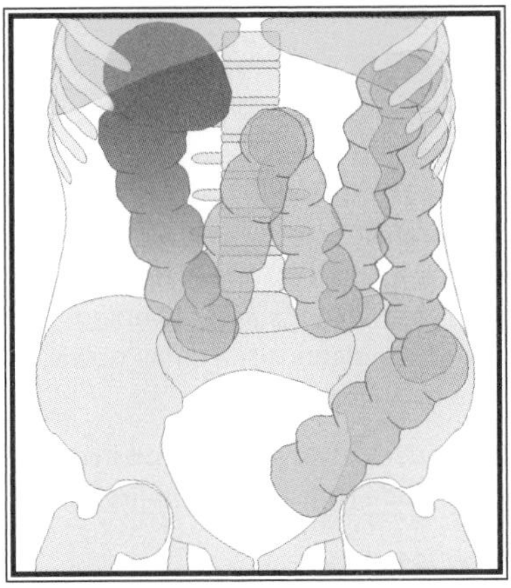

1. The large bowel is gas filled and dilated up to 6 cm in diameter down to the left side of the pelvis, where there is an abrupt cut-off. The rectum is non-distended and the small bowel collapsed. The appearances are consistent with a large bowel obstruction at the level of the sigmoid colon.
2. A CT of the abdomen is indicated to investigate further, before probable surgical intervention. This will enable the following:
   (a) confirmation of the site of obstruction
   (b) establishment of the cause of obstruction; a sigmoid tumour is most likely, although other causes include a diverticular stricture or hernia
   (c) identification of whether a perforation has occurred
   (d) in the case of the cause being a tumour, identification of any local, regional or distal metastatic disease.

Answer 2.15

➥ question on page 239

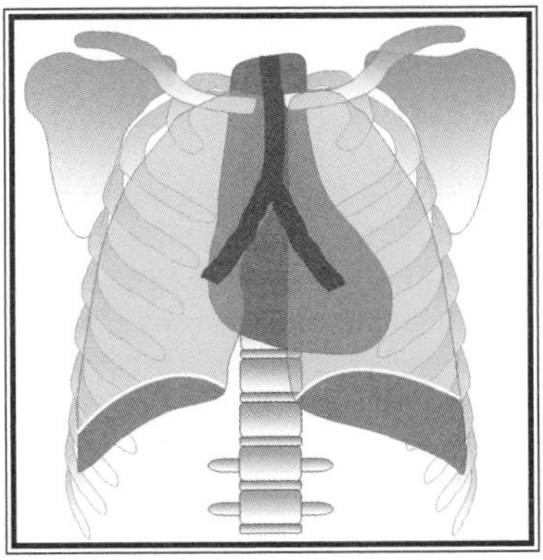

1. A radiolucent linear abnormality is noted inferior to the diaphragm bilaterally.

   Remember that gas on a plain radiograph is black so this must be gas in the abdomen.

   It is outside the bowel lumen - an abnormal finding. This is called a pneumoperitoneum.
2. This is an ERECT CXR. An erect film is invariably requested to assess for free gas within the abdomen (pneumoperitoneum).
3. The causes of pneumoperitoneum are listed on page 208 (see table 'Causes of extraluminal gas').

Answer 2.16

➥ question on page 240

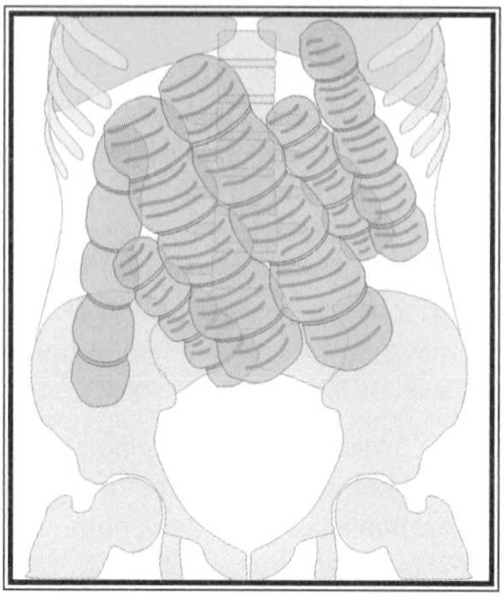

1. Multiple dilated small bowel loops. The bowel measures 4 cm in diameter and is located in the centre of the film. Multiple loops suggest that the obstruction lies in the distal small bowel. These findings are in keeping with a diagnosis of small bowel obstruction.
2. Causes of small bowel obstruction include (most common first):

- adhesions
- hernia
- obstructing mass (extraluminal causes more common than intraluminal)
- intussusception.

FEATURES OF SMALL BOWEL OBSTRUCTION
Bowel lies in centre of the film
Markings seen across the bowel wall (valvulae conniventes)
Several loops (more loops the lower the obstruction)

Answer 2.17

➥ question on page 240

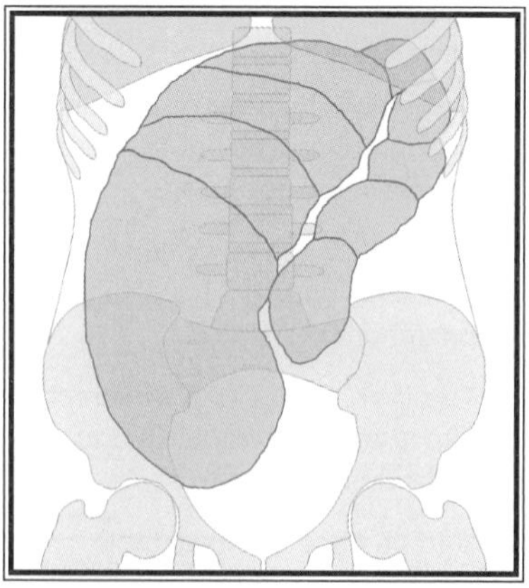

1. A large distended featureless loop of bowel arises from the pelvis into the mid/upper abdomen, with a 'coffee-bean' configuration. Proximal to this there is distended large bowel consistent with obstruction. The small bowel is collapsed. Appearances are consistent with a sigmoid volvulus.

2. The usual treatment for sigmoid volvulus is insertion of a flatus tube. A plain film is usually sufficient for diagnosis and a management decision. On occasion the volvulus might result in a section of ischaemic bowel requiring surgical resection. Sigmoid volvulus is commonly recurrent, which in itself may merit surgery. Of the three types of volvulus of the gastrointestinal tract, sigmoid is the most common, followed by caecal and gastric.

Answer 2.18

➥ question on page 241

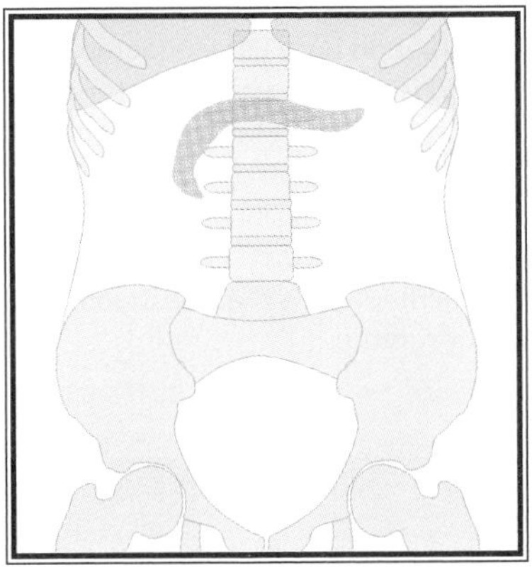

1. Extensive punctate calcification is evident in the upper abdomen, extending across the midline, conforming to the shape of the pancreas, in keeping with chronic pancreatitis.

2. Numerous complications may follow acute pancreatitis, which can be identified on imaging, in particular CT. Complications may be acute, subacute or chronic in nature, including the following:

   (a) pancreatic necrosis

   (b) pancreatic haemorrhage

   (c) pancreatic or peripancreatic abscess

   (d) pancreatic pseudocyst

   (e) pseudoaneurysm formation

   (f) thrombosis of adjacent vessels, eg the superior mesenteric vein

   (g) pancreatic calcification, which occurs in the chronic phase of pancreatitis and may involve the parenchyma or ductal components of the pancreas.

Answer 2.19

➥ question on page 241

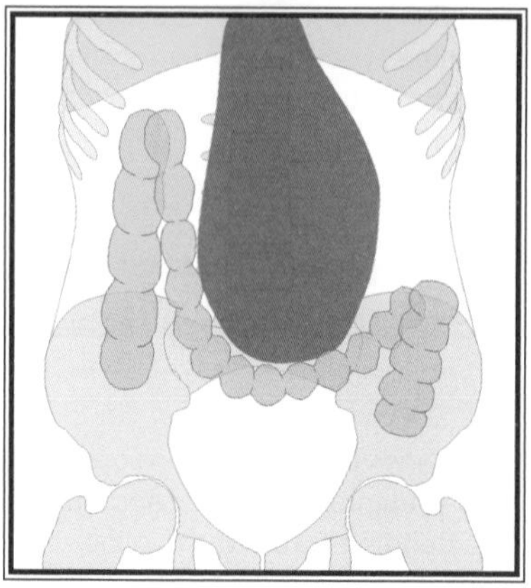

1. A large, left, paraspinal, soft-tissue abnormality is present in the mid-abdomen with a curvilinear lateral aspect, which contains a rim of calcification. The psoas shadow is separate from this. Appearances are consistent with a large abdominal aortic aneurysm.
2. Although both ultrasonography and CT can be used to assess the aorta, in this instance CT is the best choice. Ultrasonography is used for surveillance of aneurysm size. This aneurysm is large enough to warrant elective surgery and therefore full assessment with CT is merited. CT is the investigation of choice in the acute setting to assess for rupture.

Answer 2.20

➥ question on page 242

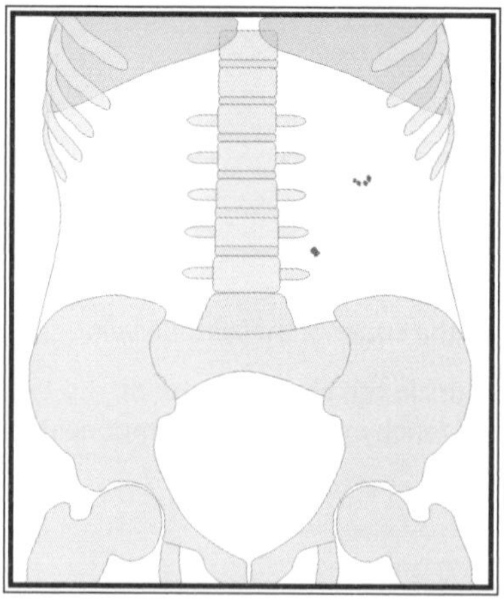

1. Multiple calcific densities project over the lower pole of the left kidney in keeping with renal calculi. An additional similar density projects between the left L3 and L4 transverse process, in keeping with a calculus within the left mid-ureter.
2. CT-KUB (kidneys, ureters and bladder) is the gold standard imaging investigation for the assessment of renal calculi, with over 99% sensitivity for calculi as small as 1 mm. This is performed without contrast with 1-mm (thin) slice acquisition. Renal calculi and the level of obstruction are identified. In addition perinephric/periureteric inflammatory change and fluid are visualised. Complications, such as hydronephrosis or pyonephrosis, can be seen. Pyonephrosis due to renal stone disease is a urological emergency and is an indication for percutaneous nephrostomy insertion.

Answer 2.21

➥ question on page 243

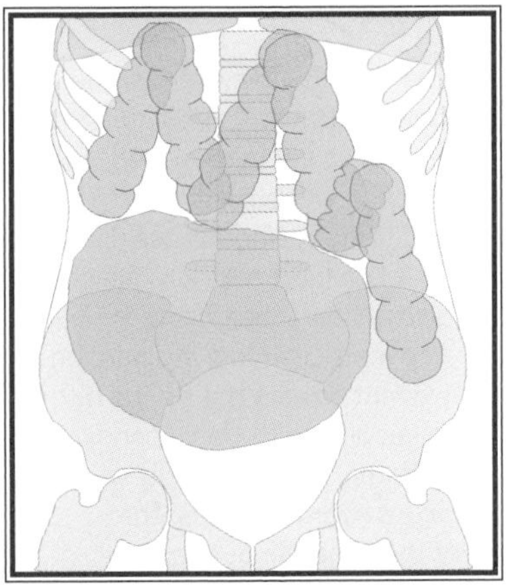

1. A large soft-tissue mass arises from the pelvis extending to the level of the umbilicus. This is well defined superiorly and is displacing the bowel into the upper abdomen. Appearances are in keeping with a pelvic mass, most likely gynaecological in origin.
2. The differential diagnosis for these appearances includes: ovarian cyst, dermoid cyst, pelvic abscess/collection and an enlarged fibroid uterus. In the first instance, assessment with ultrasonography is recommended. Depending on the findings, further cross-sectional imaging may also be required.

Answer 2.22

➥ question on page 243

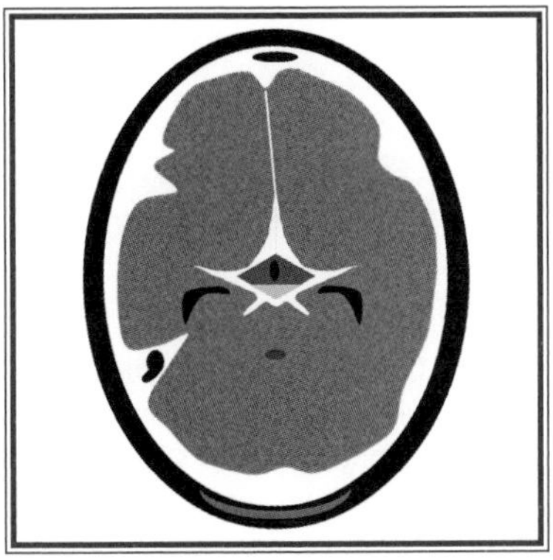

1. Extensive high-attenuation material consistent with acute blood is present within the suprasellar cistern and sulci of the brain in keeping with subarachnoid haemorrhage. The temporal horns of the lateral ventricles are dilated in keeping with early hydrocephalus.
2. Spontaneous subarachnoid haemorrhage is commonly associated with an underlying vascular abnormality, most commonly a cerebral ("berry") aneurysm. Imaging is focused on trying to identify an aneurysm, which will permit definitive treatment, such as a coil embolisation or, less commonly now, surgical clipping. This usually involves CT angiography of the circle of Willis, although catheter angiography may be performed alone or in addition to CT, especially if endoluminal treatment is to be performed.

Answer 2.23

➥ question on page 244

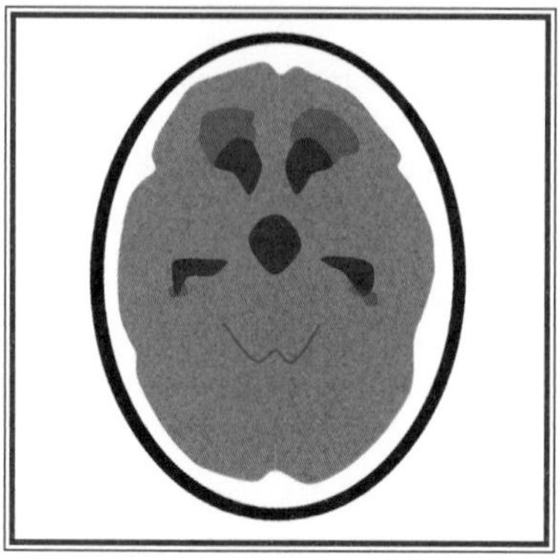

1. The ventricular system of the brain is dilated. In particular on the single image provided, note that the lateral ventricles (frontal and temporal horns) are dilated as is the third ventricle, which is also uncharacteristically round. Periventricular low attenuation is evident around the frontal horns, in keeping with transependymal oedema, which typically occurs in acute hydrocephalus (the CSF leaks across the ependymal lining of the ventricle due to high pressure within).
2. Hydrocephalus may be obstructive or non-obstructive. It may involve individual ventricles or the whole ventricular system. Causes include:
   (a) an obstructive malignant mass, such as a tumour. Potential tumours include an ependymoma
   (b) an obstructive non-malignant mass, such as a third ventricular colloid cyst
   (c) obstruction due to intraventricular debris, such as blood post-subarachnoid haemorrhage or trauma.

Answer 2.24

➥ question on page 244

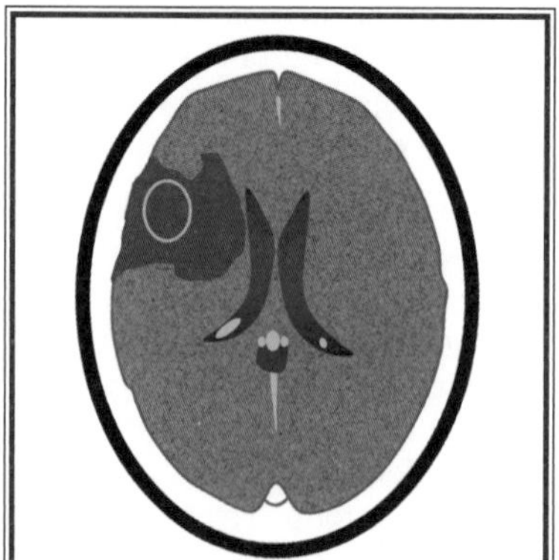

1. This CT has been performed following contrast administration. A rim-enhancing mass lies within the right frontoparietal region, with significant surrounding perilesional oedema. This is causing a mass effect, as demonstrated by sulcal effacement and mild displacement of the body of

the right lateral ventricle. In the context of the clinical history, a cerebral metastasis is the most likely diagnosis.

2. The differential diagnosis for a single rim-enhancing intraparenchymal brain mass includes:
   (a) cerebral metastasis
   (b) primary brain malignancy
   (c) cerebral abscess
   (d) tumefactive (mass like in appearance) multiple sclerosis.

Answer 2.25

➥ question on page 245

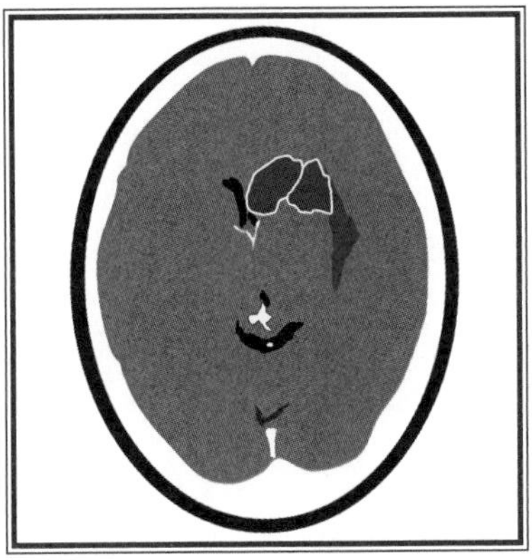

1. This scan has been performed following contrast administration. Adjacent to the frontal horn of the left lateral ventricle is an avidly rim-enhancing lesion, with a low attenuation centre. There is a moderate amount of perilesional oedema. Although there is a wide differential for a rim-enhancing solitary cerebral lesion (see Case 2.24), correlation with the clinical history makes a cerebral abscess by far the most likely cause.

2. Although not necessarily unique to those taking intravenous drugs, there are a number of conditions that occur much more commonly in this patient subgroup, including:
   (a) infective endocarditis
   (b) cerebral abscesses
   (c) groin pseudoaneurysms, which may also become infected
   (d) septic pulmonary emboli.

Answer 2.26

➥ question on page 245

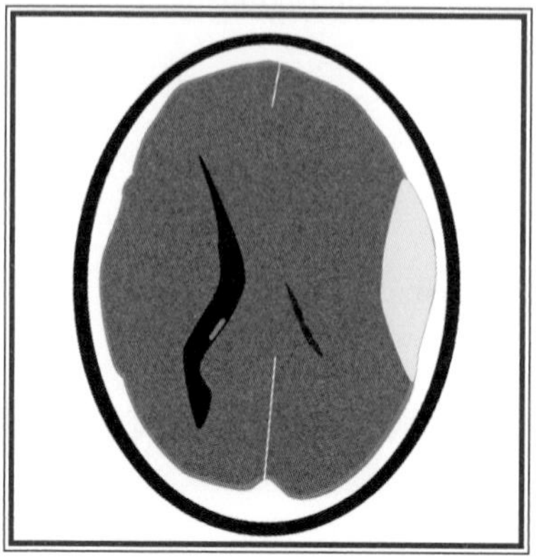

1. A high-attenuation, lens-shaped (biconvex), extra-axial abnormality is present in the left parietal region, which is causing a mass effect in the form of sulcal effacement, along with both compression and displacement of the left lateral ventricle.

   The appearances are consistent with an acute extradural haematoma.

2. Ninety-five per cent of extradural haematomas are associated with a skull fracture. The middle meningeal artery is usually the vessel damaged and is responsible for the haematoma. This differs from subdural haematomas, which are usually due to tears of the bridging veins.

Answer 2.27

➥ question on page 246

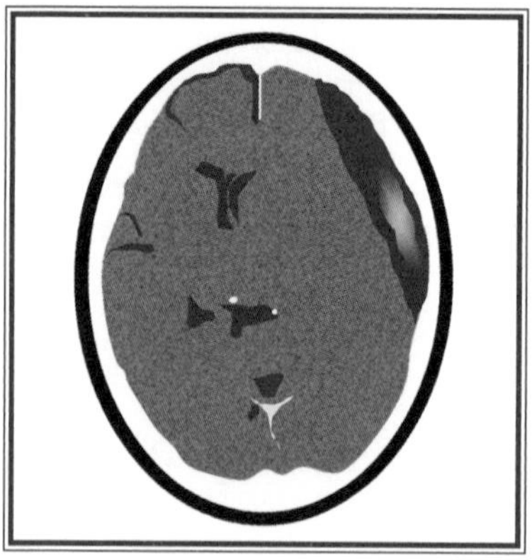

1. Blood of variable age is present within the left subdural space, in keeping with a moderate-sized subdural haematoma. Most of the haematoma content is isodense, with the brain parenchyma indicating subacute blood with some high-attenuation material within, consistent with more acute blood. The haematoma is causing significant mass effect, with displacement of the frontal horn of the left lateral ventricle and subfalcine herniation.

2. Subdural haematomas are not uncommonly found after relatively low-impact head trauma. Often, if questioned directly, patients might recall a slight blow to the head or a fall before presentation – which is often considered too trivial to be mentioned. This history may not be given, however, due to the presence of confusion.

Answer 2.28

➡ question on page 246

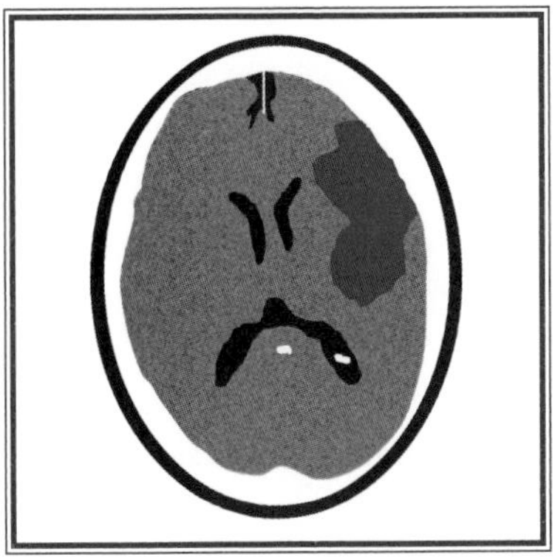

1. Extensive low attenuation is present throughout the left temporoparietal region with sparing of the head of caudate and lentiform nucleus (basal ganglia). These appearances are consistent with a left middle cerebral artery (MCA) territory infarction. No evidence of haemorrhagic transformation. No visible intra-arterial thrombus.
2. 'Time is brain' refers to the urgency with which acute stroke should be treated, where appropriate, with intravenous thrombolysis. Those patients who present to hospital within a specified time window with the clinical diagnosis of stroke, and who fulfil a number of pre-agreed criteria, should receive intravenous thrombolysis. The concept is that ischaemic, but not yet infarcted, brain (ischaemic penumbra) is reperfused and saved, resulting in a reduction in neurological deficit. At present, the time window that is adopted in many centres is 4.5 hours from the onset of symptoms. The patient must receive a CT of the head before treatment to exclude intracranial haemorrhage.

Answer 2.29

➡ question on page 247

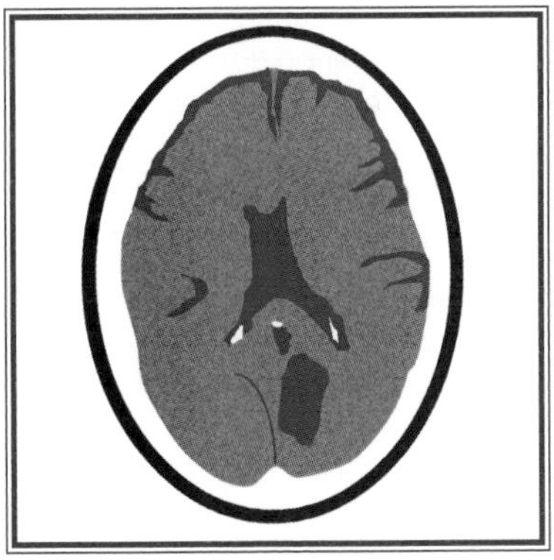

1. There is a focal area of low attenuation in the left occipital lobe. The appearances are consistent with an established posterior cerebral artery stroke involving the left occipital lobe. No acute findings to suggest an injury following trauma.
2. There are a number of factors that predispose to stroke. These include:

continued overleaf

- hypertension
- atrial fibrillation
- cardiovascular disease elsewhere ('arteriopath' status)
- diabetes mellitus
- smoking
- hyperlipidaemia
- family history of cardiovascular disease
- atheromatous plaques in the carotid or vertebrobasilar arteries
- infective endocarditis - resulting in septic emboli
- vasculitis
- dissection of the carotid or vertebrobasilar arteries (especially when stroke occurs in young people)
- procoagulant states, such as polycythaemia.

Answer 2.30

➥ question on page 248

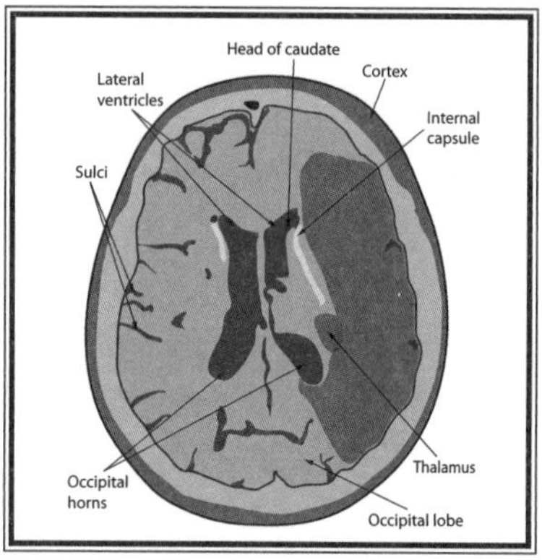

The protocol (collection of sequences) performed for different clinical queries varies in MRI. For example, the protocols for MRI of the brain in stroke, demyelination and epilepsy are different.

In this case of an acute left middle cerebral artery (MCA) infarct, the diffusion-weighted images (DWIs) and apparent diffusion coefficient (ADC) sequences are paramount. These quick-to-acquire sequences assess the movement of water molecules, which are altered in stroke due to disrupted cell membranes. They are interpreted together, to assess for the presence or absence of diffusion restriction.

In an acute infarct, intense diffusion restriction is identified. The DWI will be bright and the ADC 'mapped' on to the corresponding anatomical area will be dark.

Answer 2.31

➥ question on page 249

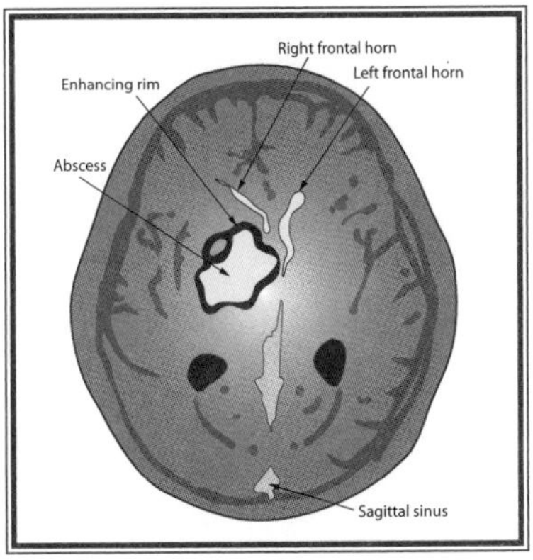

A ring-enhancing, cystic mass centred on the right basal ganglia is shown. The internal contents of the mass demonstrate avid diffusion restriction. The mass is causing effacement of the right frontal horn with mild mass effect.

Given the clinical history of fever, this is most consistent with a cerebral abscess.

Answer 2.32

➥ question on page 250

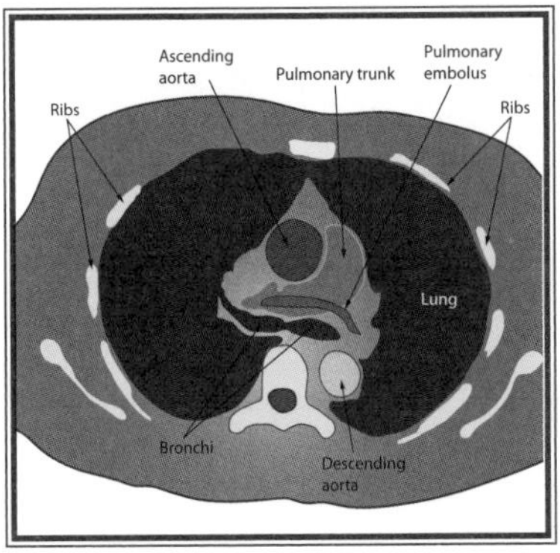

A large, linear, filling defect straddles the pulmonary trunk, extending into both main pulmonary arteries.

The appearances are those of a saddle embolus - a large central pulmonary embolus, which is associated with right heart strain. Right heart strain may be identified on echocardiography or on the CTPA as straightening of the intraventricular septum.

Answer 2.33

➥ question on page 251

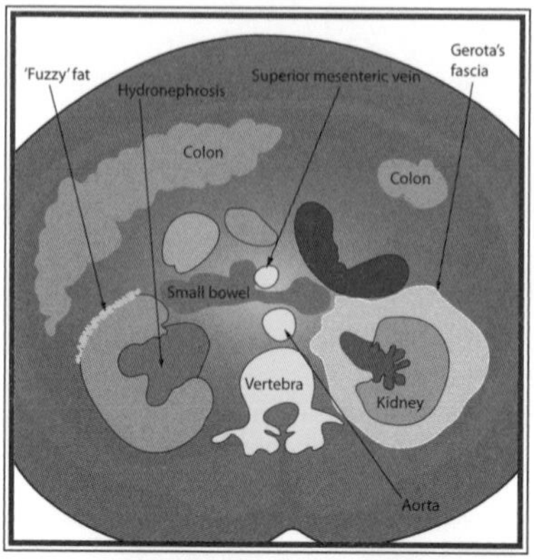

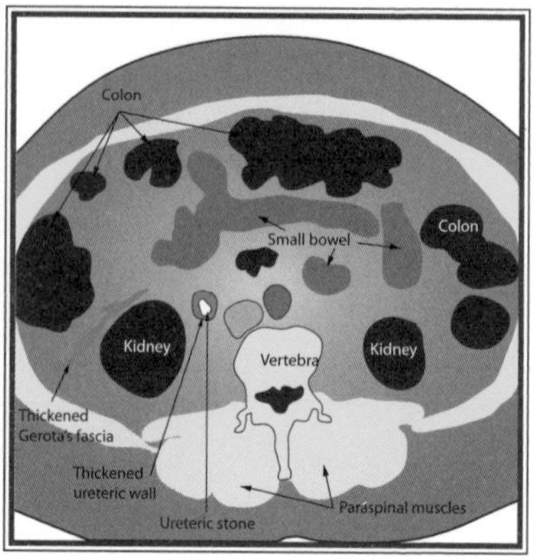

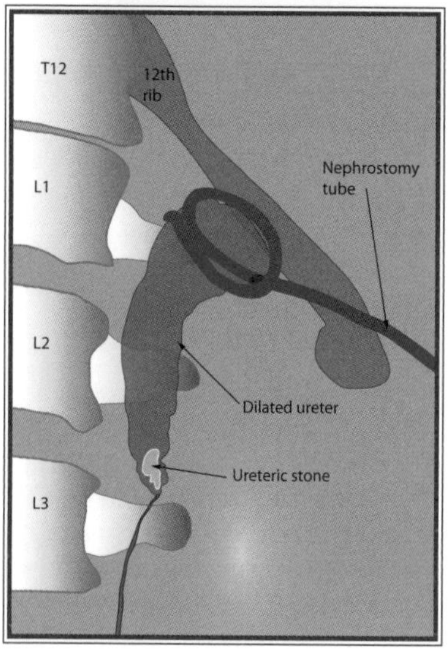

The CT demonstrates bilateral renal calculi, with a right hydronephrosis due to a proximal ureteric calculus.

A percutaneous nephrostomy insertion was requested, given the patient's swinging pyrexia.

A nephrostogram shows hydronephrosis due to almost complete obstruction from the ureteric calculus.

There is an 8-Fr nephrostomy tube in the renal pelvis.

Answer 2.34

➥ question on page 252

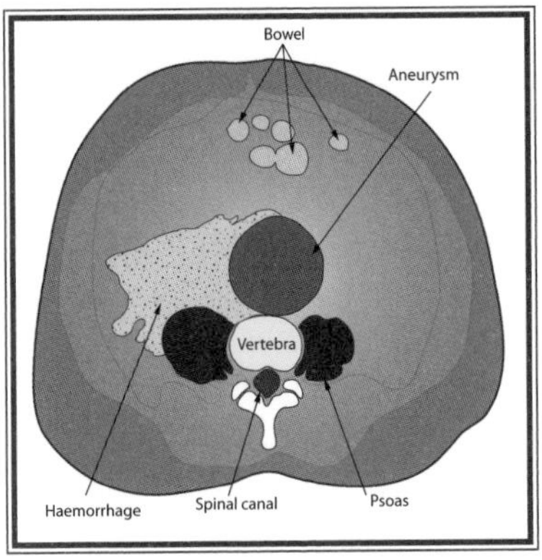

For clinical concern over a ruptured abdominal aortic aneurysm (AAA), only one thing counts - speed: speed of imaging, speed of diagnosis and speed of getting the patient to theatre.

The CT has one role - is there a retrohaemoperitoneum in the presence of an aneurysm? If there is, then get to the theatre quick. The administration of contrast just takes valuable time that the patient does not have to save his or her life. A non-contrast CT of the abdomen is sufficient.

In some circumstances contrast may well have been administered - usually when the clinician does not think this is the likely diagnosis or when other diagnoses are being queried.

Answer 2.35

➥ question on page 253

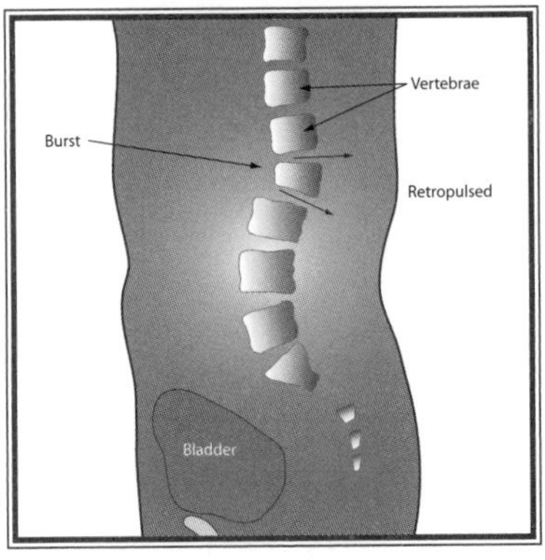

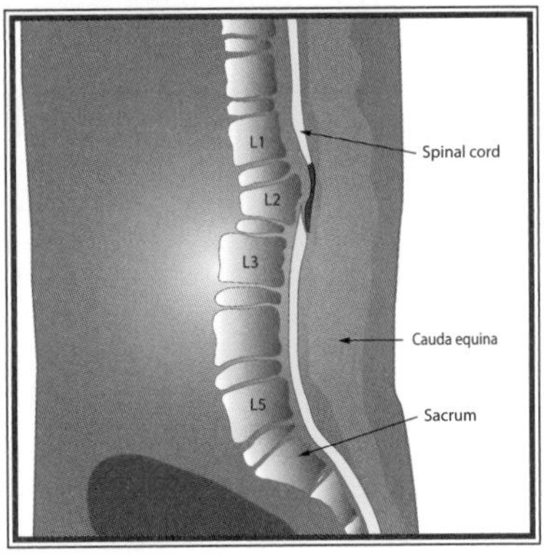

High T2 signal is evident in the L2 vertebral body, consistent with an acute fracture, with significant retropulsion severely narrowing the central canal. This is impinging on the conus/origin of the cauda equina.

There is a small L3 vertebral body fracture.

Appearances are in keeping with cauda equina compression secondary to a traumatic vertebral body fracture.

Answer 2.36

➥ question on page 254

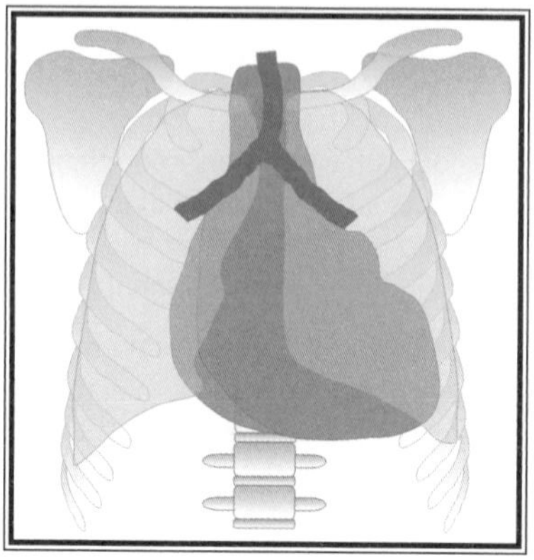

1. The heart is moderately enlarged, with prominence of the left atrial appendage. A double right heart border is evident, indicating enlargement of the left atrium. The subcarinal angle is normal; however, the other features all point towards a diagnosis of left atrial enlargement (a 'mitral heart').
2. The following are all features of cardiac failure on chest X-ray:

(a) cardiomegaly

(b) pleural effusions

(c) perihilar consolidation ('bat's wings')

(d) upper lobe venous distension

(e) interlobular septal lines ('Kerley B lines').

Answer 2.37

➥ question on page 254

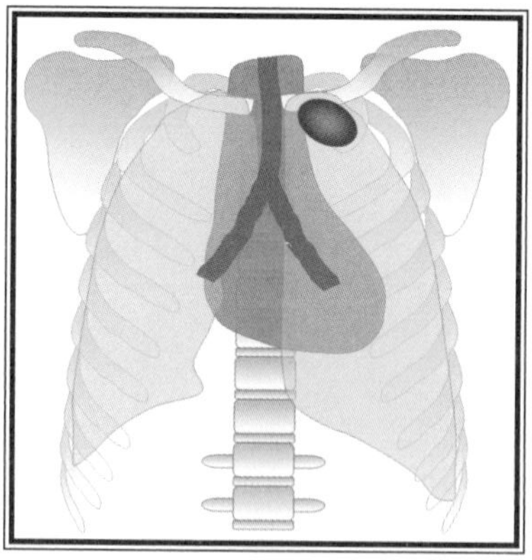

1. A lung mass on a CXR in a smoker over 50 years of age should be regarded as a bronchial carcinoma until proven otherwise. Other features that may be seen on CXR with bronchial carcinoma include:

- pleural effusion
- lung collapse (due to endobronchial tumour)
- pulmonary metastases
- bony metastases (and pathological fracture)
- secondary pneumonia

- lymphangitis carcinomatosis
- enlarged lymph nodes (hilar and paratracheal).

2. Causes of a lung mass on CXR include:
    - bronchial carcinoma
    - pulmonary metastasis
    - round pneumonia
    - lung hamartoma
    - encysted pleural effusion
    - rheumatoid nodule
    - lung abscess (usually cavitating).
3. Computed tomography of the chest would image the mass in greater detail. It will also help in the assessment of lymphadenopathy and provide evidence of local or metastatic spread

Answer 2.38

➥ question on page 255

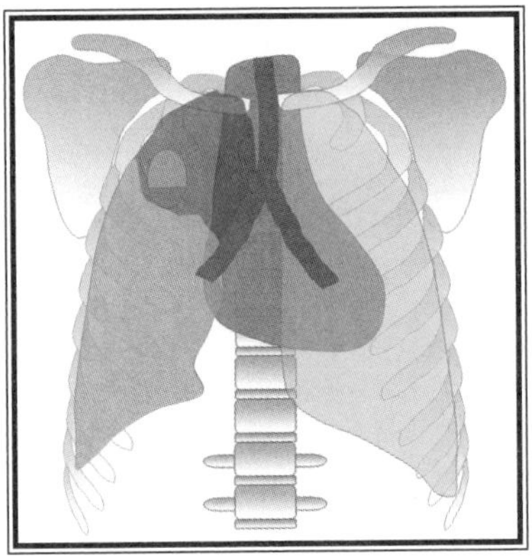

1. There is dense consolidation in the right upper lobe with an area of cavitation within. There is an air-fluid level within the cavity.
2. The differential diagnosis for a cavitating lung lesion is:
    - bronchial carcinoma (especially squamous cell carcinoma)
    - pulmonary metastasis
    - tuberculosis
    - cavitating pneumonia
    - lung abscess
    - vasculitic disease (eg Wegener's granulomatosis)
    - lung infarction
    - rheumatoid nodule.

Answer 2.39

➥ question on page 255

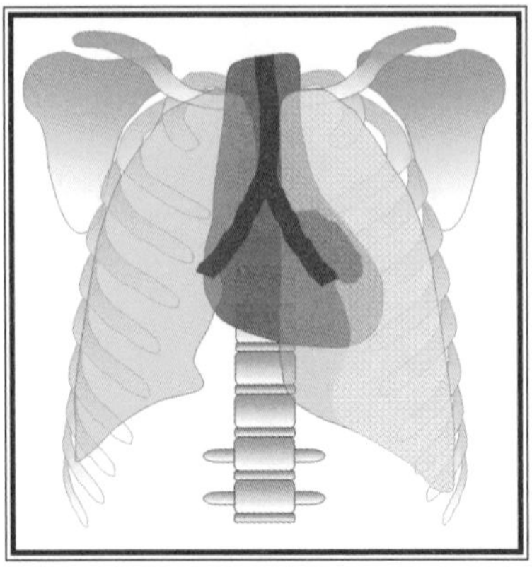

1. The left hemithorax is opacified in a 'veil-like' manner. There is the impression of a dense and enlarged left hilum. The right lung is clear.

   The appearances are in keeping with a left upper lobe collapse, with a strong suspicion of an underlying hilar mass.

2. The chest X-ray appearances are highly suspicious for a central (hilar) bronchial carcinoma, which has resulted in a left upper lobe collapse due to obstruction of the left upper lobe bronchus. This merits urgent referral to the lung cancer multidisciplinary team (MDT) for work-up and discussion. This will entail CT of the chest and upper abdomen, and bronchoscopy. With a central tumour, bronchoscopic biopsy is likely to be performed to confirm the histology and plan for treatment.

Answer 2.40

➥ question on page 256

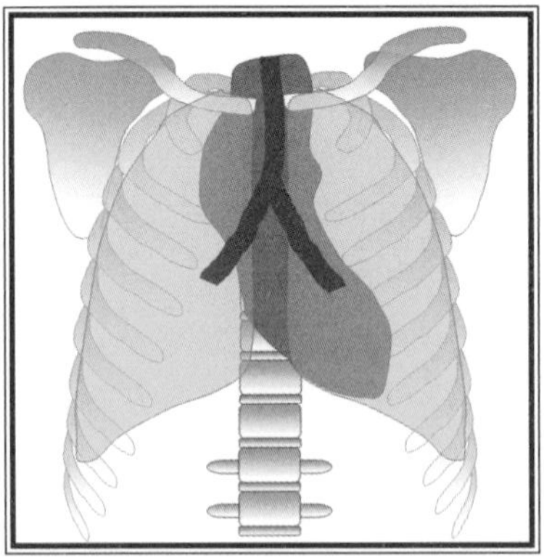

1. Large, predominantly right-sided, anterior mediastinal mass. This is causing displacement of the trachea to the left. The heart and lungs are normal in appearance.

2. The main differential diagnoses for an anterior mediastinal mass are: thyroid enlargement, thymoma, teratoma and lymphoma. CT of the chest will assist in identifying the extent of the mass and may also point towards a diagnosis, such as internal calcification in the case of a teratoma. Histological confirmation can be ascertained by CT-guided biopsy.

Answer 2.41

➥ question on page 256

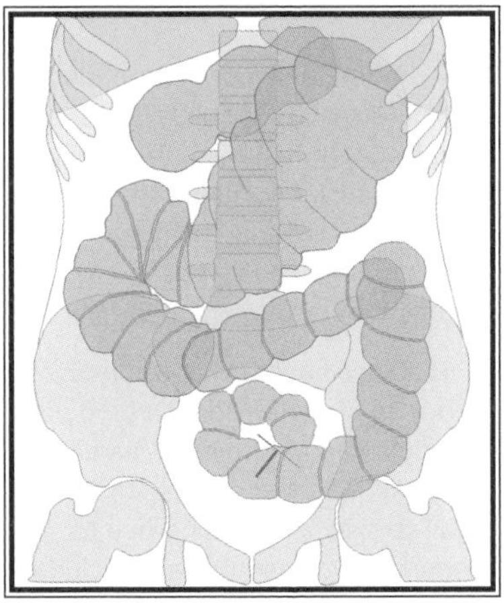

1. A large, distended, gas-filled, featureless viscus is sited in the right upper abdomen, which is separate from the collapsed stomach. The caecum is not apparent in the right iliac fossa. The small bowel is dilated. The appearances are consistent with a caecal volvulus with a resultant small bowel obstruction
2. Caecal volvulus typically occurs in young/middle-aged women with 'virgin' abdomens in comparison to sigmoid volvuli, which tend to cluster in the elderly population. Treatment is with surgery, requiring a caecopexy.

Answer 2.42

➥ question on page 257

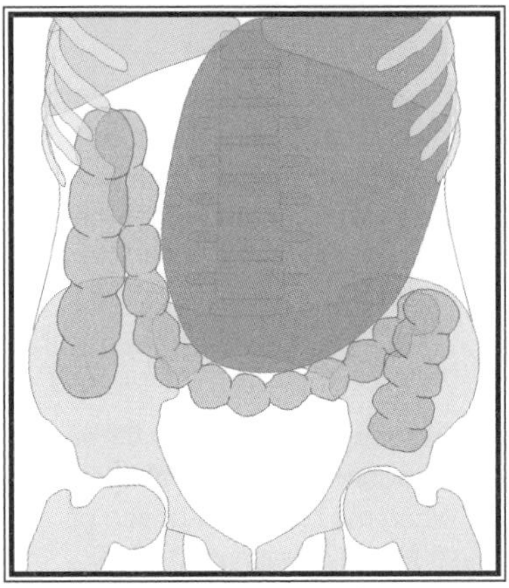

1. A large soft-tissue mass is present in the left upper quadrant extending inferomedially into the lower abdomen and upper pelvis. This is displacing both large and small bowel, consistent with being located within the peritoneal cavity. The findings are consistent with splenomegaly.
2. Potential causes of splenomegaly include: sickle cell disease, myelofibrosis and lymphoma.

Note the bilateral hip abnormalities (much more pronounced on the right) of sclerosis and collapse consistent with avascular necrosis. The unifying diagnosis is sickle cell disease. Later in the disease process the spleen may become small due to infarction.

Answer 2.43

➥ question on page 257

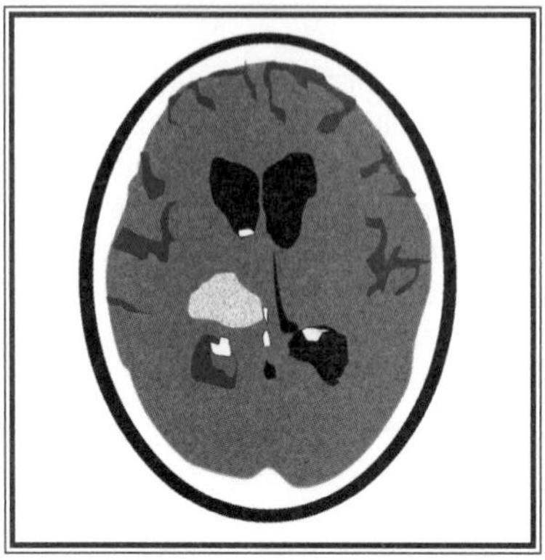

1. A moderate-sized, well-defined, high-attenuation focus is present in the right thalamus, in keeping with a thalamic haemorrhage. This is an intraparenchymal haematoma, and there is a little reactive surrounding oedema.

2. Thalamic haemorrhage is typically due to hypertension. This would be classed as a haemorrhagic stroke, which accounts for 15% of all strokes, most being due to infarction. Other typical locations for hypertensive haemorrhage include the basal ganglia and dentate nucleus of the cerebellum.

With large intraparenchymal haemorrhages there may be intraventricular extension. A small proportion of infarcts may undergo haemorrhagic transformation.

Answer 2.44

➥ question on page 258

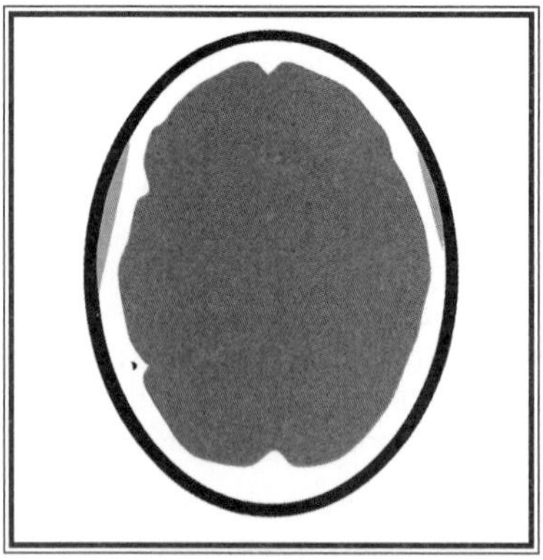

1. Throughout the visualised brain (on the single slice provided) there is diffuse loss of grey-white material differentiation of the brain parenchyma. In addition to this the basal cisterns are completely effaced. The sulci of the brain are also non-apparent.

2. The appearances of the CT are consistent with cerebral anoxia. When the brain is deprived of sufficient oxygenation for a prolonged period of time, eg during a cardiac arrest in the community with a long period of lost cardiac output, anoxia occurs. This results in the loss of grey-white matter differentiation and cytotoxic oedema.

Answer 2.45

➥ question on page 258

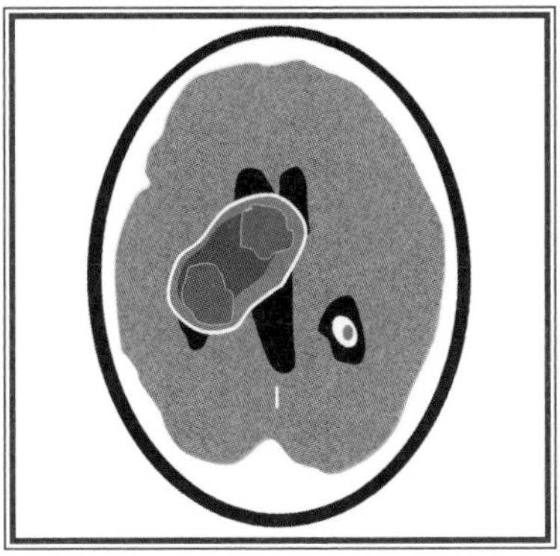

1. This post-contrast scan outlines a large heterogeneous enhancing mass in the right cerebral hemisphere bulging into and compressing the right lateral ventricle. The most likely cause for these appearances is a glioma. At present there is no evidence of hydrocephalus.
2. In adults, primary brain tumours are more common in the supratentorial than the infratentorial brain. The reverse is true in children. Potential supratentorial tumours include: glioblastoma multiforme, astrocytoma, meningioma, oligodendroglioma, neurofibroma and craniopharyngioma. Infratentorial (or posterior fossa) tumours include: ependymoma, pilocytic astrocytoma, brain-stem glioma, cerebellar haemangioblastoma and medulloblastoma, some of which are essentially unique to children.

Answer 2.46

➥ question on page 259

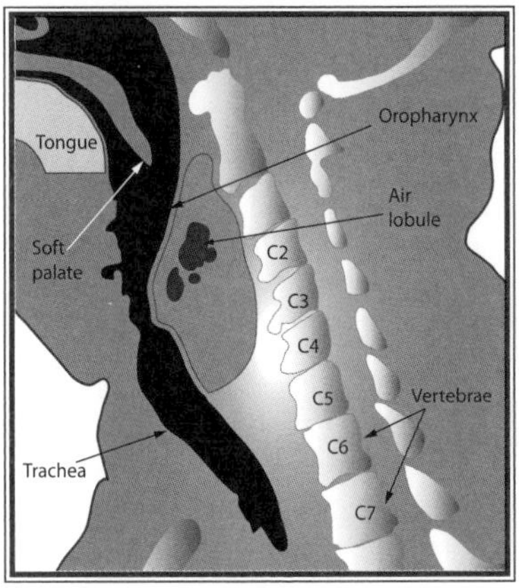

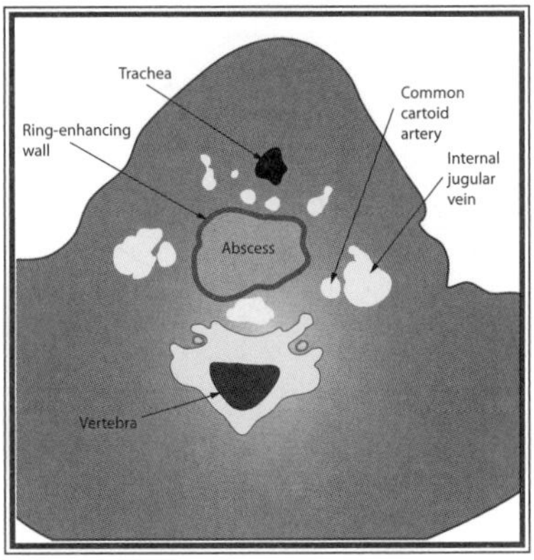

This shows a large, symmetrical, ring-enhancing cystic lesion in the retropharyneal space. This contains locules of gas, but there is no retrosternal extension and no involvement of the prevertebral space.

The appearances are in keeping with a retropharyngeal abscess.

Answer 2.47

question on page 260

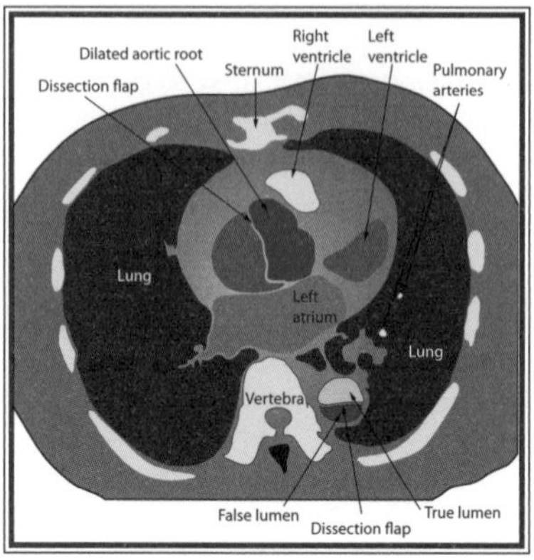

A CT thoracic angiogram has been performed to assess for an acute aortic injury. This covers the spectrum from intramural haematoma through to a frank dissection. In this case, the aortic root is dilated with a thin filling defect, representing the flap, extending from the root down into the descending aorta. One side of this (the smaller side) is the true lumen and the larger side is the false lumen. In the axial plane the appearances are similar to those of a tennis ball.

Given that the origin of the dissection is proximal to the left subclavian artery's origin from the aortic arch, this is a Stanford type A aortic dissection.

Answer 2.48

question on page 260

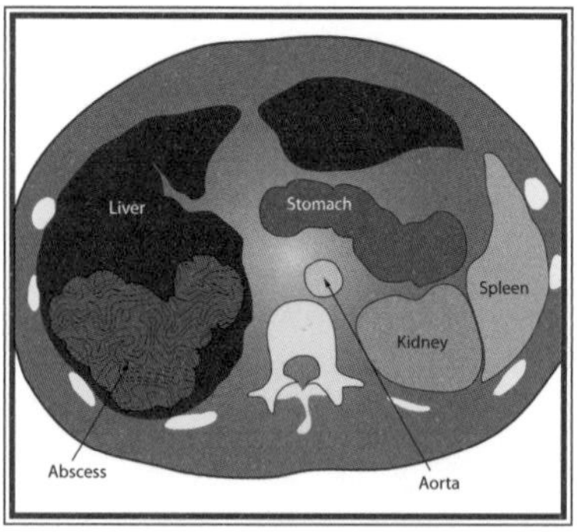

A large septated mass is seen in segments 7 and 6 of the liver. This is well defined with multiple thin septa and ring enhancement. There is no perihepatic collection. The spleen is normal in appearance.

The appearances are in keeping with a liver abscess. Given the septated nature, this is unlikely to be amenable to percutaneous drainage.

Answer 2.49

➥ question on page 261

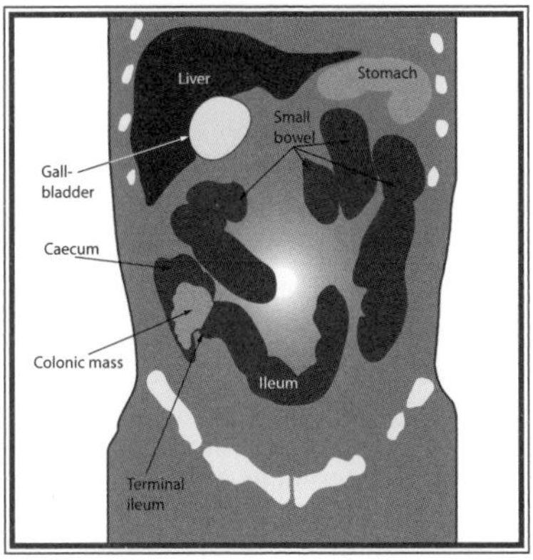

The entire small bowel is distended and fluid filled, down to the level of the ileocaecal valve. A caecal mass covers the ileocaecal valve and is the site of the obstruction. The large bowel has collapsed.

The appearances are of a high-grade distal small bowel obstruction due to an obstructing caecal malignancy.

Answer 2.50

➥ question on page 262

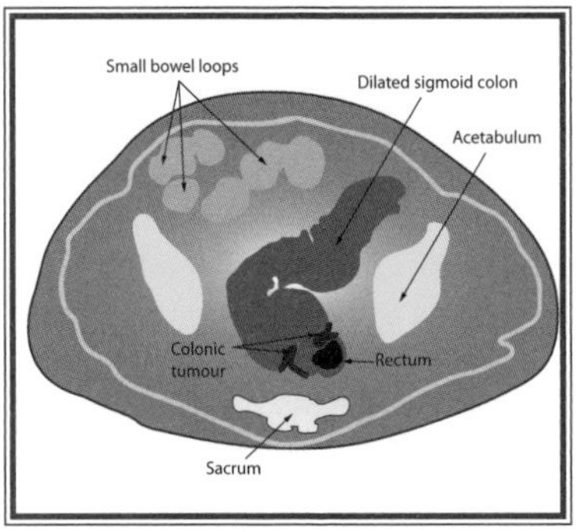

The large bowel is distended down to the level of a short stenosing tumour of the distal sigmoid colon. The rectum is collapsed.

There is no pneumoperitoneum, free fluid or collection. The appearances are those of a malignant large bowel obstruction.

Malignancy is the most common cause of a large bowel obstruction, unlike a small bowel obstruction in which malignancy features in only a small percentage of the causes for obstruction.

IV contrast is not always necessary to make the diagnosis of an obstruction on CT.

Answer 2.51

➥ question on page 262

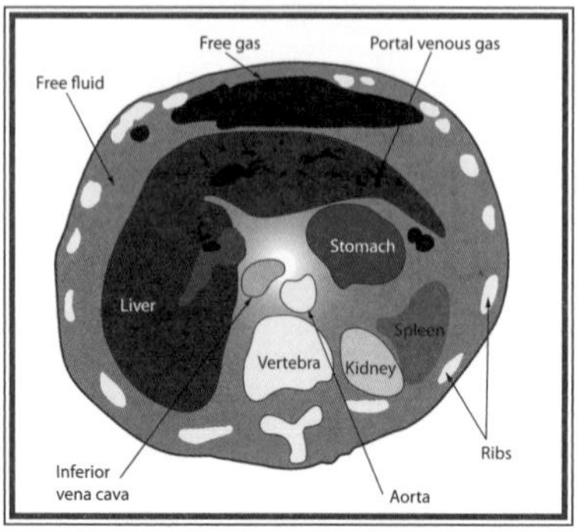

The CT illustrates a pneumoperitoneum. There is intramural gas in multiple small bowel loops. The foci of gas are in the portal vein and the hepatic vein. The small bowel wall is non-enhancing, indicating ischaemia, and there is a small volume of peritoneal free fluid.

The appearances are those of an ischaemic bowel.

Answer 2.52

➥ question on page 263

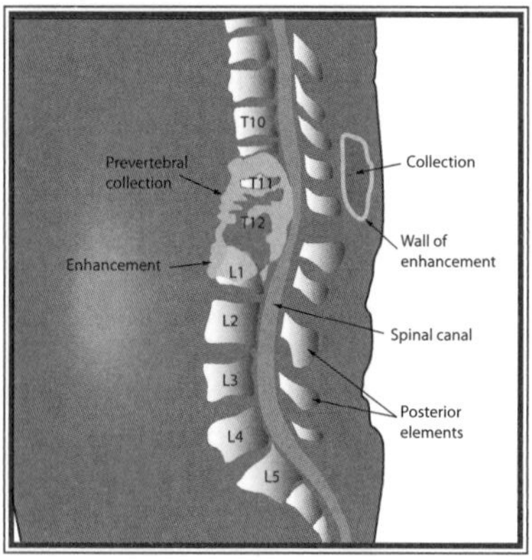

There is high T2 signal change in the T12 and L1 endplates with high T2 signal in the intervening discs. Avid contrast enhancement involves the T11–L2 vertebral bodies and the T12–L1 disc space. There is a rim-enhancing collection in the paraspinal muscles. The appearances are in keeping with spondylodiscitis.

Answer 2.53

➥ question on page 264

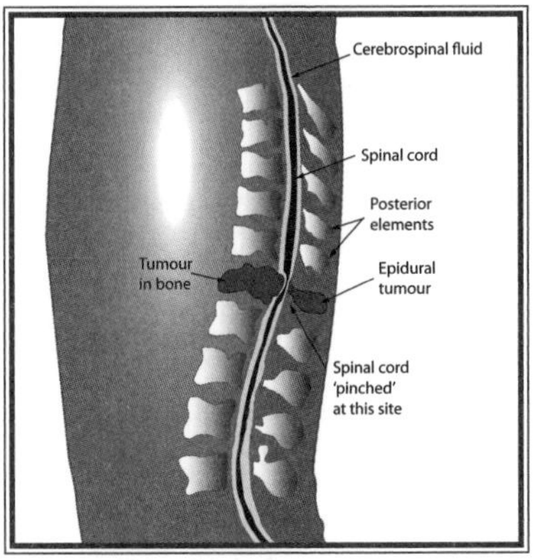

There is a metastatic deposit in the T12 vertebral body. This extends into the epidural space with displacement of the spinal cord. Further deposits are evident in the right transverse processes of L2 and L3. The appearances are those of metastatic cord compression.

Answer 2.54

➥ question on page 265

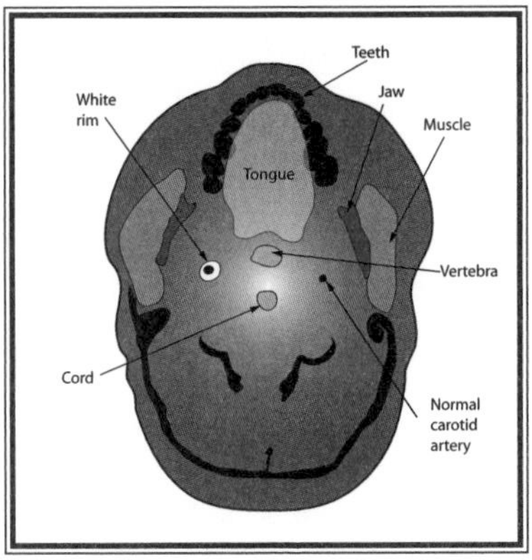

A crescenteric rim of high T2 signal surrounds the lumen of the right internal carotid artery on the T1 fat-saturated sequence, in keeping with intimal haemorrhage. The left internal carotid artery is normal.

Appearances are in keeping with a carotid artery dissection . Since anatomical structures often exist in pairs, comparison of the two structures is a useful way of detecting pathology.

Answer 2.55

➥ question on page 265

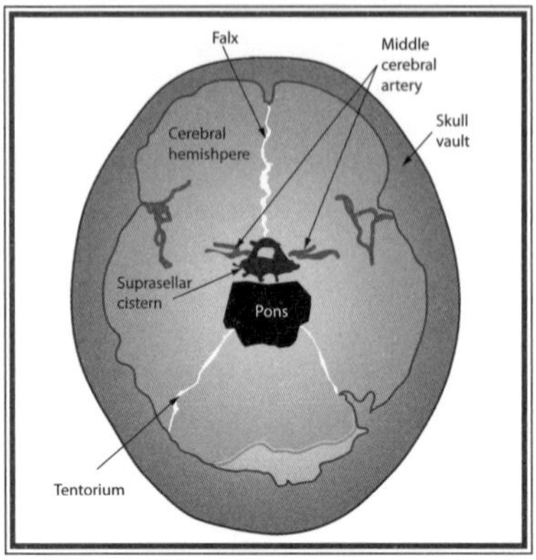

On a CT, acute blood has a high attenuation, so it can appear similar to contrast. This is one reason why, if there is any remote chance of haemorrhage or thrombus being clinically queried, a plain CT study should also be performed before the administration of contrast.

A dense, linear, high-attenuation abnormality is evident peripherally in the left side of the posterior fossa, parallel to the skull vault. This is asymmetrical compared with the right side and is consistent with a left transverse sinus thrombosis.

There are no changes in the left cerebellar hemisphere to suggest end-organ damage.

A CT or MR venogram would confirm this finding. The thrombus will appear as a filling defect within the contrast-filled sinus.

Answer 2.56

➥ question on page 266

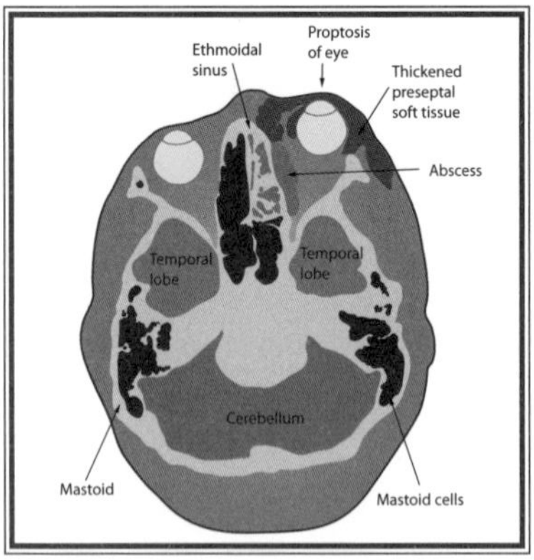

The CT shows a left-sided preseptal oedema. The maxillary sinuses are opacified with fluid, which is indicative of sinusitis.

A lentiform, rim-enhancing collection is evident on the medial aspect of the left orbit, displacing the medial rectus muscle laterally. The underlying lamina papyracea (the paper-thin bone that forms the medial orbit wall) is breeched.

This is the typical appearance of a subperiosteal collection secondary to sinusitis.

Answer 2.57

➥ question on page 266

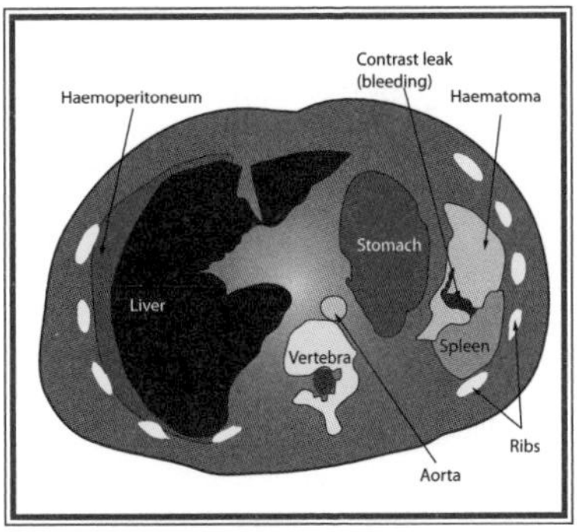

The use of contrast, often in multiple phases, is required in the assessment of haemodynamic instability in cases of trauma. This is required to accurately review for solid organ injuries.

Abnormal perfusion of the spleen with a large central laceration, along with perisplenic haematoma, indicates a case of high-grade splenic injury. In fact, contrast is extravasating from the splenic hilum, indicating active bleeding.

Answer 2.58

➥ question on page 267

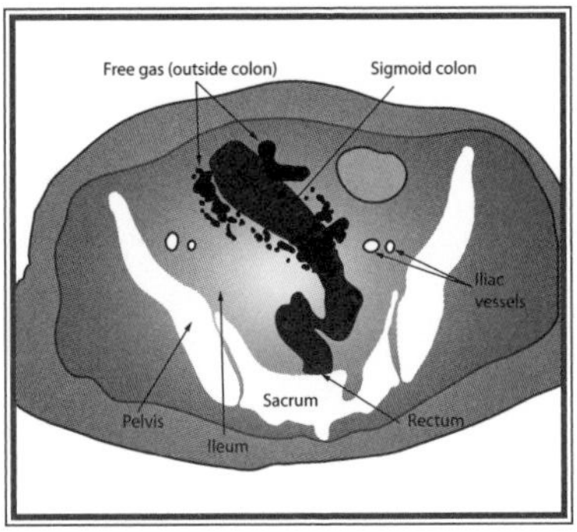

The distal sigmoid colon is thickened with an associated large amount of extraluminal gas and semisolid mass. There are multiple small loculi of gas adjacent to the sigmoid loop in the pelvis.

The appearances are of a sigmoid colon perforation – the mass represents a faeculoma, consistent with a stercoral performation.

Answer 2.59

➥ question on page 268

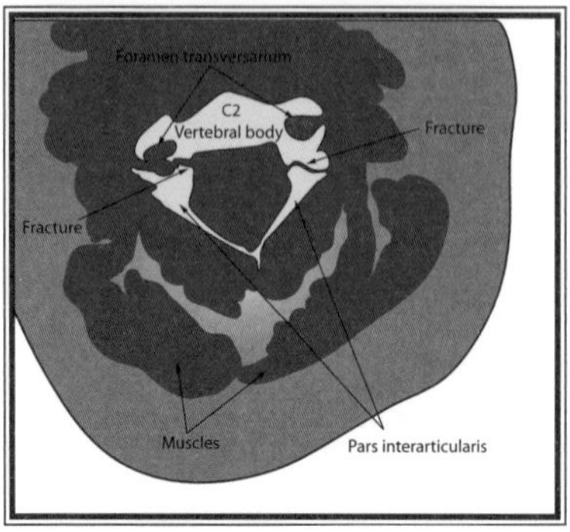

The CT of the cervical spine demonstrates bilateral pars interarticularis fractures of the C2 vertebra. The right pars interarticularis fracture extends into the foramen transversarium.

The C2–3 disc height is mildly increased with subtle anterolisthesis of C2. The atlantodental and atlantoaxial spaces are normal.

There is no significant paraspinal haematoma or spinal cord compression. The appearances are those of a Hangman's fracture.

3

AT THE BEDSIDE AND IN THE CLINIC

11

OBSERVATION CHARTS

The most easily measured and readily available data on a patient lie at the bedside on a series of observation charts. Nursing staff dutifully complete a number of observations on a regular basis. The nature of these and the frequency at which they are taken vary, depending on the clinical status of the patient. Analysis and interpretation of bedside chart data are an extension of the clinical assessment of a patient, and may provide the first evidence of a downward trend in clinical condition. The best way to learn from bedside charts is to pick them up and try to interpret them during your clinical attachments.

DON'T FORGET

Data interpretation begins at the end of the bed.

Vital signs

The so-called 'vital signs' represent the basic set of observations that are recorded regularly for all patients and include the parameters listed in the box below.

BASIC OBSERVATIONS MEASURED (WITH NORMAL RANGES)

Pulse rate	60–100 beats/min
Blood pressure	Abnormally high - >140 mmHg systolic or >90 mmHg diastolic Abnormally low - <90 mmHg systolic or a drop of 20 mmHg or more systolic from the patient's baseline
Respiratory rate	14–18 breaths per minute
Oxygen saturation	96–100% on room air
Temperature	36.5–37.5°C

Looking at how a particular physiological parameter varies with time can be highly informative. For example, taking a one-off temperature recording may or may not be useful in a patient with a particular symptom, but much more useful is the way in which the patient's temperature varies with time. In the example in Fig 11.1, the temperature can be seen to be 'swinging' and this pattern is highly suggestive of a serious infection or inflammatory process.

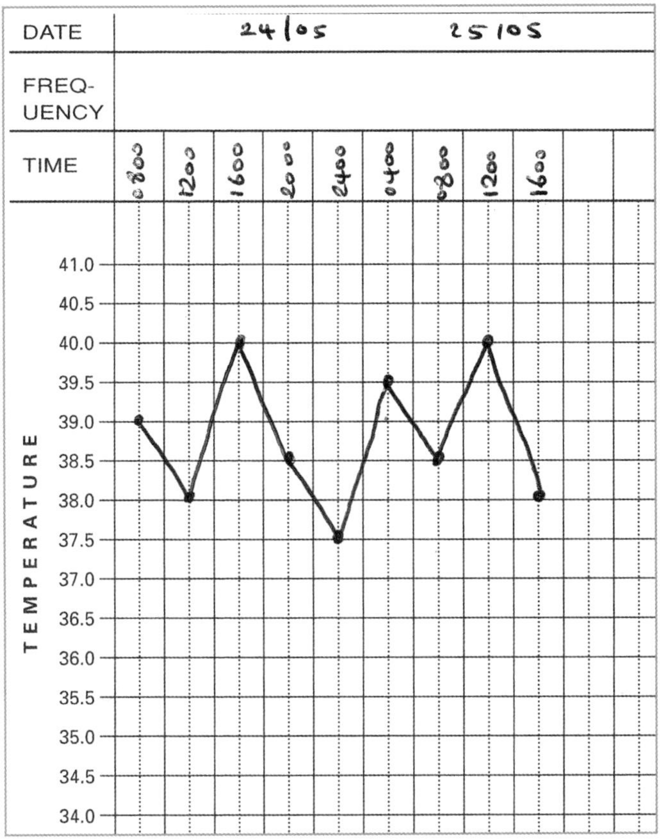

Fig 11.1: Swinging fever.

Similarly, a steadily rising respiratory rate or pulse rate, or a falling blood pressure, can highlight evolving physiological changes much more readily than can a snapshot recording at one moment in time.

Early warning scores

'Early warning scores' are now commonplace in clinical areas, with the National Early Warning Score (NEWS) being favoured in many hospitals. To calculate such a score, weightings are given for deviations in set physiological parameters away from normality. The higher the deviation, the greater the score. An example is shown in the table below. There are several advantages to such a system. A patient with seemingly minor abnormalities in several parameters will be identified as acutely unwell because their score will be quite high. Also, nursing staff who might not be confident in knowing when to call for medical assistance can be assured that a high score equates to a seriously unwell patient who requires urgent help from a senior doctor. As with any vital sign measurement, a change in early warning score is more informative than a one-off reading.

	3	2	1	0	1	2	3
Pulse (beats/min)		<40	41-50	51-90	91-110	111-130	≥131
Respiratory rate (breaths/min)	≤8		9-11	12-20		21-24	≥25
Temperature (°C)	≤35		35.1-36.0	36.1-38.0	38.1-39.0	≥39.1	
Systolic BP (mmHg)	≤90	91-100	101-110	111-219			≥220
SaO_2 (%)	≤91	92-93	94-95	≥96			
Inspired O_2				Air		Supplemental O_2	
CNS (use AVPU scale)				Alert (A)			Voice (V) Pain (P) Unresponsive (U)

Royal College of Physicians. *National Early Warning Score (NEWS)*. London: RCP, 2012.

Neurological observations

Neurological observations are recorded at intervals in patients who are at risk of deterioration in their level of consciousness. Two commonly used systems are described.

1. AVPU

This is a quickly recorded summary measure of neurological status. The patient is graded as:

A - if they are **A**lert
V - if they respond to **V**oice
P - if they respond only to **P**ain
U - if they are **U**nresponsive.

2. Glasgow Coma Scale (GCS)

This is more time-consuming to measure than the AVPU score, but also provides more information. It is scored out of 15, with a minimum score of 3 and a maximum of 15. The patient's best response at the time of assessment should be recorded.

TASK	PERFORMANCE	SCORE
Eyes open	Spontaneously	4
	To speech	3
	To pain	2
	None	1
Best verbal response	Oriented	5
	Confused	4
	Inappropriate words	3
	Incomprehensible sounds	2
	None	1
Best motor response	Obeys commands	6
	Localises pain	5
	Flexion withdrawal	4
	Abnormal flexion	3
	Extension to pain	2
	None	1

Figure 11.2 shows a GCS chart from a patient who exhibits a sudden drop in GCS at 11am.

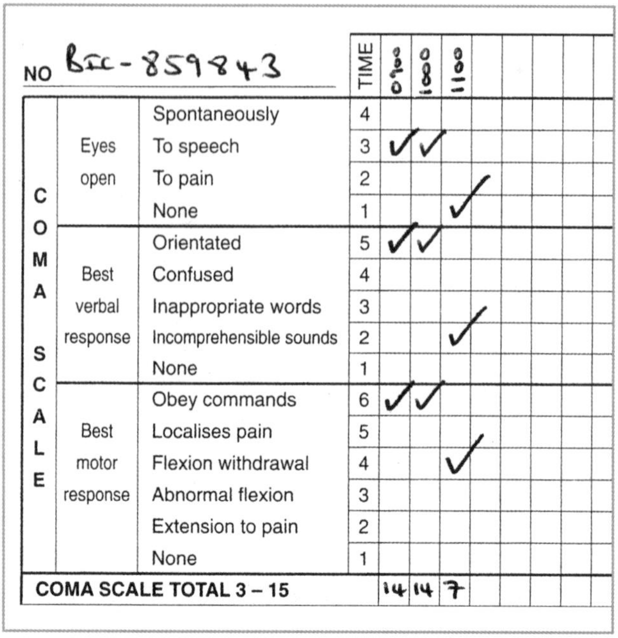

NO BCC-859843

			TIME	0700	1000	1100
COMA SCALE	Eyes open	Spontaneously	4			
		To speech	3	✓	✓	
		To pain	2			
		None	1			✓
	Best verbal response	Orientated	5	✓	✓	
		Confused	4			
		Inappropriate words	3			
		Incomprehensible sounds	2			✓
		None	1			
	Best motor response	Obey commands	6	✓	✓	
		Localises pain	5			
		Flexion withdrawal	4			✓
		Abnormal flexion	3			
		Extension to pain	2			
		None	1			
COMA SCALE TOTAL 3 – 15				14	14	7

Fig 11.2: Sudden drop in GCS.

Fluid balance

A carefully completed fluid balance chart can be extremely helpful in making management decisions for patients. In essence, these charts record the quantity and type of all fluid entering and leaving the body.

Examples of fluid entering the body:

- Food and drink taken orally
- Intravenous fluid
- Nutrition given enterally (eg via a nasogastric or percutaneous gastrostomy tube) or parenterally (ie intravenous feeding)
- Blood products (eg packed red cells, platelets, cryoprecipitate, fresh frozen plasma)
- Intravenous drugs.

Examples of fluid leaving the body:

- Urine
- Bowel motions
- Blood (from any orifice, including blood loss during surgery)
- Fluid from drains (eg chest drain).

One should also bear in mind insensible fluid loss. This refers to fluid that is lost but not normally recorded, and includes moisture lost in expired air and sweat. A general rule of thumb is that, in normal circumstances, a patient loses approximately 500 ml/day of fluid through insensible losses. These losses can increase massively, eg if a patient has extensive burns or if they have a fever.

Interpreting a fluid balance chart should incorporate several steps:

1. Compare total input with total output, remembering to account for insensible losses. Are they equal, or is there a positive or negative fluid balance? A positive fluid balance means that more fluid has entered the patient than has left, and would be entirely appropriate, for example, in a patient being treated for dehydration. A negative fluid balance means that more fluid has left the patient than has entered, and would be entirely appropriate, for example, in a patient with heart failure who is fluid overloaded and being treated with diuretics. Is the total volume of fluid entering the patient too little, adequate or too much for requirements? This will depend on the age, sex and weight of the patient, and also on the state of health (particularly current illnesses, cardiac and renal function).
2. Look at the type of fluid that the patient has received and correlate this with the clinical circumstances.
3. Think about electrolytes. Is the patient receiving enough electrolyte replacement to account for his or her body's daily requirements as well as compensating him or her for any abnormal electrolyte losses. For example, an elderly person might require 40 mmol potassium per day to maintain potassium equilibrium when healthy. If he develops severe diarrhoea, however, he will lose a lot of potassium from the gut and may well need much more than 40 mmol potassium per day to prevent him becoming hypokalaemic. Output from drains can often be important sources of electrolyte losses and can easily be overlooked.

Drug charts

A great deal of information about a patient can be gleaned by examining their drug chart. Errors are common and doctors at all levels should be vigilant and watch for potentially dangerous mistakes or oversights in drug prescriptions.

Other bedside data

Stool chart

Patients with altered bowel activity often have bowel movements recorded using a stool chart based on the 'Bristol Stool Chart' (Fig 11.3). Although not very appealing, a chart such as this allows staff to record the frequency and nature of bowel activity.

Bristol Stool Chart

Type 1	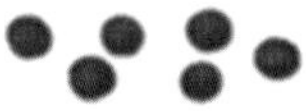	Separate, hard lumps, like nuts (hard to pass)
Type 2	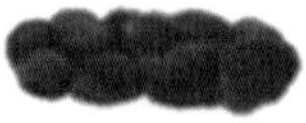	Sausage-shaped but lumpy
Type 3	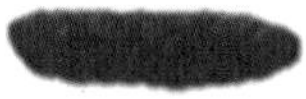	Like a sausage but with cracks on its surface
Type 4	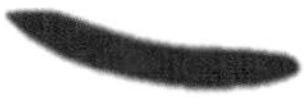	Like a sausage or snake, smooth and soft
Type 5		Soft blobs with clear-cut edges (passed easily)
Type 6	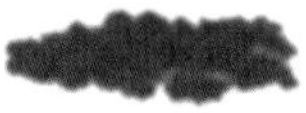	Fluffy with ragged edges, a mushy stool
Type 7	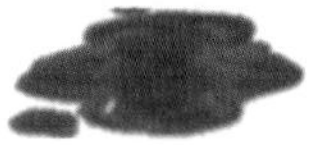	Watery, no solid pieces. **Entirely liquid**

Fig 11.3: Bristol Stool Chart. (From Lewis SJ, Heaton KW. Stool form scale as a useful guide to intestinal transit time. *Scand J Gastroenterol* 1997;**32**:920–4.)

Weight chart

It is often helpful to monitor a patient's weight with time. Malnourished patients might be monitored for weight gain after the establishment of a feeding programme, whereas patients with fluid overload are often monitored for weight loss as they are treated with diuretics and their oedema improves. Sudden dramatic changes in weight are, however, uncommon. Unless the patient has had a procedure (eg a large quantity of fluid drained or limb amputation), be wary that a sudden change in weight might simply be an error.

Blood glucose (and ketones)

Patients with diabetes mellitus will have their blood glucose level checked frequently during their stay using finger-prick blood draws and glucometers. Adjustments to their treatment may be required if they have either hyper- or hypoglycaemia. Patients with diabetic ketoacidosis (and some other patients too) will also have measurements taken of ketone levels in the blood or urine. Blood ketone levels are increasingly being measured with bedside ketometers, which work much like glucometers. Urinary ketones are measured using urinalysis strips. As treatment for ketoacidosis is administered, ketone levels should fall into the normal range.

Blood glucose recording is not limited to patients with diabetes, however. Other examples of patients who should have blood glucose measured include:

- Patients who have been treated with insulin for hyperkalaemia
- Patients who are malnourished and are at risk of hypoglycaemia
- Patients with liver failure who are at risk of hypoglycaemia
- Patients on high doses of corticosteroids who are at risk of hyperglycaemia.

Respiratory function

Patients with respiratory difficulty often have simple respiratory tests performed at regular intervals. The most common example would be the peak expiratory flow rate (PEFR) in patients with obstructive airway diseases such as asthma. In addition, patients at risk of neuromuscular weakness affecting respiration should have their vital capacity checked regularly. A falling vital capacity can indicate the need for assistance with ventilation. (See Chapter 13 for more information.)

Cardiac telemetry

Patients with cardiac disease and critical illness are at risk of cardiac arrhythmia and cardiac arrest, and their heart's electrical activity is often monitored using a bedside ECG machine. Interpretation of such data is included in Chapter 12. A useful function of many telemetry machines is that the heart rhythm strips are stored for several days. Patients who exhibit intermittent cardiac arrhythmias can have their heart rhythms analysed retrospectively, thus allowing the identification of serious problems.

Other information at the bedside

The area around a patient's bed often has a wealth of additional information for the astute observer to note. Therapists who have assessed a patient may record information such as the following on signs around the bed:

- Details about mobility, including devices to be used when mobilising or how many staff members will be required to help a patient mobilise.
- Communication difficulties: patients with deafness, dysphasia or who do not speak the native language may therefore be identified.
- Swallowing difficulties: signs such as 'nil orally' or 'yoghurt consistency foods only' might be seen.
- Dietary and fluid requirements such as fluid restrictions, salt restrictions, etc.

OBSERVATION CHARTS – WHAT YOU NEED TO KNOW

- When reviewing real patients, take time to review the wealth of data that is recorded on bedside charts.
- Trends are usually much more informative than one-off readings.
- A high early warning score is usually an indication of a very unwell patient who requires urgent attention.
- Make sure that you know how to assess level of consciousness on the AVPU scale and Glasgow Coma Scale.
- Do not forget to account for insensible losses when assessing fluid balance data.
- Sudden rapid changes in weight are usually due to error, fluid shifts or a medical procedure.

12

INVESTIGATIONS IN CARDIOLOGY

Electrocardiography

The electrocardiogram (ECG) is one of the most important commonly requested tests in medical practice.

DON'T FORGET

If possible, always compare ECGs with previous tracings.

Components of an ECG tracing

A standard ECG comprises 12 individual tracings (called leads). An ECG machine produces these tracings by comparing electrical signals from 10 sensors. Six are placed on the chest and one on each of the four limbs. By convention, the tracings are given standard names, with each representing an electrical signal from a particular part of the heart. V1, V2, V3, V4, V5 and V6 'look at' the heart in a horizontal plane. Each of these tracings represents the electrical signal detected at one of the chest sensors; aVL, aVF, aVR, I, II and III look at the heart in a vertical plane.

LEAD	LOOKS AT
V1, V2, V3 and V4	Anterior surface (right ventricle and septum)
V5, V6, aVL and I	Lateral surface (left ventricle)
II, III and aVF	Inferior surface
aVR	Right atrium

In a patient having an acute myocardial infarction, it is therefore possible to determine which part of the heart is affected by assessing which leads show changes.

If any individual lead is examined in detail, various peaks and troughs will be noted. These represent electrical activity at various times in the cardiac cycle. It is sometimes difficult to see every detail on each tracing. Names are attached to particular parts of the tracing as follows.

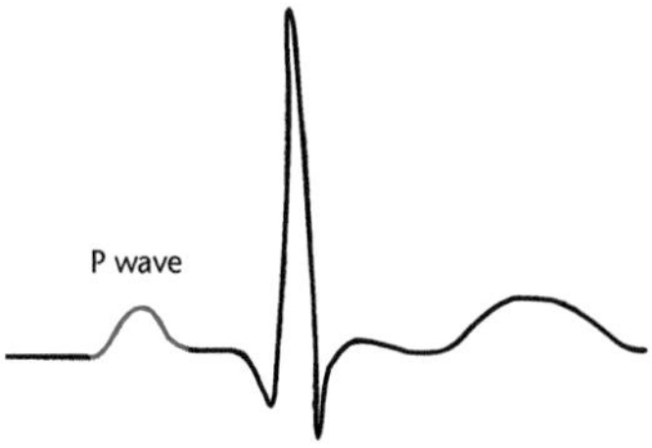

Fig 12.1: The P wave.

The first bump in a tracing is called a 'P wave'. This represents the electrical activity associated with depolarisation of the atria. There is a further electrical signal associated with atrial repolarisation, but this cannot usually be seen on an ECG, since the small electrical signal is overshadowed by the much more powerful ventricular activity.

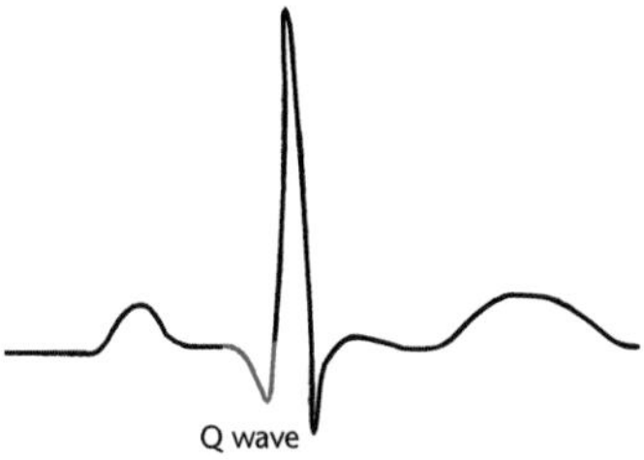

Fig 12.2: The Q wave.

Following along from the P wave, a downward dip in the tracing is known as a Q wave. This may or may not be present.

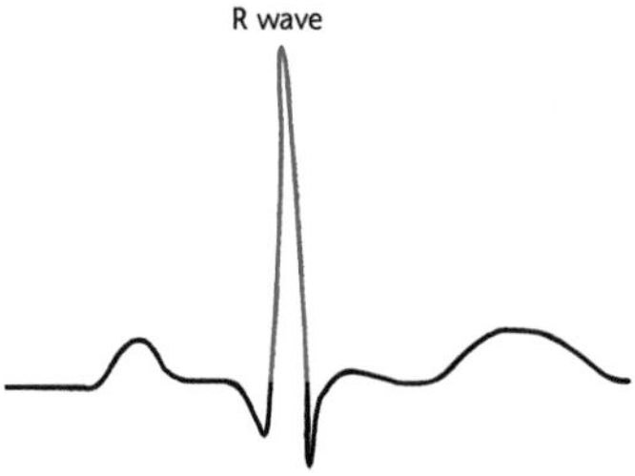

Fig 12.3: The R wave.

The first upward peak after the P wave is known as an R wave.

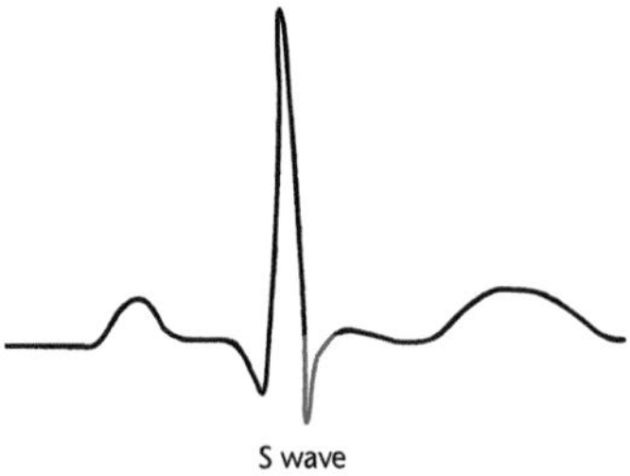

Fig 12.4: The S wave.

Any dip below the baseline following an R wave is called an S wave.

The Q, R and S waves are known collectively as the QRS complex. This represents ventricular depolarisation.

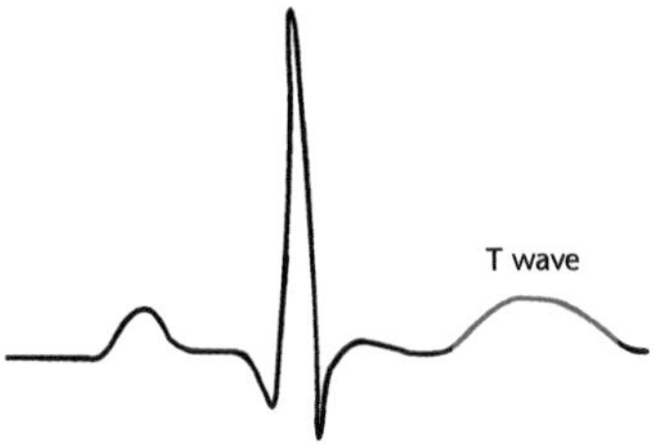

Fig 12.5: The T wave.

Following the QRS complex, an upward deflection in the tracing is known as a T wave. This represents ventricular repolarisation. T waves are followed by P waves, and the cycle is complete.

Interpreting an ECG

The following aspects should be addressed when interpreting an ECG:

Heart rate	QRS complexes
Heart rhythm	ST segment
Cardiac axis	Q-T interval
P waves	T waves

Heart rate

ECGs are printed on squared paper. This paper usually runs through the ECG machine at a standard rate (25 mm/s). If, for some reason, the machine is set to run at a different speed, interpretation is more difficult.

DON'T FORGET

Always check that the paper speed is at 25 mm per second.

At this speed, on a horizontal axis, each small square represents 0.04 second, and each large square (which is five small squares wide) represents 0.2 second.

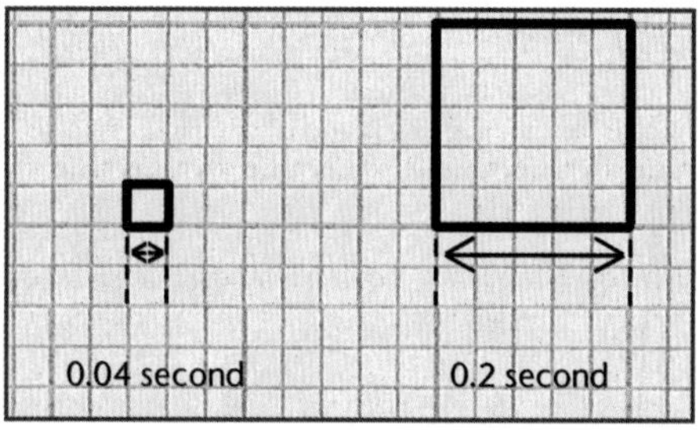

Fig 12.6: Standard squared paper used when recording ECGs.

The ventricular rate is calculated by looking at the distance between consecutive QRS complexes. Usually the distance between R waves is analysed.

When there are a number of large squares between each R wave, the ventricular rate is most easily calculated by counting the number of large squares between each R wave and dividing this number into 300.

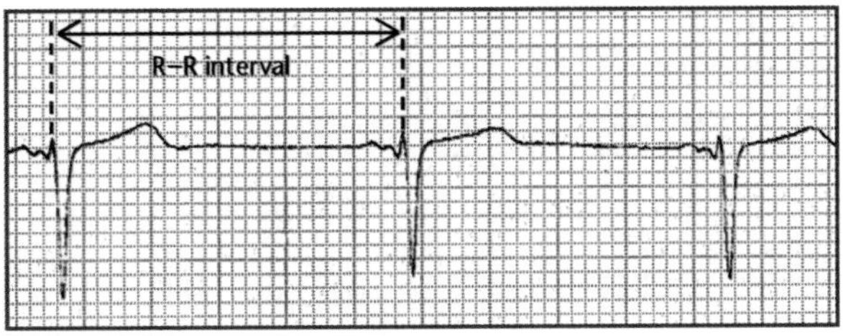

Fig 12.7: Measuring the R-R interval.

In the ECG shown, there are approximately five large squares between each R wave. The ventricular rate is therefore 300 ÷ 5 = 60 beats/min.

When the ventricular rhythm is more rapid, counting large squares can prove difficult. In such instances, the number of small squares between consecutive R waves is counted, and this number divided into 1500.

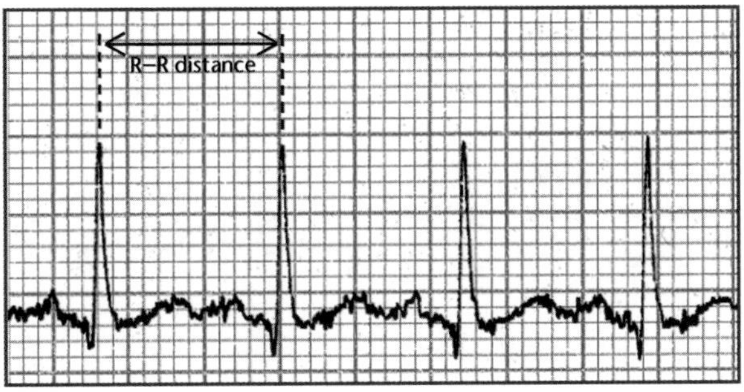

Fig 12.8: Measuring the R-R interval with a faster heart rate.

In the example, there are 12 small squares between each R wave. The ventricular rate is therefore 1500 ÷ 12 = 125 beats/min.

Ventricular rate (beats per minute) = 300 ÷ number of large squares between R waves

OR

Ventricular rate (beats per minute) = 1500 ÷ number of small squares between R waves

Both approaches give the same answer, but the second approach tends to be easier if the heart rate is rapid.

A heart rate of less than 60 beats/min is termed **bradycardia**. A rate of greater than 100 beats/min is **tachycardia**.

If the heart rhythm is irregular, calculate the rate using the number of squares between several R waves. Divide the answer to obtain an average R-R interval.

For example, if there are 40 large squares between the first and the eleventh R wave, the average R-R interval is 4 large squares and the heart rate is approximately 300 ÷ 4 = 75 beats/min.

Heart rhythm

There are several heart rhythms that you will be expected to recognise. To assess rhythm, look for P waves and their relationship to QRS complexes. Remember that normally one P wave should be followed by one QRS complex. Good leads for assessing P waves are leads II, V1 and V2.

Sinus rhythm

Sinus rhythm describes a normal heart rhythm in which electrical signals begin in the sinus node. A P wave should precede each QRS complex, and be at a normal, fixed interval from it. The P-R interval is used to measure the interval between P waves and QRS complexes. It is measured by counting the number of squares between the start of the P wave and the start of the QRS complex. This distance should be between three and five small squares.

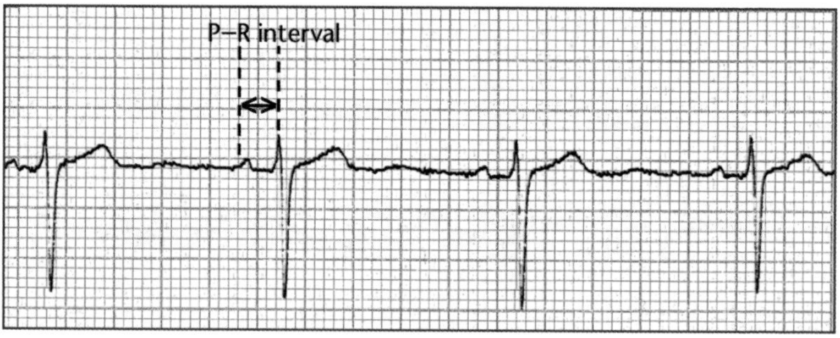

Fig 12.9: Normal sinus rhythm illustrating the P-R interval.

- Sinus tachycardia describes sinus rhythm at a rate of over 100 beats/min.
- Sinus bradycardia describes sinus rhythm at less than 60 beats/min.
- Sinus arrhythmia is the term used to describe the normal variation in heart rate with respiration. Normally, the heart rate increases on inspiration.

MEMORY AID

In sinus arrhythmia, the heart rate INcreases on INspiration.

SINUS RHYTHM CHECKS

To diagnose sinus rhythm, all of the following criteria should be met:
1. P wave preceding every QRS complex
2. P-R interval is normal
3. P-R interval is constant

Atrial fibrillation

This is the term used to describe erratic electrical activity in the atria. In this condition, no P waves are seen, and the ECG baseline commonly shows irregularity. QRS complexes occur irregularly.

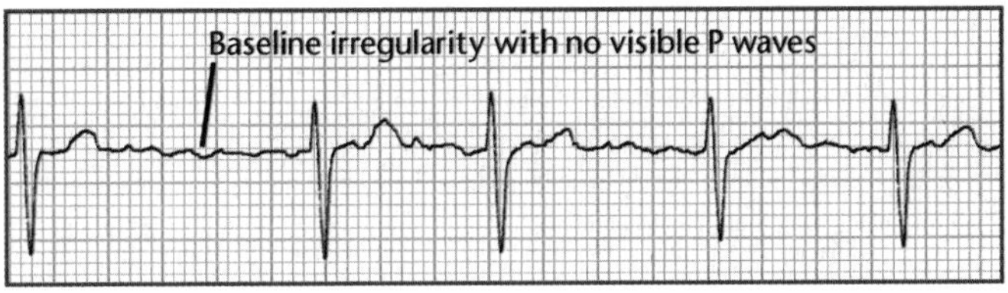

Fig 12.10: Atrial fibrillation.

This tracing fails sinus rhythm check 1, as no P waves are visible.

Atrial flutter

This condition is similar to atrial fibrillation in many ways. However, the ECG shows the presence of F waves (flutter waves). The baseline of the ECG therefore adopts a 'saw-toothed' appearance. Atrial flutter may occur with a fixed degree of atrioventricular block, eg three-to-one block. This means that, for every three flutter waves, there would be one QRS complex. Alternatively, the rhythm may have variable block, where the number of flutter waves preceding each QRS complex varies from beat to beat.

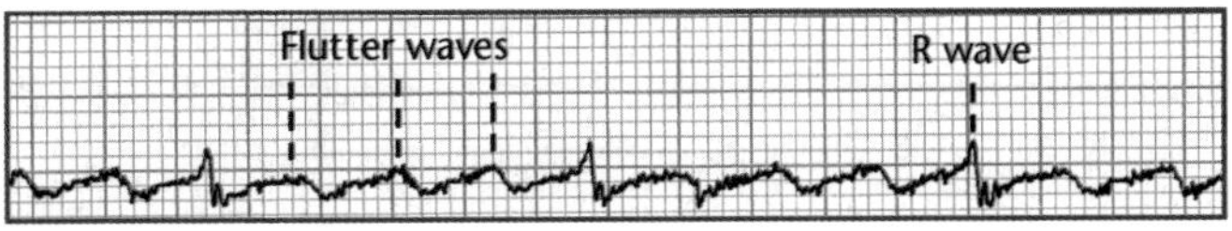

Fig 12.11: Atrial flutter.

This tracing fails sinus rhythm check 1, as no P waves are visible. You should be able to instantly recognise atrial flutter on account of its distinctive appearance.

Heart block

Heart block describes a problem with conduction between the atria and ventricles. There are various types.

First-degree heart block

In first-degree heart block, a P wave precedes each QRS complex, but the P–R interval is prolonged (more than five small squares). The P–R interval remains constant from beat to beat.

In simple terms, imagine first-degree heart block as a condition in which the wiring of the heart is still intact, but is a little slow. It therefore takes longer than normal for electrical signals to travel from the atria to the ventricles.

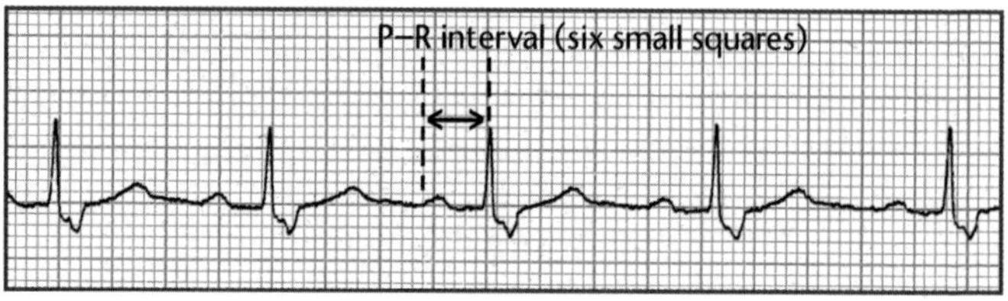

Fig 12.12: First-degree heart block.

You will appreciate that this example is not normal sinus rhythm because, although there is a P wave before every QRS complex (check 1), the P–R interval is prolonged (six small squares).

Second-degree heart block

Second-degree heart block describes the spectrum of conduction problems that are more severe than first-degree, but less severe than third-degree, heart block.

There are three main types:

1. Mobitz type I (Wenckebach phenomenon)
   This rhythm runs in cycles, and will be identified if the tests for sinus rhythm are checked. The first P–R interval in a cycle is often normal. With each successive heart beat, the P–R interval lengthens. Eventually, there will be a P wave with no following QRS complex. The cycle then begins again.

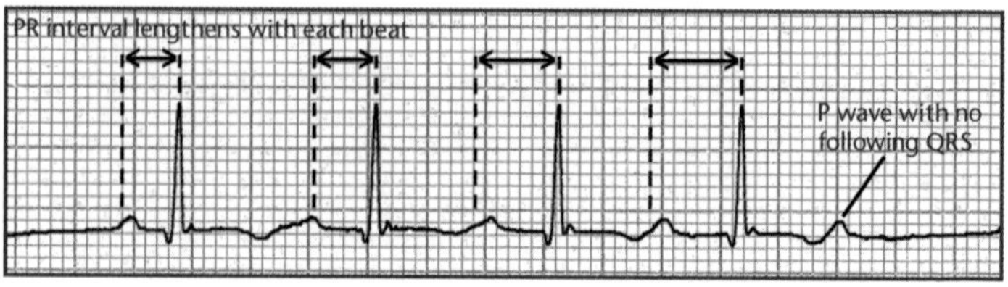

Fig 12.13: Mobitz type I heart block.

2. Mobitz type II
   Again, you will diagnose this rhythm if you check the requirements for sinus rhythm. In this rhythm, the P–R interval is constant. Its duration may be normal or prolonged. However, periodically there will be no conduction between the atria and ventricles, and there will be a P wave with no associated QRS complex.

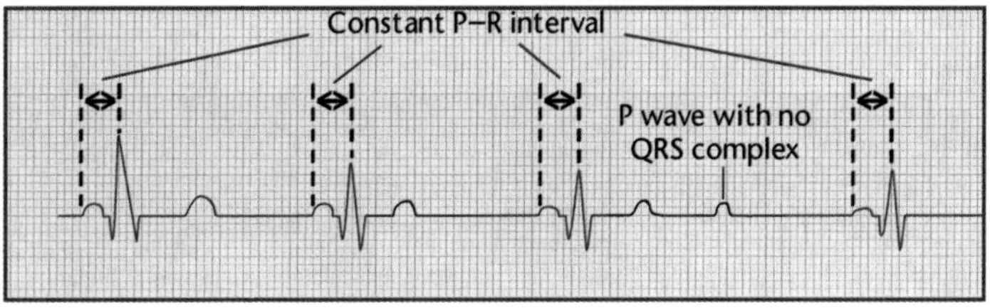

Fig 12.14: Mobitz type II heart block.

3. Fixed degrees of atrioventricular block
   These rhythms are described as two-to-one, three-to-one, four-to-one block, etc. In two-to-one block, for example, two P waves are found for every QRS complex.

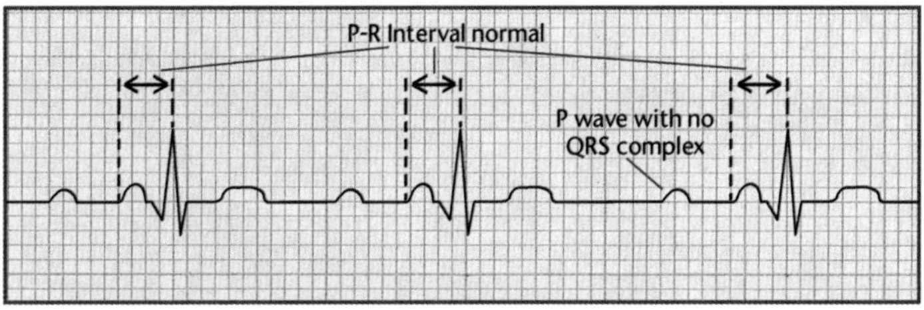

Fig 12.15: Two-to-one atrioventricular block.

Third-degree heart block

In this condition, there is no functioning electrical connection between the atria and ventricles. You may like to think of this as a state in which the 'wires' between atria and ventricles have been 'cut'. P waves and QRS complexes will be seen, but these will have no constant relationship to each other. If you suspect this rhythm, take a sheet of paper and lay it alongside the ECG in question. Mark on the paper the position of the P waves. Next, move your paper so that the first mark you have made lines up with the first QRS complex. You will see that the P waves and QRS complexes are completely dissociated. The QRS complex arises because of intrinsic pacemaker activity below the atrioventricular node.

Note that QRS complexes can be normal in width or wide (see below).

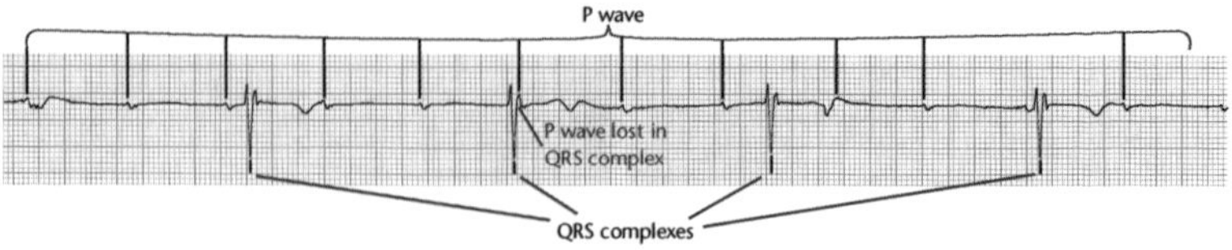

Fig 12.16: Third-degree heart block.

Cardiac axis

The cardiac axis is an arbitrary concept used to describe the average direction of electrical activity in the heart. Normally, the average flow of electrical energy is from the upper right heart border towards the apex. In various disease states, the cardiac axis can shift.

There are several methods for assessing axis, but students often find this a difficult exercise. One method relies on looking at leads I, II and III, and determining whether the QRS complexes are predominantly upgoing or downgoing. QRS complexes in a particular lead are upgoing if average electrical flow (axis) is towards that lead, and downgoing if it is away from the lead (Fig 12.17).

A good rule of thumb is to assess the QRS complexes in leads I and II and, if both are predominantly upgoing, the axis is normal as shown in Fig 12.19. In right axis deviation, the axis shifts clockwise and, as a result lead I becomes downgoing because average electrical flow is away from it. In left axis deviation, the axis shifts anti-clockwise and, as a result, leads II and III become downgoing. Figure 12.18 illustrates the standard convention for quantifying the cardiac axis. Figure 12.19 illustrates all three scenarios.

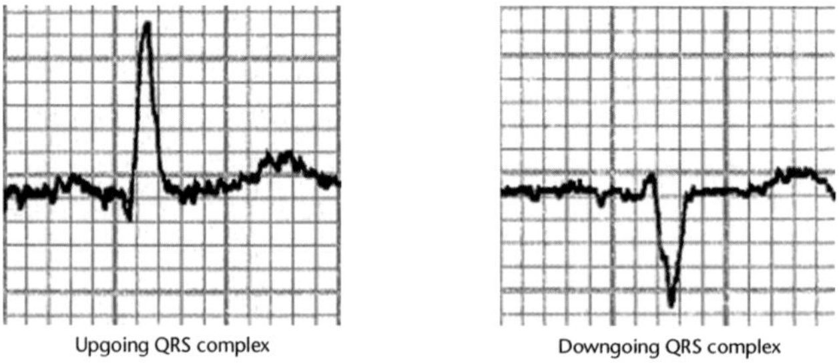

Fig 12.17: Upgoing and downgoing QRS complexes.

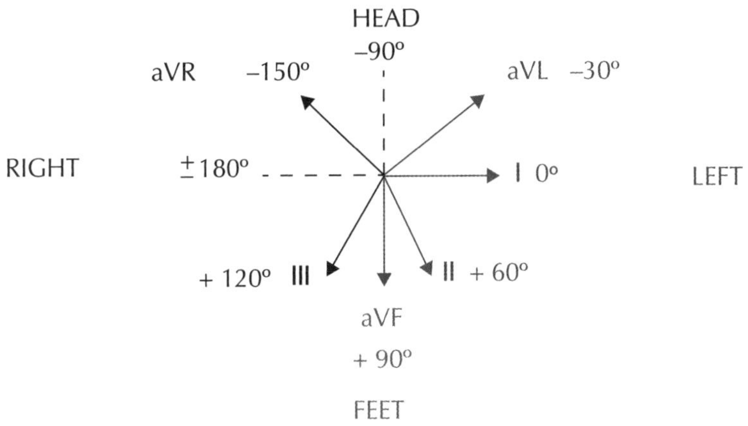

Fig 12.18

AXIS	LEAD I	LEAD II	LEAD III
Normal	Upgoing	Upgoing	Upgoing (or downgoing)
Right axis deviation	Downgoing	Upgoing	Upgoing
Left axis deviation	Upgoing	Downgoing	Downgoing

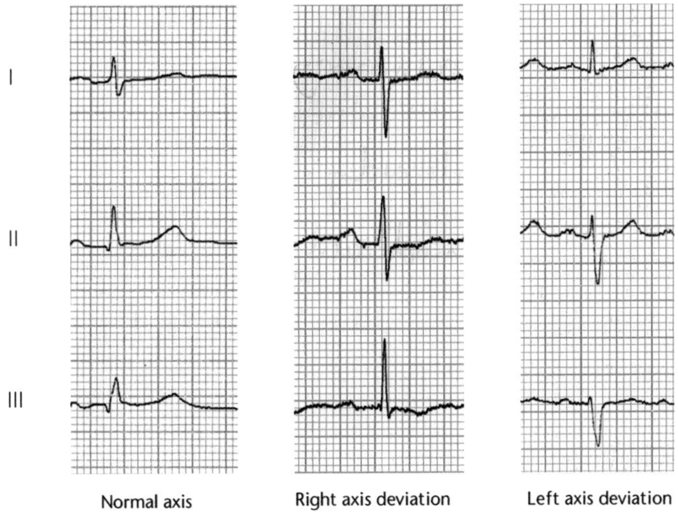

Fig 12.19: Leads I, II and III showing a normal axis, right axis deviation and left axis deviation.

P waves

Look at leads II, V1 and V2 for the best views of P waves. Assess their size and shape. P waves should not exceed the maximum dimensions shown in Fig 12.20. Always make sure that an ECG has been correctly calibrated before commenting on the heights of peaks. The standard calibration is 10 mm = 1 mV.

DON'T FORGET

Always check that an ECG is calibrated to 10 mm = 1 mV.

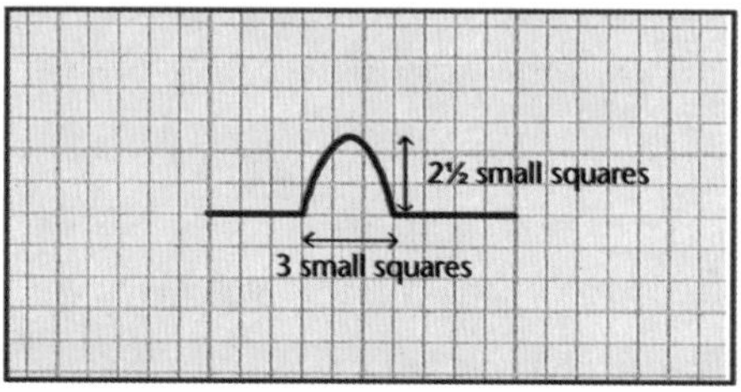

Fig 12.20: Normal P-wave dimensions.

- P pulmonale describes tall, peaked P waves. These occur in conditions when the right atrium becomes enlarged.
- P mitrale describes wide P waves that are often bifid. This may be seen in patients with mitral stenosis.

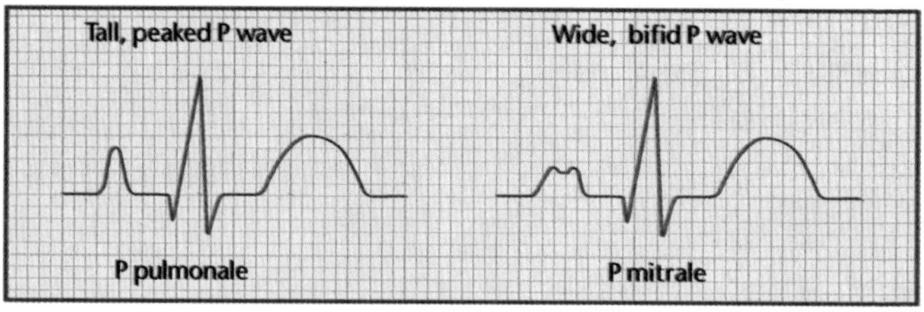

Fig 12.21: P pulmonale and P mitrale.

MEMORY AID

In P **P**ulmonale, the P waves are **P**eaked.

In P **M**itrale, the P waves are bifid and look like the letter **M**.

QRS complexes

Q waves

Look at the location and size of Q waves. The maximum dimensions of Q waves should not exceed those shown in Fig 12.22.

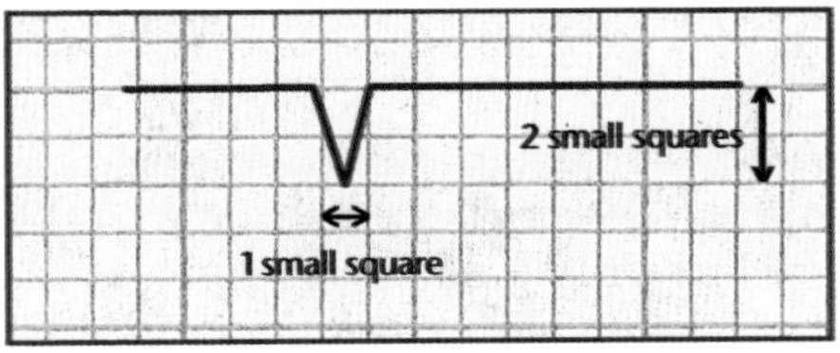

Fig 12.22: Q-wave maximum dimensions.

Because of the direction taken by electrical signals in the heart, small Q waves may normally be seen in leads looking at the lateral aspect of the heart (V5, V6, aVL and I). Large Q waves or Q waves in other locations are abnormal, and indicate the presence of scar tissue in the heart (eg after a myocardial infarction).

Height of R and S waves

Much information can be gleaned by looking at the height of R and S waves. The most common abnormality detected is left ventricular hypertrophy. There are many ECG criteria for predicting whether hypertrophy is present. One method involves finding the sum of the height of the S wave in V1 (in mm) and the height of the R wave in V6 (in mm). If greater than 35 mm, it is probable that left ventricular hypertrophy is present. An echocardiogram is necessary to confirm hypertrophy.

There are several causes of very small complexes, the most common being pericardial effusions, pericarditis and emphysematous lungs.

QRS duration

A normal QRS complex should be less than three small squares wide.

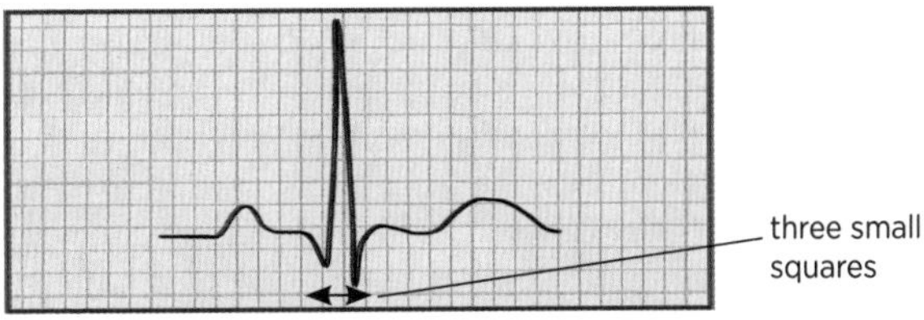

Fig 12.23: Normal maximum QRS complex duration.

Wide complexes indicate abnormal conduction through the ventricles. Normally, electrical signals are carried through the ventricular muscle in specialised conducting tissue – the bundle of His and its left and right branches. Problems in this conducting tissue result in electrical impulses being carried more slowly through non-specialised cardiac tissue. This results in widening of the QRS complex. You should be able to recognise the typical ECG features of problems in both the left and right bundle branches (named left and right bundle-branch block). Problems with QRS duration and other ECG abnormalities can be seen in tricyclic antidepressant toxicity - see page 53 for details.

In right bundle-branch block (RBBB), two upward deflections (ie two R waves) are seen in the QRS complex in V1. This is known as an RSR pattern. A deep S wave is normally seen in V6.

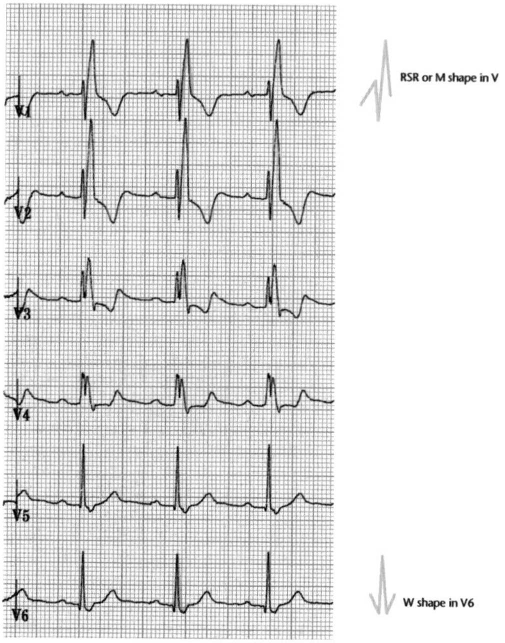

Fig 12.24: Right bundle-branch block.

In left bundle-branch block (LBBB), the ECG is typically highly bizarre in appearance. An RSR pattern may be seen in V6. Conduction is so disordered in LBBB that many of the normal morphological features of an ECG are not distinguishable. After establishing heart rate, rhythm, axis and that LBBB is present, analysis of the ECG should stop. Confusion often arises in practice when students attempt to comment on what appear to be highly abnormal ST segments and T waves. It is important to be able to identify LBBB, because, if it develops in a patient, it can be a sign of myocardial infarction.

Do not attempt to comment on the ST segment when LBBB is present.

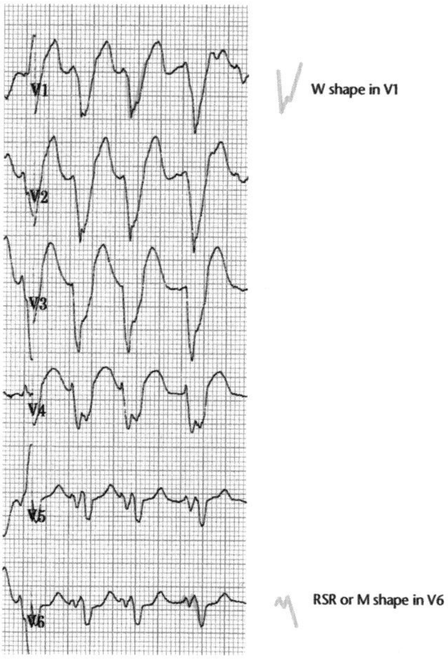

Fig 12.25: Left bundle-branch block.

Remember the name William Morrow, to remind you that:

In LBBB, there is a W shape to the QRS complex in V1 and an M shape to the complex in V6

In RBBB, there is an M shape to the QRS complex in V1 and a W shape to the complex in V6

	V1						V6
LBBB	W	I	L	L	I	A	M
RBBB	M	O	R	R		O	W

ST segment

The ST segment is that part of a tracing that lies between the QRS complex and the T wave.

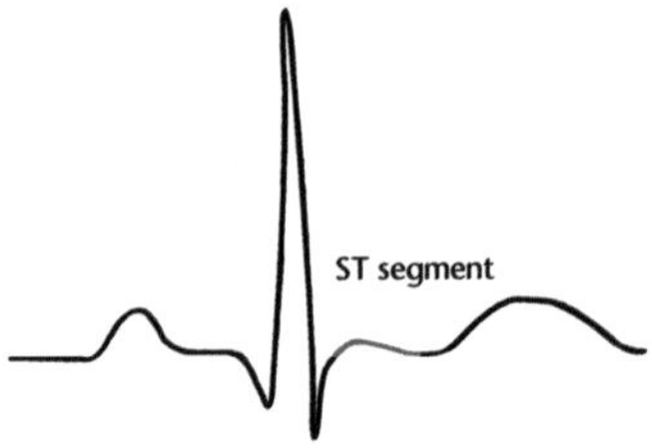

Fig 12.26: The ST segment.

Normally, the ST segment should be horizontal and isoelectric (ie lying on the baseline of the tracing). Abnormalities include elevation and depression.

The ST segment may be elevated. The most common causes for this are myocardial infarction (where ST elevation occurs in the heart leads 'looking at' damaged parts of the heart) and pericarditis (where ST elevation occurs in most or all ECG leads). The ST elevation associated with myocardial infarction is typically convex upwards, whereas it is concave (saddle-shaped) in pericarditis.

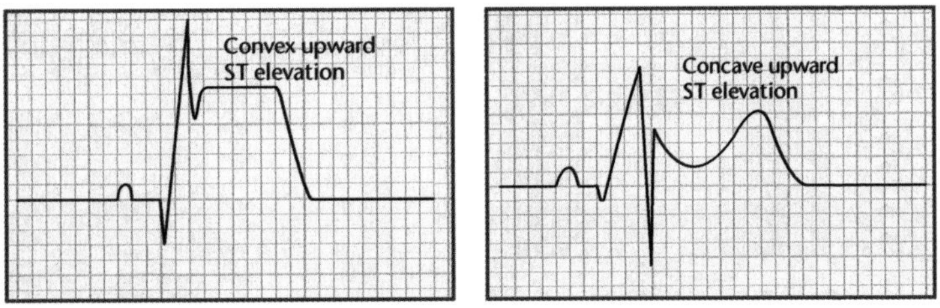

Fig 12.27: Convex and concave ST elevation (exaggerated for clarity).

ACUTE MYOCARDIAL INFARCTION REQUIRING URGENT REPERFUSION
1. ST segment elevation (convex upwards) in keeping with acute myocardial infarction, or 2. New LBBB: in a patient with typical chest pain

ST elevation that persists over weeks and months after a myocardial infarction may signify the presence of a ventricular aneurysm.

Horizontal ST depression can represent cardiac ischaemia, and may be seen during episodes of angina pectoris. ST depression may also indicate a non-ST elevation myocardial infarction (NSTEMI), which can be distinguished from ischaemia only by measuring biochemical markers of cardiomyocyte damage (see page 36 for details).

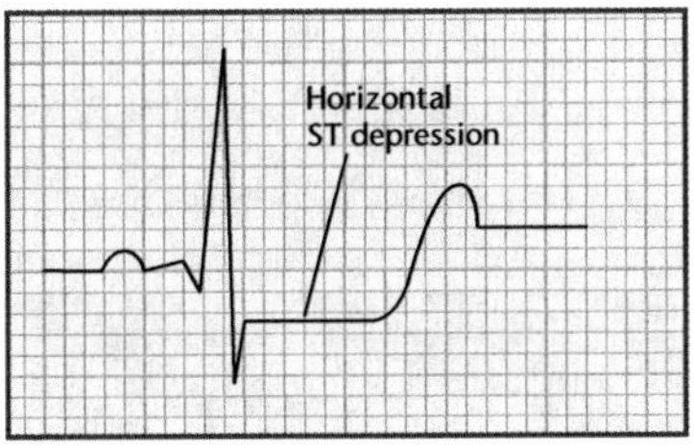

Fig 12.28: Horizontal ST depression.

When ST depression in lateral chest leads is seen alongside features in keeping with left ventricular hypertrophy, this is called a strain pattern, and is a feature of marked left ventricular hypertrophy. It can be difficult to differentiate from changes associated with ischaemia.

Down-sloping ST depression (often called 'reverse tick' ST depression) is seen in patients on digoxin.

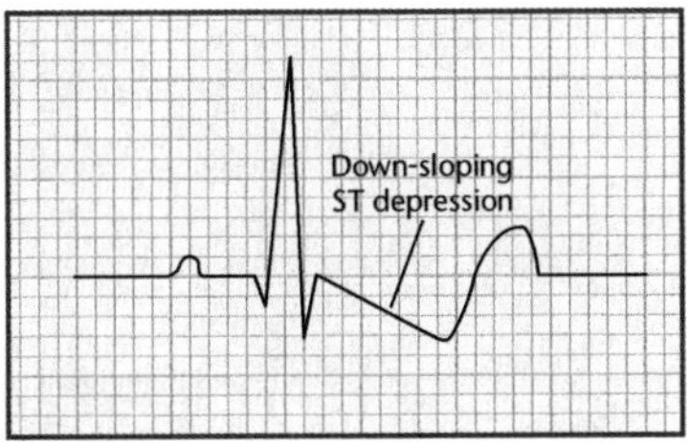

Fig 12.29: Down-sloping ST depression.

Q-T interval

The Q-T interval is the distance from the start of the QRS complex to the end of the T wave. Long Q-T intervals predispose to cardiac dysrhythmias. The Q-T interval varies with heart rate, but should in general not be more than two large squares in duration.

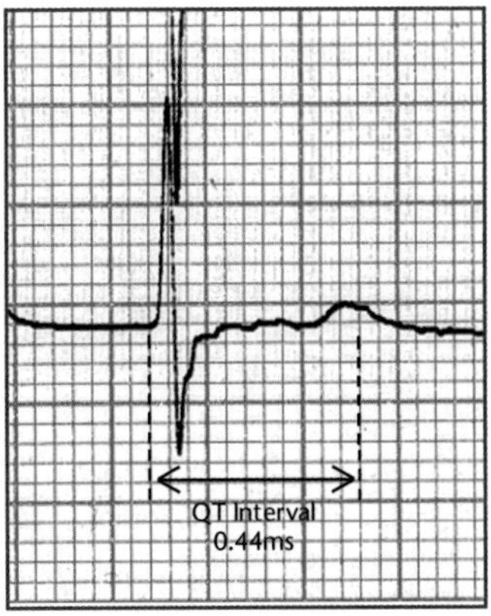

Fig 12.30: Prolonged Q-T interval.

To make matters a little more complicated, the Q-T interval increases as the heart rate slows. Thus bradycardia can be associated with an apparently long Q-T interval. To correct for this, the Bazett correction is applied to the Q-T interval to take the heart rate into account. The corrected Q-T interval (Q-Tc) is calculated as follows:

$$Q\text{-}Tc = \frac{Q\text{-}T}{\sqrt{R\text{-}R}}$$

where R-R is the number of seconds between consecutive R waves.

This value should generally be less than 0.45 second.

T wave

The final stage in ECG interpretation should be to look at the T waves. T waves may be upright or inverted (upside down). They are generally less than two-thirds of the height of their neighbouring R wave, and should not be more than two large squares tall.

Inverted T waves are normally seen in leads aVR and III. They may also be seen in lead V1 ± V2, but not V2 alone. T-wave inversion in other leads may be of little consequence, but is often a sign of cardiac ischaemia, or of NSTEMI.

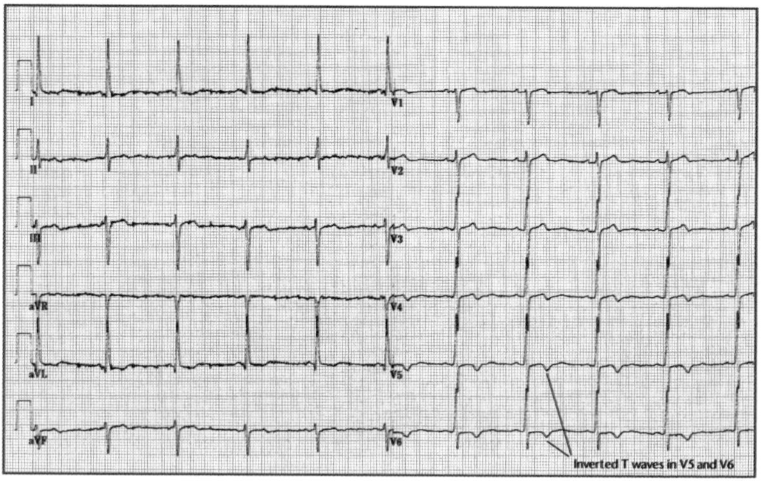

Fig 12.31: 12-lead ECG with T-wave inversion in the lateral chest leads.

T-wave changes often accompany changes in the serum potassium level. Typical findings are shown in the table.

HYPERKALAEMIA	HYPOKALAEMIA
Tall, tented T waves Loss of P waves QRS complex broadening Sine-wave-shaped ECG Cardiac arrest rhythms	Flat, broad T waves ST depression Long Q-T interval Ventricular dysrhythmias

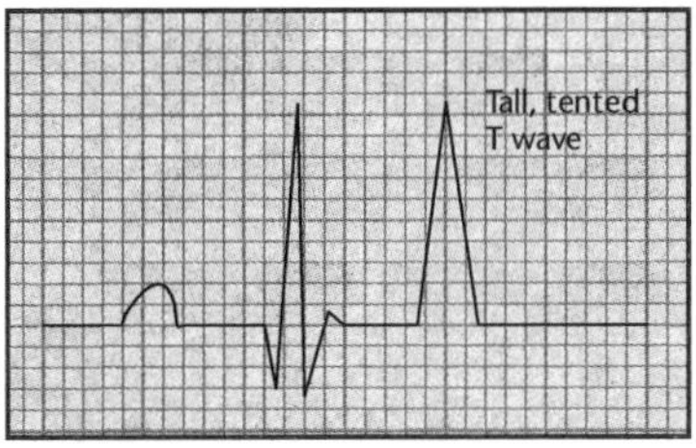

Fig 12.32: T waves in hyperkalaemia.

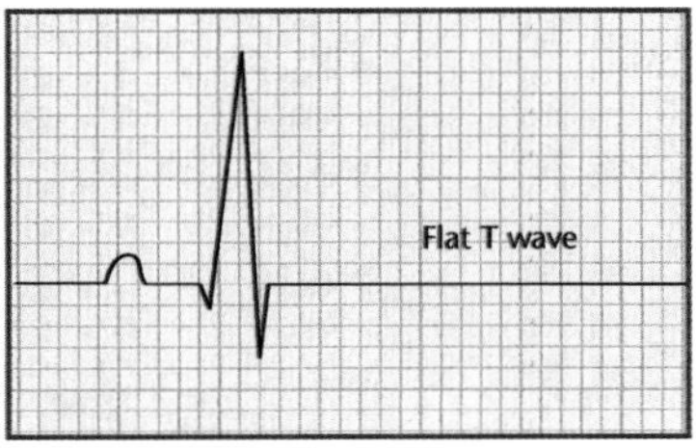

Fig 12.33: T waves in hypokalaemia.

Summary

When interpreting an ECG, always use the following headings:

Heart rate Heart rhythm Cardiac axis P waves	QRS complexes ST segment Q-T interval T waves

Cardiac arrest rhythms

When a patient has a cardiac arrest, the heart stops pumping blood around the body. The electrical activity in the heart does not always stop immediately, however, and the immediate advanced management of patients with cardiac arrest is largely determined by exactly what is happening to the heart rhythm. It is imperative that you are able to identify each of the following rhythms.

'Shockable' rhythms

If one of these rhythms is identified, the priority in treatment is to deliver electricity to the heart using a defibrillator.

Ventricular fibrillation (VF)

This is identified by the erratic nature of the electrical activity. It is random and unpredictable. It is sometimes classified as being fine or coarse depending on whether the electrical activity is of small (fine) or large (coarse) amplitude.

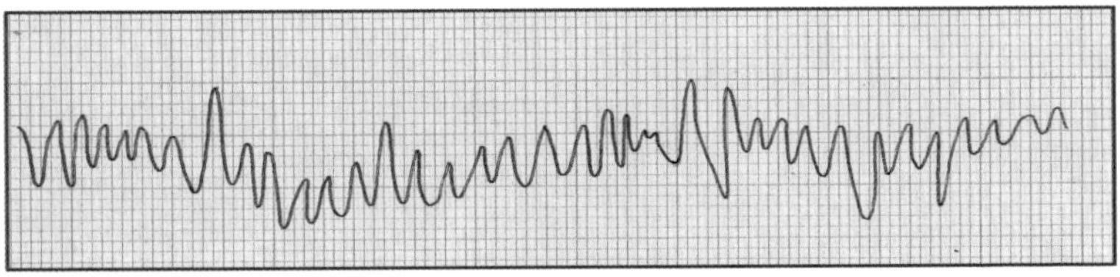

Fig 12.34

Ventricular tachycardia (VT)

This is a broad QRS complex tachycardia that has a very distinctive appearance on an ECG monitor. It is not always associated with cardiac arrest, but is always a significant arrhythmia.

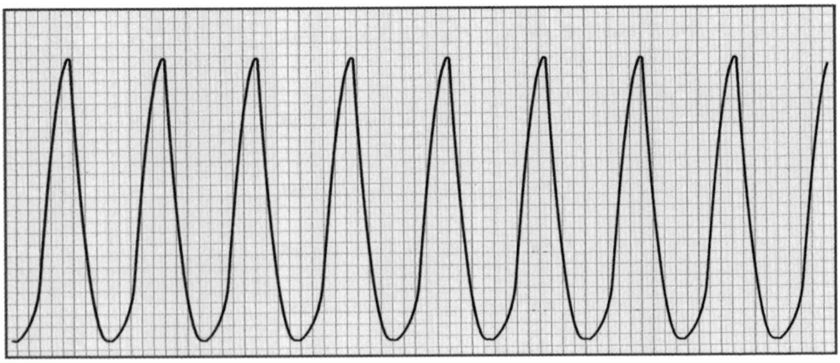

Fig 12.35

'Non-shockable' rhythms

Defibrillation will not be helpful to patients with one of these rhythms. Cardiopulmonary resuscitation should be administered and attempts made to reverse the cause of the cardiac arrest.

Pulseless electrical activity (PEA) (also known as electromechanical dissociation or EMD)

The heart rhythm is indistinguishable from a heart rhythm normally compatible with life.

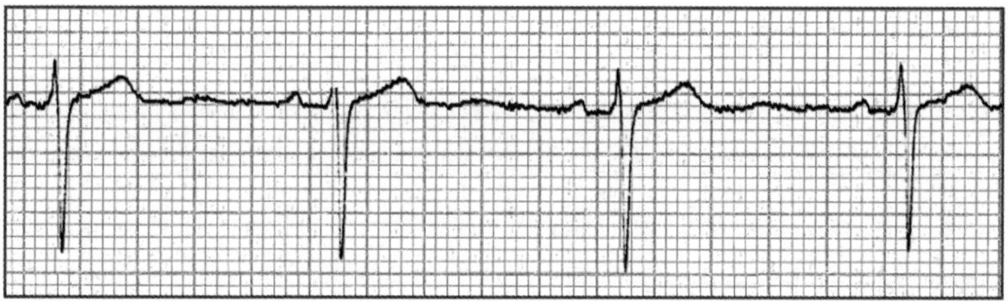

Fig 12.36

Asystole

There is no identifiable cardiac electrical activity. It is important to adjust the gain on the ECG monitor to ensure that 'fine' ventricular fibrillation is not missed.

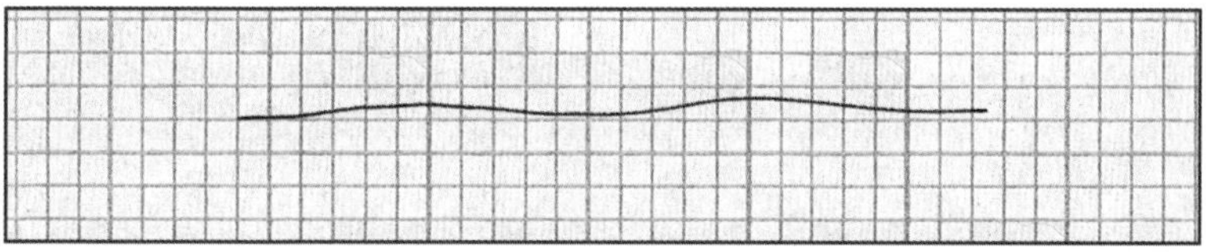

Fig 12.37

P-wave asystole

In this rhythm, only P waves are seen. There is no ventricular activity. This rhythm may respond to cardiac pacing.

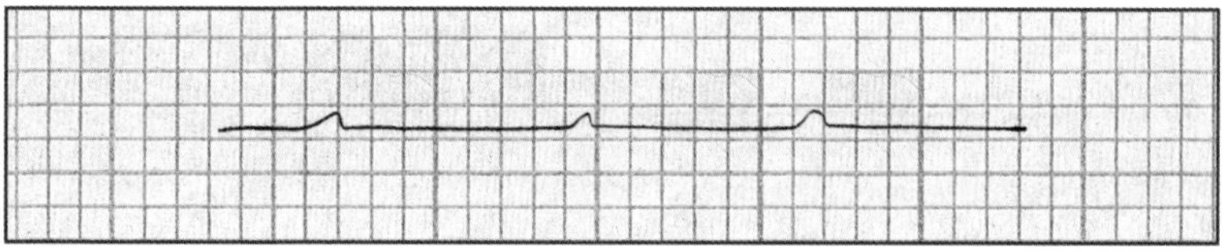

Fig 12.38

Cardiac imaging

Echocardiography

It is unlikely that you will be required to have detailed knowledge of echocardiography at undergraduate level. However, it is important that you are familiar with echocardiographic reports and understand how to interpret them.

You may find it helpful to use the following headings when reading echocardiographic reports. Common abnormalities and points to bear in mind are also listed.

COMPONENT OF REPORT	COMMENT
Size of heart chambers (atria and ventricles)	The normal maximum diameter of the left atrium is 4.5 cm. Enlargement of the left atrium is particularly significant in patients with atrial fibrillation. The normal maximum diameter of the left ventricle in diastole is 5.5 cm - this will be increased in abnormally enlarged left ventricles, eg with dilated cardiomyopathy
Ventricular septal thickness	This should be less than 1.2 cm. A thickened septum should raise suspicions of hypertrophic obstructive cardiomyopathy (HOCM)
Left ventricular function	Hypokinesis refers to walls that contract poorly. Akinesis refers to walls that do not appear to contract at all. The left ventricular ejection fraction is normally around 65%
Details about each valve	Stenotic or regurgitant valves will often be described in terms of severity as trace, mild, moderate or severe. Often pressure gradients across valves and valve areas are documented. For the aortic valve, severe stenosis is present if there is a pressure gradient of more than 50 mmHg across the valve, or if the valve area is less than 1 cm^2
Vegetations or tumours	Bear in mind that a small vegetation may be missed with transthoracic echocardiography. Transoesophageal echocardiography is more reliable
Estimated pulmonary artery pressure	A pressure >35 mmHg suggests pulmonary hypertension. Note that this is an estimated pressure reading only
Pericardial effusion	Present or absent

Other imaging modalities

Increasingly, computed tomography (CT) and magnetic resonance imaging (MRI) of the heart are being performed in patients with suspected cardiac disease. CT assessment of the coronary arteries, including an assessment of calcification (calcium scoring), is increasingly used in the non-invasive assessment of patients with chest pain. MRI of the heart can provide detailed information on many aspects of cardiac structure and function. Interpretation of such images is in the territory of a specialist cardiologist and is certainly beyond the scope of this book. Thankfully the written reports from such imaging investigations are usually self-explanatory.

Dynamic tests in cardiology

Dynamic heart testing is commonly used to investigate chest pain and known ischaemic heart disease. In the resting state, a patient with significant coronary artery atherosclerosis may have a normal ECG. However, when the heart is put under stress by increasing its rate, its energy requirements increase. If sufficient blood cannot be supplied to the myocardium under such circumstances, the tissue becomes ischaemic and the ECG will change.

Features that would be in keeping with ischaemic heart disease include horizontal or down-sloping ST-segment depression or elevation, particularly if these are associated with angina or a reduction in blood pressure.

Other dynamic tests are used to assess cardiac function in particular patient groups. In patients who are unable to exercise, pharmacological agents (eg dobutamine) can be administered to increase the heart rate and put the heart under stress. Cardiac function can then be assessed by performing echocardiography or by nuclear imaging techniques which look at the uptake of isotopes by cardiac muscle. By so doing, areas of the heart that pump defectively or have inadequate blood supply can be identified.

Ambulatory blood pressure monitoring

Ambulatory blood pressure monitoring (ABPM) is being increasingly used as an investigative tool in the management of people with high blood pressure. It gives a lot more information than a one-off office blood pressure measure, and can help identify people with various blood pressure patterns, such as:

- White-coat hypertension: blood pressure 'artificially' high when measured by a doctor or nurse, ie ABPM lower than clinic pressure.
- Masked hypertension: blood pressure 'artificially' low when measured by a doctor or nurse, ie ABPM higher than clinic pressure.

- Nocturnal dipping: it is normal for the blood pressure to drop overnight when sleeping. The mean arterial pressure should drop by at least 10 mmHg.
- Non-dipping: blood pressure that does not fall in sleep.
- Reverse dipping: blood pressure that increases during sleep.

To interpret an ABPM results summary take the following steps:

- Look at how many of the attempted readings were successful. If the vast majority of readings were successful, the study is useful. If only a few readings were successful, the results of the study are of questionable value.
- Compare the average daytime pressure with the most recent clinic readings and decide if the patient is 'normal', or has 'white-coat' or 'masked' hypertension. Bear in mind that most people's blood pressure will be lower at home. Make a conclusion about whether the daytime pressure is normal, high or low.
- Look at the overnight blood pressure. Compare the mean arterial pressure overnight with that obtained during the day. If the blood pressure does not dip normally, the patient should be questioned. A poor night's sleep or obstructive sleep apnoea is a common cause for blood pressure failing to dip at night. If the patient slept well on the night of the study, one can use the ABPM result to classify them into having normal-, non- or reverse-nocturnal dipping.

An ABPM record can also provide much more information, such as detail about the pulse pressure and heart rate at various times of the day. These data may also be helpful in stratifying a patient's cardiac risk.

INVESTIGATIONS IN CARDIOLOGY – WHAT YOU NEED TO KNOW

- It is critical to learn which surface of the heart each lead assesses.
- Until you become expert at ECG interpretation, take your time and look at the following, in order: rate, rhythm, axis, P waves, QRS complexes, ST segment, Q–T interval and T waves.
- Ensure that the machine is set at 25 mm per second before interpreting an ECG.
- Ventricular rate (beats per minute) = 300 ÷ number of large squares between R waves, OR 1500 ÷ number of small squares between R waves.
- To diagnose sinus rhythm, all of the following criteria should be met: 1. P wave preceding every QRS complex. 2. P–R interval is normal. 3. P–R interval is constant.
- Atrial fibrillation is the commonest cause of an irregularly irregular rhythm.
- Look at leads I, II and III to determine the cardiac axis.
- The normal QRS duration is less than three small squares, ie less than 0.120 second.
- The mnemonic 'WiLLiaM MoRRoW' is helpful in differentiating right and left bundle-branch block.
- New left bundle-branch block can indicate acute myocardial infarction.
- Ventricular fibrillation and ventricular tachycardia are the 'shockable' cardiac arrest rhythms.

13

RESPIRATORY INVESTIGATIONS

Pulmonary function tests

Peak expiratory flow rate

Peak expiratory flow rate (PEFR) is a simple bedside test that gives a useful insight into the respiratory function of a patient. The PEFR is measured in litres per minute using a basic plastic device. An average recording of three attempts is documented on a peak flow chart. The trend in PEFR and its relationship to symptoms are a guide to the severity of illness and the effectiveness of treatment.

Some patients with asthma will keep records of their PEFR. For comparative purposes recordings should be taken at the same time each day. This will eliminate changes due to normal diurnal variation. There is a normal variation in PEFR in people with asthma, with a typical dip first thing in the morning.

It is important to appreciate when interpreting values that the normal PEFR varies with age, height and sex.

PATIENT	HEIGHT (cm)	NORMAL PEFR (l/min)
25-year-old man	175	630
25-year-old woman	175	505
60-year-old man	160	545
60-year-old woman	160	445

DON'T FORGET

PEFR varies with age, sex and height.

Spirometry

Spirometry provides a wealth of information about lung volumes and function. Spirometry reports can appear confusing. However, by looking at four indices, most of the important patterns of lung disease can be distinguished.

KEY RESULTS IN SPIROMETRY		
INDEX	ABBREVIATION	INTERPRETATION
Forced expiratory volume in 1 second	FEV_1	The volume of air that can be expired in 1 second
Forced vital capacity	FVC	The volume of air expired in a complete expiration
Ratio of FEV_1 to FVC	FEV_1/FVC	-
Carbon monoxide transfer coefficient	*K*CO	A measure of the rate of diffusion of carbon monoxide from the alveoli into the capillary blood

Values obtained by spirometry should always be compared with age- and sex-matched control values. Often results are converted into percentages of the predicted value in order to simplify interpretation.

Arguably the most useful index is the FEV_1/FVC. This test can be used to distinguish between obstructive airway disease (eg asthma, COPD) and restrictive lung disease (eg pulmonary fibrosis). In an obstructive defect, the FEV_1/FVC will be less than 70%. The percentage is greater than 80% with a restrictive defect.

COMMON PATTERNS OF FEV_1/FVC
<70% in obstructive airway disease >80% in restrictive lung disease

The theory underlying these patterns is easily understood. In a patient with obstructive airway disease, airway obstruction makes expiration slow (and usually wheezy). The FEV_1 is therefore typically low, since only a small volume of air can be expired in 1 second. These patients also 'trap air' so the FVC will usually be high. A low FEV_1 and a high FVC combine to give a low FEV_1/FVC. In other words, the volume of air in the lungs is normal or high, but it is not easily forced out.

In restrictive lung disease, on the other hand, there is no airway obstruction. The FEV_1 is therefore typically higher than with an obstructive defect (although it is still usually reduced compared with normal). Small lung volumes contribute to a low FVC. A relatively high FEV_1 and a low FVC combine to give a high FEV_1/FVC. Put simply, the patient can force air out of their lungs, but as the lung volume is reduced there is less of it to force out.

The three main patterns of lung function (normal, obstructive and restrictive) are shown pictorially on Fig 13.1.

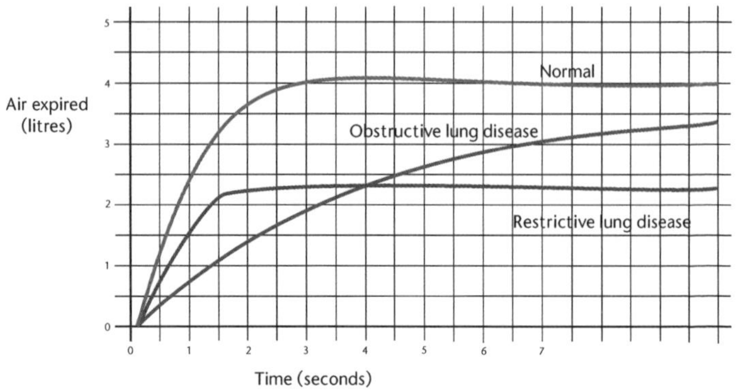

Fig 13.1

The *K*co measures the ease of diffusion of carbon monoxide from alveolar air to capillary blood. Anything that hinders gas transfer from alveolus into blood will therefore result in a low *K*co. Common causes of low *K*co are shown in the box below.

CAUSES OF A LOW *K*CO
Interstitial lung disease
Emphysema
Pulmonary oedema
Pulmonary embolism
Anaemia

In rare cases, the *K*co can be raised. In such circumstances, gas transfers more easily than normal from alveolus into blood. Examples include polycythaemia (see page 77) or in cases of pulmonary haemorrhage (eg Goodpasture syndrome).

Note that anaemia is the classic case where a patient will have a low *K*co with normal spirometry. The *K*co is low because there is less haemoglobin present to carry gas away from the alveoli.

14

OTHER TESTS

Urine examination

Inspection

A brief inspection of a patient's urine can provide important information, as shown in the box.

APPEARANCE	POSSIBLE CAUSE
Bloody	Bleeding in the urinary tract
Orange	Use of rifampicin (anti-tuberculous drug)
Red, becoming purple/brown on exposure to light	Porphyria
Reddish brown	Myoglobin, seen in rhabdomyolysis

Urinalysis

Dipstick urinalysis is an inexpensive and convenient test that can be performed in a matter of minutes and inform the operator about the potential presence of a number of disease states. You should be familiar with common causes of the most commonly occurring abnormalities, as shown in the box.

APPEARANCE	POSSIBLE CAUSE
Bilirubin	Seen in liver disease
Blood	Seen with glomerular damage, and in multiple pathologies along the length of the urogenital tract. It can also be seen if urine is contaminated with blood from menstruation
Glucose	The presence of glucose is called glycosuria and can be seen in uncontrolled diabetes mellitus, and sometimes in pregnancy
Ketones	Found in ketoacidosis, fasting, pregnancy
Leukocytes	Seen in urinary tract infection
Nitrite	Seen in urinary tract infection. Note that it is nitrite, not nitrate, that is tested
pH	Very variable. Checking urinary pH can be helpful in patients with renal stones and in those suspected of having renal tubular acidosis
Protein	Seen in glomerular damage, abnormal tubular protein resorption, Bence Jones proteinuria, urinary tract infection and structural disease of the urinary tract
Specific gravity (SG)	A measure of the degree of concentration of the urine. A SG of 1.00 would indicate that the urine was effectively water – SG is therefore always >1
Urobilinogen	Seen in liver disease and haemolysis

Lumbar puncture

Cerebrosinal fluid (CSF) is obtained by performing a lumbar puncture. A wide variety of tests can be performed on CSF as detailed below.

COMPONENTS OF A ROUTINE CSF ANALYSIS	
Opening pressure Appearance (Gram stain + culture if infection suspected)	Total protein Glucose Microscopy for cell counts

Important information on a patient's condition can be gleaned at the bedside during the process of lumbar puncture, even before fluid is sent for analysis.

Opening pressure

Once a needle has been passed and CSF is draining, a manometer can be attached to measure the 'opening pressure'. This is meaningful only if the patient is in the 'standard' lateral decubitus position (lying on their side) at the time of puncture. If lumbar puncture is performed with the patient upright, the opening pressure will be artificially elevated. Reference ranges for adults for opening pressure are variably quoted between texts, but a pressure of between 8 and 20 cmCSF is probably normal.

COMMON CAUSES OF ABNORMAL OPENING PRESSURE	
Abnormally low	**Abnormally high**
CSF leak Recent lumbar puncture	Meningitis Tumour Intracranial haemorrhage Idiopathic intracranial hypertension

CSF appearance

The gross appearance of CSF can give an early indication of fluid composition. Textbooks list many subtle colour variations of CSF, which are quite difficult to appreciate unless you are experienced in this area. The most abnormal CSF appearances are listed in the box overleaf.

CHARACTERISTIC CSF APPEARANCE	
Appearance	**Characteristic of**
Clear	Normality
Cloudy or purulent	Meningitis
Bloody	Traumatic tap or subarachnoid haemorrhage

The inadvertent puncture of a blood vessel during the process of lumbar puncture will result in blood-stained fluid being drained. The operator will not know with any certainty, however, that a blood vessel has been hit, and one must therefore be able to distinguish between CSF that is truly blood stained and CSF that appears blood stained only because of the puncture of a vessel. One simple method for doing this at the bedside involves collecting three separate CSF samples. If the fluid remains blood stained to the same degree in all samples, it is likely that the CSF is truly blood stained. If, however, the fluid becomes less blood stained with time, it is more likely that the lumbar puncture has been a traumatic tap. Laboratory testing of the CSF for the presence of xanthochromia provides another, much more robust method of distinguishing between these two possibilities and is discussed below.

Laboratory tests

Microscopy

CSF microscopy permits the counting of cells in the fluid. An elevated red cell count is most commonly seen as a result of the lumbar puncture needle puncturing a blood vessel en route to the subarachnoid space. It will also be seen in cases of intracranial haemorrhage. However, a measure of the red cell count in three consecutively collected specimens of CSF can help differentiate between these two possibilities, similar to the bedside test described above.

An elevated white cell count (>5 cells/mm^3) suggests central nervous system infection (ie meningitis or encephalitis), but can also be found in other conditions such as inflammatory diseases and cancer. If puncture of a small blood vessel has occurred during lumbar puncture, the white cell count will also be elevated falsely due to the presence of these cells in the blood. The particular type of white cells present can also be informative. In infection, a predominance of neutrophils suggests bacterial meningitis. Lymphocytes predominate in other infective causes of meningitis (eg viral, tuberculosis or fungal).

Microbiological testing

Microscopy after Gram staining (for bacterial infection), Ziehl-Neelsen staining (for tuberculosis), culture and genetic techniques (eg polymerase chain reaction [PCR] techniques to detect bacterial or viral DNA) can all be useful in the analysis of CSF when infection is suspected. Refer to Chapter 5 for further details. It is worth bearing in mind that, as it is imperative that antimicrobial treatment should be administered as soon as possible in patients with suspected bacterial meningitis, lumbar puncture is often (rightly) performed after treatment has been started. This can change the CSF constituents such that 'textbook' patterns may not be seen, and a high index of suspicion is necessary. More specialised microbiological testing can be performed if an unusual organism (eg syphilis, cryptocococci, human immunodeficiency virus [HIV]) is suspected.

Protein measurement

Normal CSF contains between 0.15 and 0.45 g/l of protein approximately, but the precise reference range varies depending on the laboratory used. Abnormally elevated CSF protein is a good pointer that some pathological process is active in the central nervous system, but it is impossible to be sure about causality using the protein measure alone. The box below lists some of the more common conditions that are associated with elevated CSF protein, but this list is by no means exhaustive.

COMMON CAUSES OF RAISED CSF PROTEIN	
Meningitis	Neoplastic disease
Brain abscess	Guillain-Barré syndrome
Intracerebral haemorrhage	Multiple sclerosis

Glucose measurement

Interpretation of the CSF glucose concentration in isolation is meaningless – it must be interpreted in relation to the blood glucose concentration. A blood sample for glucose measurement must always be sent at the time of lumbar puncture.

DON'T FORGET

Always interpret CSF glucose results in the context of blood glucose levels.

CSF glucose should be around 40–60% that of the level in blood. An abnormally high glucose level will be seen with simultaneous high blood sugar level (ie in poorly controlled diabetes) and is not a pointer to CSF pathology. An abnormally low CSF glucose level is, however, highly important and is suggestive of, but not limited to, bacterial, fungal or tuberculous infection. Viral infections of the CNS do not characteristically lower the CSF glucose concentration significantly.

Other tests

There are a multitude of specialised tests that can be performed on CSF in certain circumstances. The most commonly requested of these are detailed below.

Spectrophotometry

The term 'xanthochromia' describes a yellow discoloration of CSF. This can sometimes be detected by inspecting CSF, but is more reliably quantified in a laboratory using spectrophotometry. A positive test indicates that bilirubin is present in the fluid, and will therefore be found in patients with significant jaundice. Assuming that the patient does not have jaundice, xanthochromia is tested for most commonly in patients who are suspected to have had a subarachnoid haemorrhage (SAH), because blood in the CSF breaks down to form bilirubin. CT scanning of the head should be performed first, with lumbar puncture being performed if SAH is suspected but no evidence of it is seen on the scan. It is necessary to wait at least 12 hours after the onset of symptoms to ensure that any blood in the CSF has had time to break down into bilirubin.

The presence of xanthochromia in a sample can also be helpful in distinguishing blood-stained CSF from a traumatic tap in addition to the methods used above. In a traumatic tap, blood will only have entered the CSF at the time of lumbar puncture, and will not break down into bilirubin. Testing for xanthochromia will therefore be negative in these circumstances.

Oligoclonal bands

The presence of oligoclonal bands in CSF is often tested for in patients who are suspected of having multiple sclerosis (MS). Oligoclonal bands are due to the presence of immunoglobulins in the CSF and are detected when CSF is tested using electrophoresis. Although characteristic of MS, the finding of oligoclonal bands is not diagnostic, because they can be found in a variety of rare neurological diseases.

Cytological examination

Cytological examination of the CSF can be helpful in the diagnosis of neurological malignancy. The specifics of the tests used are beyond the scope of this text, but a cytological report normally incorporates a cytologist's overall impression and is therefore relatively easy to interpret.

Ankle-brachial pressure index

The ankle-brachial pressure index (ABPI) is an easily measured clinical parameter that is often used to assess the adequacy of blood flow to the lower limbs.

The patient should lie flat on a bed when having an ABPI measured. The systolic blood pressure in the brachial artery is measured using a stethoscope and sphygmomanometer. The systolic blood pressure at the ankle is then measured using a sphygmomanometer wrapped around the calf and a Doppler probe positioned over the posterior tibial or dorsalis pedis artery. Cuff pressure is inflated until blood flow to the foot is cut off. Flow is slowly re-established by deflating the cuff, and the pressure at which the first Doppler signal is obtained is noted.

After performing these tests, the observer will have two figures - the systolic blood pressures in the brachial artery and at the ankle. The ABPI is calculated simply by finding their ratio. In health, the ratio should be greater than or equal to 1. As the value decreases, symptoms and signs of arterial insufficiency to the lower limbs would be expected. Values lower than 0.5 may result in critical ischaemia. ABPIs of lower than 0.2 can be associated with ulceration and gangrene.

ABPI	INTERPRETATION
>1	Normal
<0.5	At risk of critical ischaemia
<0.2	At risk of ulceration and gangrene

One potentially complicating factor relates to the fact that some patients (particularly those with long-standing diabetes mellitus) have calcified arteries which cannot be compressed with a blood pressure cuff. In such cases, Doppler signals will be obtained even when the cuff is inflated to very high pressures. ABPIs cannot be reliably measured in these patients.

DON'T FORGET

The ABPI must be interpreted with caution in patients with diabetes mellitus.

Schirmer test

Keratoconjunctivitis sicca is the term used to describe dry eyes. This phenomenon can occur in isolation (primary Sjögren syndrome) or in association with many other rheumatological conditions.

The test is performed by attaching a specially shaped piece of filter paper to the lower eyelid. This is left for 5 min, and the distance that has become wet is then measured. Normally 10 mm or more of the paper will become wet.

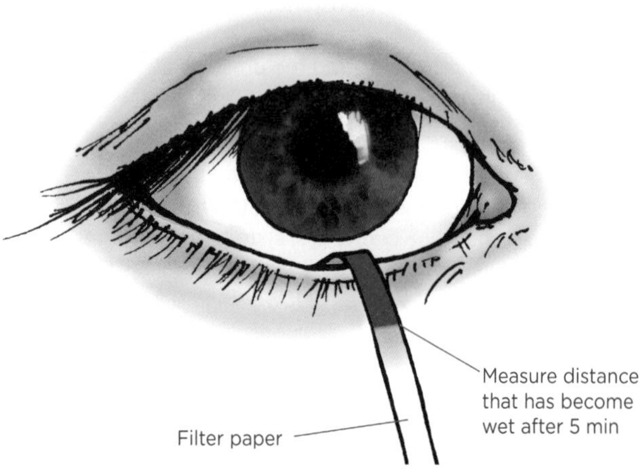

Fig 14.1

It is important to bear in mind, however, that normal tear production is reduced in old age. Also, drugs with anticholinergic properties, such as tricyclic antidepressants, reduce tear production and may result in a false-positive Schirmer test.

Audiography

Audiograms illustrate, in graphic form, how well a person can hear noises at different frequencies. A healthy ear can hear sounds transmitted in the air better than those conducted by bone. This is because the ossicles in the middle ear amplify sound waves in the air.

Several patterns of abnormalities should be recognised.

1. **Conductive deafness**
   Anything that impedes the progression of sound waves down the ear canal can result in conductive deafness. The classic example of this is the patient with severe ear wax. In these conditions, sounds conducted by bone will be heard louder than those conducted by air. The audiogram will show a gap between the hearing level for air and bone conduction. This is termed a wide air-bone gap.

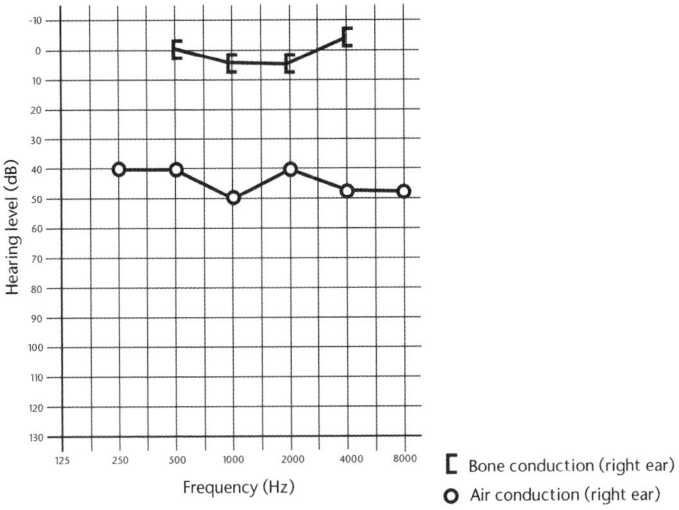

Fig 14.2: Audiogram illustrating conductive deafness.

2. **Sensorineural deafness**
   A patient with unilateral auditory nerve damage (eg due to an acoustic neuroma) will have reduced hearing for both air conduction and bone conduction.

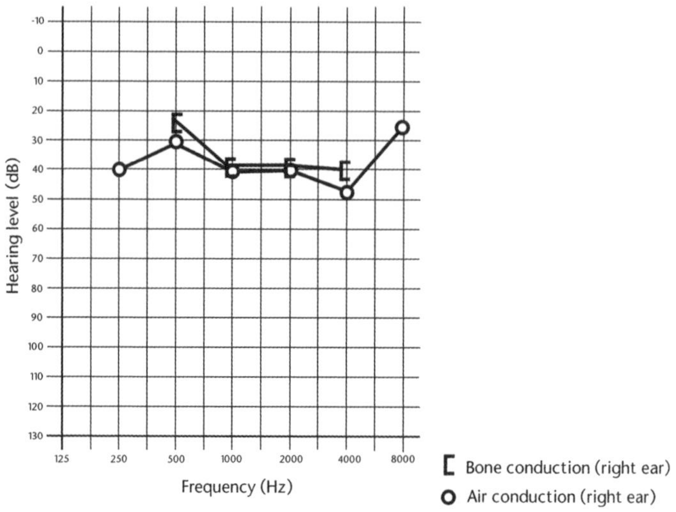

Fig 14.3: Audiogram illustrating sensorineural deafness.

3. **Presbyacusis**
   This describes the loss of hearing of sounds at high frequencies that is a common finding in elderly patients. It represents a form of sensorineural deafness.

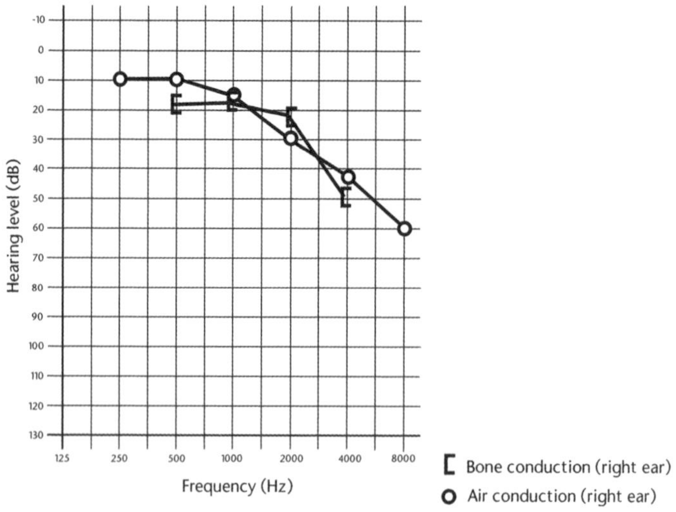

Fig 14.4: Audiogram illustrating presbuacusis.

4. **Noise-induced hearing loss**
   Patients with noise-induced hearing loss typically have difficulty hearing sounds with a frequency around 4000 Hz. Their audiograms usually have a trough at this frequency level.

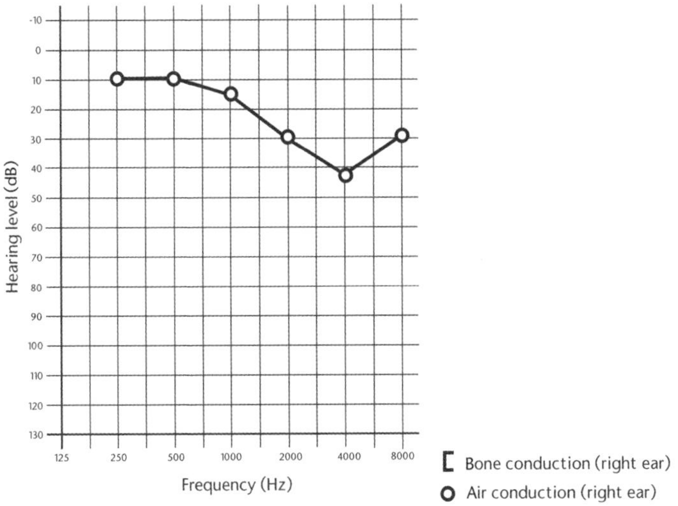

Fig 14.5: Audiogram illustrating noise-induced hearing loss.

Risk calculations

Cardiovascular risk

The quantification of cardiovascular risk can assist in deciding which patients 'qualify' for risk-reducing therapies such as lipid- or blood pressure-lowering agents. There are a number of methods used to estimate risk. One popular method is to use an online risk calculator called QRISK®2 (https://www.qrisk.org/2016/). After typing in some details about a patient, a summary of risk is given, such as the example presented in Fig 14.6.

'QRISK®2 score' is an estimate of the risk of stroke or myocardial infarction over the next 10 years. The 'relative risk' is how many times higher this patient's risk is compared with a healthy person of the same age, sex and ethnicity - in this case the patient is four times more likely to have a cardiovascular event than one of his peers. The 'Healthy Heart Age' is an indication of what age a healthy person would have to be to have an equivalent risk to the patient in question. In this case, the 64-year-old patient has the risk of a typical person aged >84 years. At the time of this book going to print, QRISK®3 has just become available.

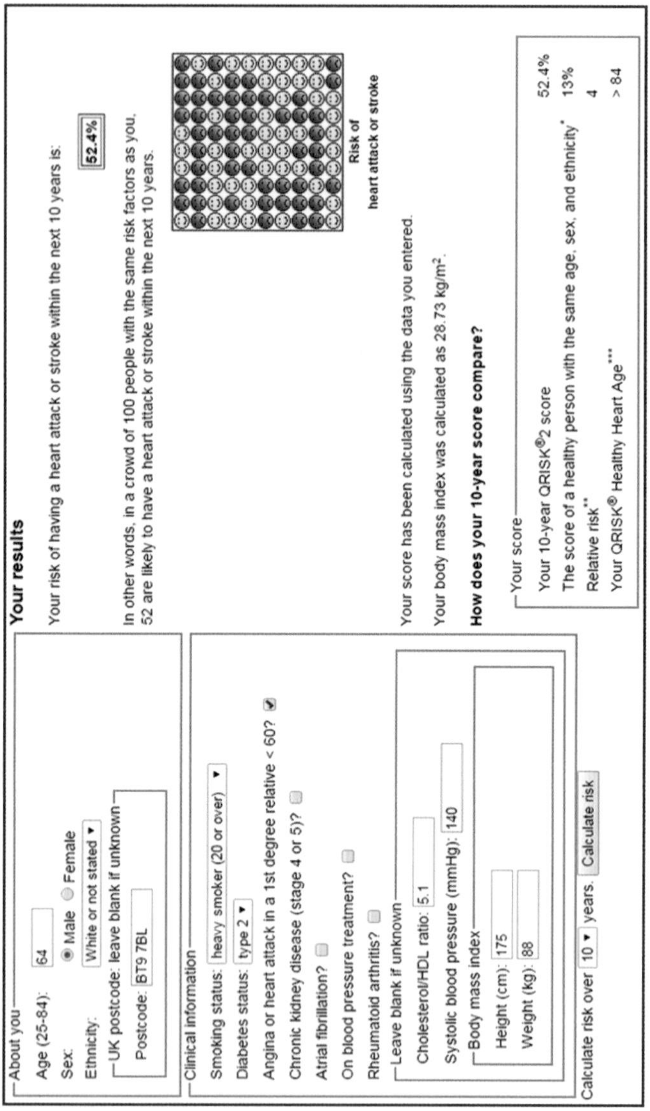

Fig 14.6: Using QRISK®2 to estimate cardiovascular risk.

Fracture risk

A patient's risk of fracturing a bone can be estimated in a process similar to estimating their cardiovascular risk. The FRAX® WHO Fracture Risk Assessment Tool (https://www.shef.ac.uk/FRAX/) is commonly used for this purpose. See Fig 14.7.

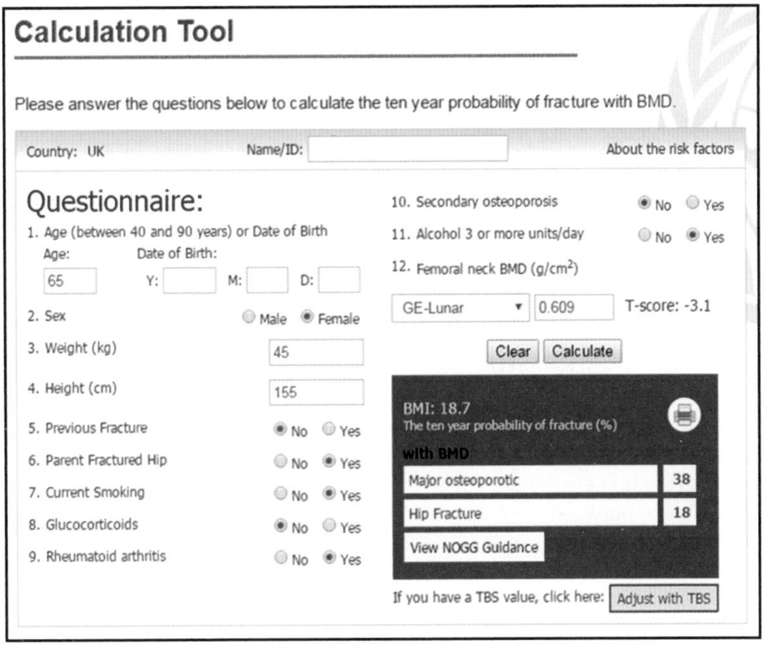

Fig 14.7: Using FRAX® to estimate fracture risk.

In this example, the patient has an 18% chance of having a hip fracture in the next 10 years, and a 38% chance of sustaining a major osteoporotic fracture of any type.

Neurophysiology

Neurophysiology is a specialist domain within neurology. Only a brief understanding of the common investigations is necessary for an undergraduate. Likewise, knowledge of the key findings in classic conditions will suffice. It is unlikely that one would be expected to interpret neurophysiological investigations.

MAIN NEUROPHYSIOLOGICAL INVESTIGATIONS
Nerve conduction studies
Electromyography
Visually evoked responses
Electroencephalography

Nerve conduction studies

Nerve conduction studies (NCS) measure how well individual nerves transmit electrical signals. The nerve of interest is stimulated, usually electrically, with surface electrodes placed on the skin. One electrode stimulates the nerve and the resulting electrical activity is recorded by the other electrodes. The distance between electrodes and the time taken for electrical impulses to travel between electrodes are used to calculate the nerve conduction velocity.

The most common reason for NCS to be requested is for suspected carpal tunnel syndrome. In this condition, the median nerve is entrapped within the confines of the carpal tunnel.

Electroencephalography

Electroencephalography (EEG) is the recording of electrical activity from the brain using a series of scalp electrodes. Usually, recordings over a period of several minutes are taken. Broadly speaking, EEG can be used to diagnose epilepsy and diffuse brain disease. In epilepsy, it is most valuable if a recording takes place during a seizure since it is not unusual to obtain a normal recording between seizures.

In difficult cases, EEG recording can take place over several hours or days in a supervised room in hospital with video recording. EEG may also be invaluable in diagnosing non-convulsive status epilepticus and distinguishing true seizures from pseudoseizures. In non-convulsive status epilepticus, a patient is having ongoing seizures, despite these not manifesting themselves clinically. Prompt diagnosis by EEG may prevent permanent neurological deficit.

Electromyography

Surface or needle electrodes are used to detect muscle action potentials following controlled electrical stimulation. The electrical stimulation provokes action potentials within the nerves which in turn stimulate a magnified response in muscles.

Electromyography (EMG) may be modified for some indications. The most important to know is single-fibre EMG and EMG with repetitive stimulation used when myasthenia gravis is clinically suspected.

Visually evoked responses

In this test, the eye is stimulated in order to evoke a response within the occipital cortex. It is performed by placing a series of electrodes over the scalp in the occipital area while asking the patient to observe a series of visual patterns. The response is recorded via the electrodes. Two indices are noted:

1. The speed of response of the nerve (termed 'P100 latencies')
2. The height of the waveform obtained.

This test is usually performed in patients in whom multiple sclerosis is suspected. In multiple sclerosis, the waveform will be preserved, but the speed of response will be delayed because of optic nerve demyelination.

Classic neurophysiological disease associations

TEST	RESULT	DISEASE
EEG	Spike and wave	Primary generalised epilepsy
EEG	Periodic complexes	Creutzfeldt-Jakob disease
EMG	Short polyphasic motor potentials Sometimes spontaneous fibrillation and high-frequency repetitive discharges	Polymyositis
EMG (single fibre)	Fatiguability following repetitive stimulation	Myasthenia gravis
EMG	Repetitive single motor unit potentials all low amplitude. Short duration polyphasic motor unit potentials	Myotonic dystrophy
EMG	Spontaneous fibrillations	Motor neuron disease
NCS	Delay in conduction of median nerve	Carpal tunnel syndrome (entrapment neuropathy)
Visually evoked responses (VERs)	Delayed P100 latencies, without amplitude loss	Multiple sclerosis

AT THE BEDSIDE AND IN THE CLINIC: CASES

3

Case 3.1

A 25-year-old man experiences an extremely severe headache of rapid onset. It settles somewhat after around 12 hours, and he fails to seek medical attention until 7 days have passed. The A&E doctor is concerned about the possibility of a subarachoid haemorrhage (SAH). A CT scan of the head is unremarkable. Lumbar puncture is performed, and a sample sent for spectrophotometry. The following interpreted report is returned:

> 'Oxyhaemoglobin is present in sufficient quantity to impair the ability to detect bilirubin. SAH not excluded.'

What is the next-line investigation, and why was it not requested initially?

➥ answer on page 388

Case 3.2

A 21-year-old soldier complains of a headache for the past 2 days and a dislike of light. He is feverish. He has recently returned from deployment in Germany. Examination did not reveal any focal neurological signs or signs suggestive of raised intracranial pressure. The CSF opening pressure at the time of lumbar puncture was normal (17 cmCSF). Lumbar puncture is performed, and the following results obtained.

Appearance	Clear. No organisms seen	
WCC	101/mm^3 (>95% lymphocytes)	(<5/mm^3)
RCC	9/mm^3	(0/mm^3)
Glucose	3.9 mmol/l	(Approx. 40–60% of plasma glucose)
Total protein	0.62 g/l	(0.15–0.45 g/l)
Plasma glucose	5.8 mmol/l	(Random 4.0–8.0 mmol/l)
Plasma total protein	72 g/l	(60–80 g/l)

Interpret this CSF sample and give a differential diagnosis of the cause.

➥ answer on page 388

Case 3.3

A 74-year-old woman attends the diabetes clinic for a routine appointment. Her medical history includes type 2 diabetes (diagnosed 15 years previously), two previous myocardial infarctions and previous varicose vein surgery. She has noticed an ulcer on her left leg. Examination reveals the presence of varicose eczema, and a shallow ulcer of diameter 4 cm affecting the medial aspect of the left leg.

1. **How would you manage this woman?**

The ABPI was 0.9.

2. **What treatment should the patient receive?**

→ **answer on page 389**

Case 3.4

DAILY WEIGHTS

DATE	TIME	WEIGHT
10/06/05	0800 HRS	125 KG
11/06/05	0800	124 KG
12/06/05	0800	123.1 KG
13/06/05	0800	122.2 KG
14/06/05	0800	115.4 KG
15/06/05	0800	115.9 KG
16/06/05	0800	116.6 KG
17/06/05	0800	118.1 KG

1. **Explain the findings on this daily weight chart for this patient with liver cirrhosis and ascites.**
2. **What could be the reason for the sudden loss of nearly 7 kg on 14/06/05?**

→ **answer on page 389**

Case 3.5

A 39-year-old man is admitted to the neurology ward following a short illness. He is unable to move his legs. He was previously well, although he did have a short bout of diarrhoea a week ago after his return from holiday in Turkey.

Lumbar puncture was performed. The CSF opening pressure at the time of lumbar puncture was 18 cmCSF.

Appearance	Clear. No organisms seen	
WCC	5/mm^3	(<5/mm^3)
RCC	2/mm^3	(0/mm^3)
Glucose	3.6 mmol/l	(Approx. 40–60% of plasma glucose)
Total protein	2.1 g/l	(0.15–0.45 g/l)
Plasma glucose	4.7 mmol/l	(Random 4.0–8.0 mmol/l)
Plasma total protein	65 g/l	(60–80 g/l)

1. **What are the significant findings and what condition could cause this?**
2. **What other test might help in coming to a diagnosis?**

➥ **answer on page 390**

Case 3.6

HOSPITAL

AFFIX LABEL HERE OR ENTER

SPECIAL TEMPERATURE PULSE AND RESPIRATION CHART

FULL NAME Paul Bell

ADDRESS 1 The Crescent, Bishop Stepford

D.O.B. 22/01/79 WD./O.P.D. 5

HOSPITAL NO. BIC 02 - 1234

TIME	1000	1200	1400	1600	1800	2000	2200	2400	0200	0400	0600	0800
SpO$_2$	97% RA	99% RA	97% RA	98% RA	99% RA	96% RA	98% RA	91% RA	86% RA	84% RA	89% RA	99% RA

MONTH / DATE / FREQUENCY

41.0 40.5 40.0 39.5 39.0 38.5

Give your impression of the problem in this patient.

➥ **answer on page 391**

Case 3.7

A 52-year-old male shop assistant presents as an emergency to his general practitioner complaining of central chest pain. This has been present for 30 minutes. He is sweaty and short of breath, and complains of nausea. His risk factors for ischaemic heart disease include smoking and hypertension.

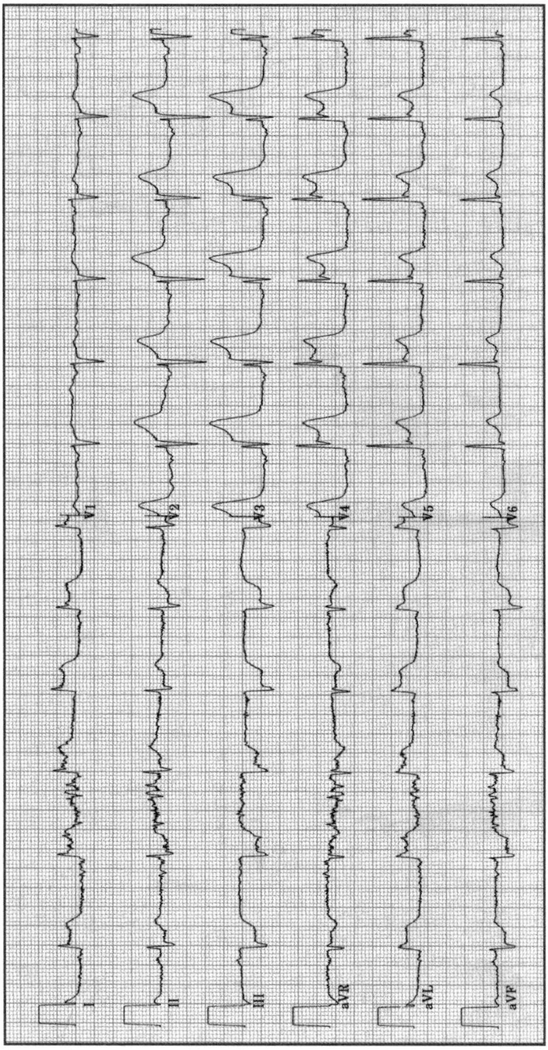

His ECG is shown. How would you interpret it?

➥ answer on page 392

Case 3.8

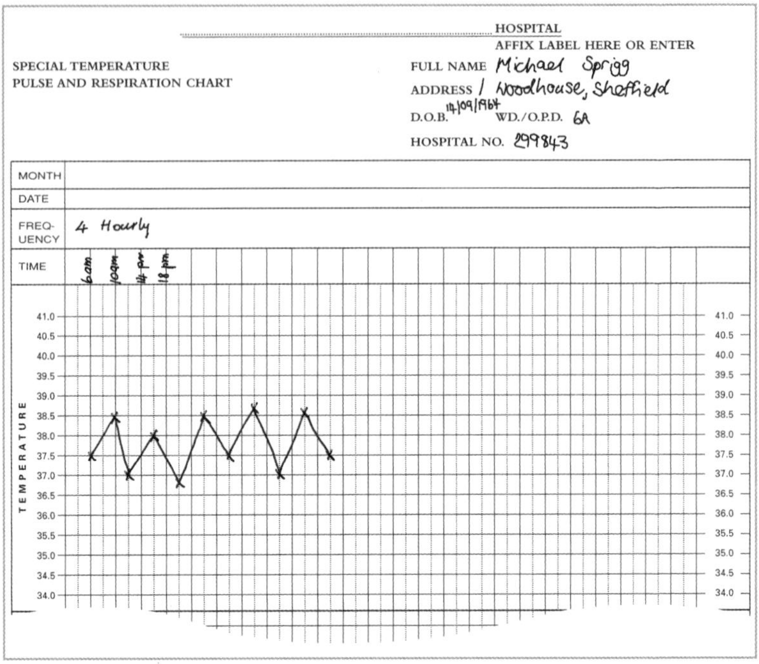

Describe the findings on this chart.

➥ answer on page 394

Case 3.9

Start date 19/02/05

Drug Prescription and Administration Record (DPAR1)

Tim Scott

Patient details
Affix label

ADC 542219 DOB 11/03/69

Drug allergies:

ASPIRIN

Weight		Date		Signature	
Weight		Date		Signature	[signature]

For the safety of the patient, please read the following instructions:

- Use generic names;
- Do not alter existing instructions;
- Discontinue a drug by drawing a line through it and signing.
- All drugs given must be initialled in the appropriate box.
- Write in CAPITALS and BLACK ink;
- Changes must be ordered by a new prescription;

REGULAR PRESCRIPTIONS

Date, month and year →

Drug	Frequency	Dose	Route	Start date	Stop date	Signature	Stop signature	Additional information	Times
CLOPIDOGREL	OD	75MG	PO	19/02		[signature]			08
AMLODIPINE	OD	10MG	PO	19/02		[signature]			08
WARFARIN								SEE INR CHART	
PARACETAMOL	QDS	1G	PO	19/02	21/02	[signature]	[signature]		08, 12, 16, 22
ERYTHROMYCIN	QDS	250MG	PO	19/02		[signature]			08, 12, 16, 22

continued overleaf

Tim Scott
ADC 542219 DOB 11/05/69

Date	INR result	Warfarin dose	Prescribed by	Given by	Time	Date	INR result	Warfarin dose	Prescribed by	Given by	Time
19/02	2.35	4 mg	[illegible]	CM	2200						
20/02	–	4 mg	[illegible]	CM	2200						
21/02	2.98	3 mg	PKH	EFF	2200						
22/02	–	3 mg	[illegible]	KRT	2200						
23/02	3.99	2 mg	PKH	NHY	2200						

What has caused the fluctuation in the INR?

➥ **answer on page 395**

Case 3.10

A 67-year-old woman is reviewed in the cardiology clinic 2 months after a myocardial infarction. She complains of shortness of breath on walking 100 metres on the flat, which she did not have before her heart attack. On further questioning, she reports having to sleep on five pillows to prevent shortness of breath. An echocardiogram is requested.

Aortic root diameter is 3.3 cm
Morphologically normal aortic valve. No restriction of aortic valve leaflet opening. Aortic regurgitation (trace)
Left ventricular cavity size and wall thickness are normal. Left ventricular diastolic cavity diameter is 5.1 cm. Septal diastolic thickness is 1.1 cm
Posterior wall thickness is 1.1 cm. Severely hypokinetic anterior wall. Left ventricular ejection fraction is 25%
Morphologically normal mitral valve. Mitral regurgitation (trace)
Normal left atrial dimensions
Estimated pulmonary artery systolic pressure is 22 mmHg
Normal right ventricular cavity dimension. Right ventricular systolic function is normal. Normal tricuspid valve
Normal inferior vena cava and hepatic vein size indicating normal venous pressures
Technically fair study. Other cardiac valves and chambers appear normal. No pericardial effusion. No evidence of bacterial endocarditis on this study

How would you explain this woman's symptoms?

➥ **answer on page 397**

Case 3.11 +

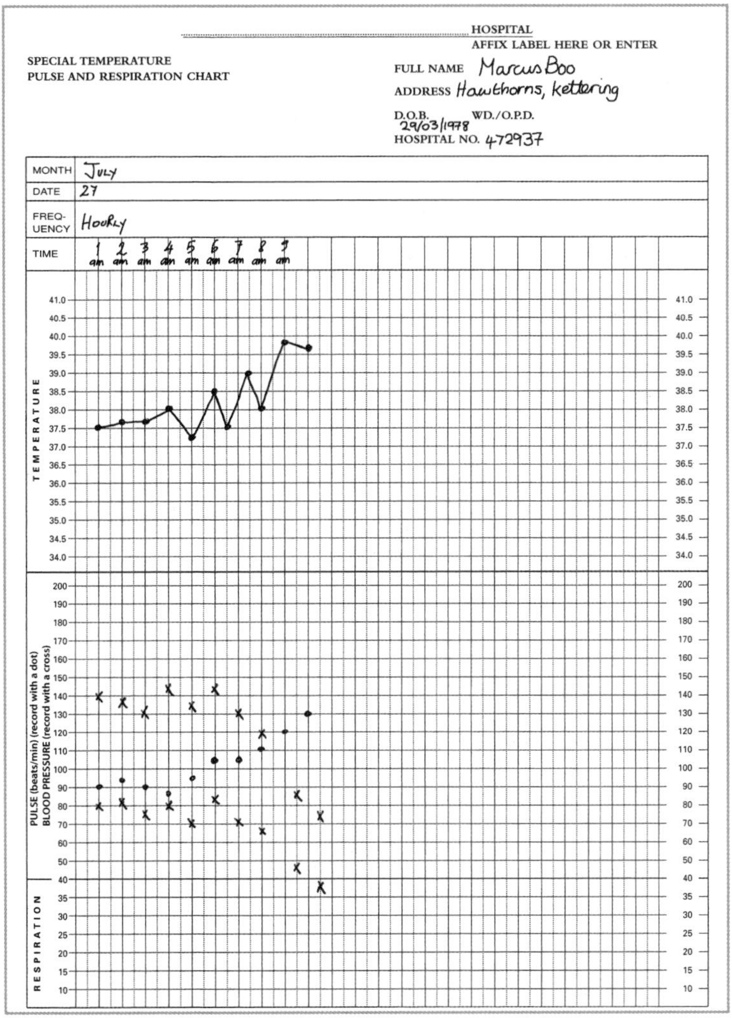

1. Describe each abnormality on the observation chart and the overall impression.
2. Where should this patient be cared for?

➥ answer on page 398

Case 3.12 +

A 29-year-old bank clerk has become known to local neurologists over the past year following several presentations to both the hospital and the outpatient clinic with a variable constellation of neurological symptoms. Initially a complaint of numbness over the lateral aspect of the left leg was mentioned. This resolved. Of late, she has had an episode of loss of vision in the right eye lasting 4 weeks. Examination reveals global hyperreflexia and a mild cerebellar gait.

The patient attends the ward for a series of tests including lumbar puncture. The CSF opening pressure was 17 cmCSF.

Appearance	Clear. No organisms seen	
WCC	2/mm^3	(<5/mm^3)
RCC	1/mm^3	(0/mm^3)
Glucose	3.9 mmol/l	(Approx. 40–60% of plasma glucose)
Total protein	0.46 g/l	(0.15–0.45 g/l)
Oligoclonal bands	Present	
ACE level	Normal	

A blood sample was taken at the same time:

Plasma glucose	5.1 mmol/l	(Random 4.0–8.0 mmol/l)
Plasma total protein	68 g/l	(60–80 g/l)
Oligoclonal bands	Absent	

What is the likely diagnosis?

➥ **answer on page 399**

Case 3.13

A 50-year-old manager presents to the accident and emergency department complaining of chest pain. He is very worried that he may be having a heart attack, since his brother had one last year. He has no other risk factors for cardiac disease. On further questioning, he describes doing heavy work in his garden on the previous day. Examination reveals an anxious man with tenderness on either side of the sternum. An ECG is performed.

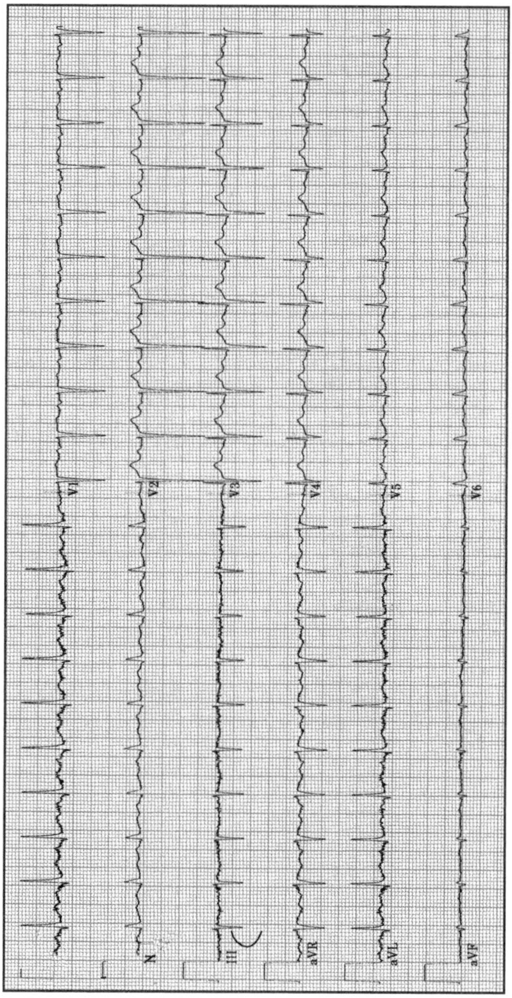

What is your interpretation?

➥ answer on page 400

Case 3.14

NAME Roger Hales

WARD 2F

NO 998877

COMA SCALE			DATE / TIME					
Eyes open	Spontaneously	4	✓				
	To speech	3		✓	✓	✓	
	To pain	2					✓
	None	1					
Best verbal response	Orientated	5	✓	✓	✓		
	Confused	4				✓	
	Inappropriate words	3					
	Incomprehensible sounds	2					✓
	None	1					
Best motor response	Obey commands	6	✓	✓	✓	✓	
	Localises pain	5					
	Flexion withdrawal	4					
	Abnormal flexion	3					✓
	Extension to pain	2					
	None	1					

Explain what action one should take on becoming aware of these observations.

➥ **answer on page 402**

Case 3.15

A 70-year-old man with a long history of rheumatoid disease is reviewed at clinic. He complains that he is unable to make it to the newsagents any longer without having to stop to catch his breath. He has no history of chest or cardiovascular disease. He has no other symptoms. On examination, fine end-inspiratory crepitations are heard at both lung bases. Spirometry is requested.

FEV_1	68% predicted
FVC	50% predicted
FEV_1/FVC	85%

1. **Outline the abnormal findings in the results above.**
2. **What is the most likely cause for these abnormalities in this patient?**
3. **What imaging test would be most useful here?**

➥ **answer on page 403**

Case 3.16

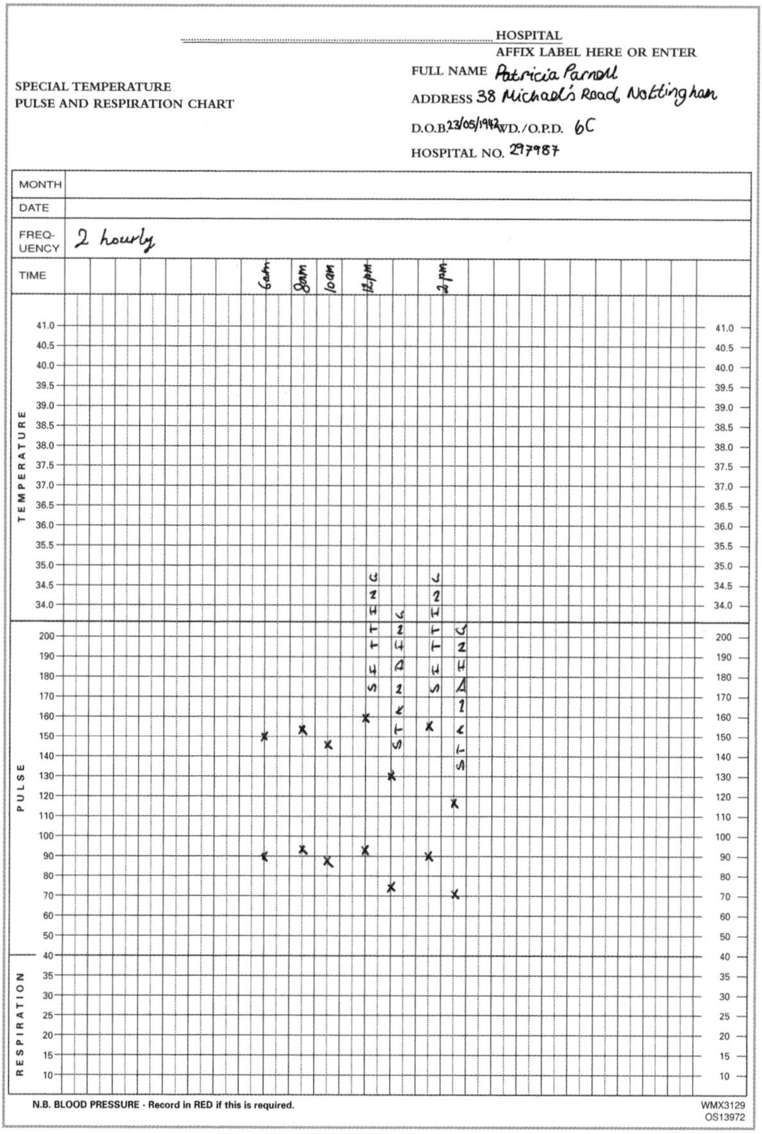

1. What abnormality is seen?
2. Suggest a list of potential underlying diagnoses.

➥ answer on page 404

Case 3.17

The following chart plots changes in PEFR of a patient with asthma during her hospital stay.

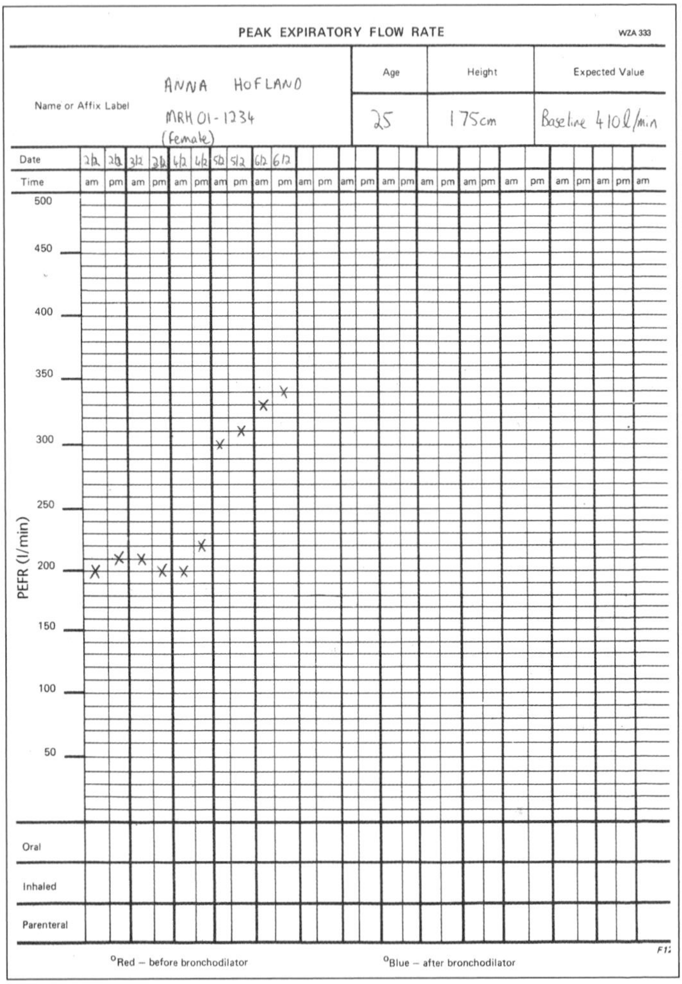

How would you interpret this chart?

➥ answer on page 405

Case 3.18

Start date 22/09/2005

Drug Prescription and Administration Record (DPAR1)

Andrew Brown

Patient details
Affix label
BIC 293949
DoB 22/06/1959

Drug allergies: NKDA

Weight | Date | Signature
Weight | Date | Signature

REGULAR PRESCRIPTIONS

Date, month and year →	Times ↓	22/09	23/09	24/09	25/09										
Drug: ATENOLOL; Frequency: OD; Dose: 50 MG; Route: PO; Start date: 22/09/05; Stop date: ; Signature: [signature]; Stop signature: ; Additional information:	08	TB	RA	SM	EM										
Drug: SPIRONOLACTONE; Frequency: OD; Dose: 100 MG; Route: PO; Start date: 22/09/05; Stop date: ; Signature: [signature]; Stop signature: ; Additional information:	08	GM	GM	SM	EM										
Drug: LISINOPRIL; Frequency: OD; Dose: 5 MG; Route: PO; Start date: 23/09/05; Stop date: ; Signature: [signature]; Stop signature: ; Additional information:	08	/	GM	SM	EM										
Drug: SLOW-K; Frequency: BD; Dose: ii; Route: PO; Start date: 24/09; Stop date: ; Signature: [signature]; Stop signature: ; Additional information:	08			SM	EM										
	22			TRJ	RMT										
Drug: LACTULOSE; Frequency: BD; Dose: 10 MLS; Route: PO; Start date: 24/09; Stop date: ; Signature: [signature]; Stop signature: ; Additional information:	08			SM	EM										
	22			TRJ	RMT										

What electrolyte is likely to be deranged in this patient?

➥ **answer on page 406**

Case 3.19

A 19-year-old university student complains of a headache of 8 h duration accompanied by a dislike for lights. She has vomited twice. She is sweaty to the touch. No rash is apparent. The A&E officer was concerned enough to request a CT scan of the brain which was reported as normal. She proceeds to lumbar puncture. The CSF pressure was normal at the time of lumbar puncture.

Appearance	Cloudy. No organisms seen	
WCC	228/mm^3 (predominantly neutrophils)	(<5/mm^3)
RCC	4/mm^3	(0/mm^3)
Glucose	2.1 mmol/l	(Approx. 40–60% of plasma glucose)
Total protein	0.96 g/l	(0.15–0.45 g/l)
Plasma glucose	5.9 mmol/l	(Random 4.0–8.0 mmol/l)
Plasma total protein	69 g/l	(60–80 g/l)

Describe the CSF, and state the most likely diagnosis.

→ **answer on page 407**

Case 3.20

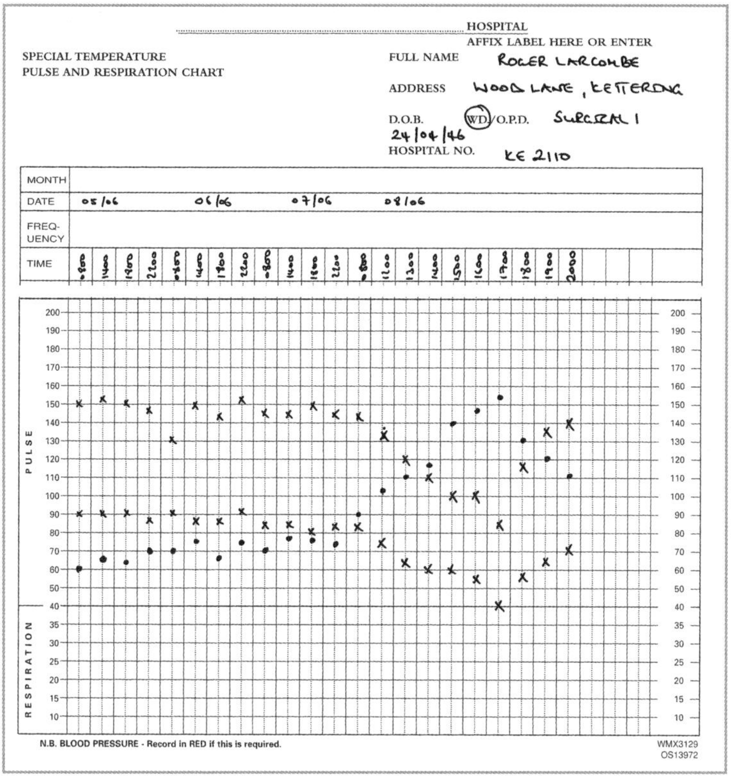

NAME	ROGER LARCOMBE	HOSPITAL NUMBER	KE2110
DATE OF BIRTH	24/04/1946	WARD	SURGICAL I

DATE	TIME	AMOUNT	CONSISTENCY	BLOOD	MUCUS	PUS	SIGN
5/6	08 00	SMALL	4				[signature]
	16 00	MODERATE	5				[signature]
6/6	10 00	SMALL	5	DARK			[signature]
	20 00	SMALL	4	DARK			[signature]
7/6	0900	MODERATE	5	DARK			[signature]
	1300	SMALL	4				[signature]
	21 00	MODERATE	4	DARK			[signature]
8/6	06 00	LARGE	5	BLACK+FOUL			[signature]
	07 00	MODERATE	5	"			[signature]
	09 00	LARGE	5	"			[signature]
	13 00	MODERATE	5	"			[signature]
	1700	MODERATE	5	"			[signature]

Describe the findings on these charts and what investigation(s) are needed to confirm the cause.

➥ **answer on page 408**

Case 3.21

You are called to a cardiac arrest. Nursing staff have attached ECG electrodes, and the following rhythm is noted on the monitor.

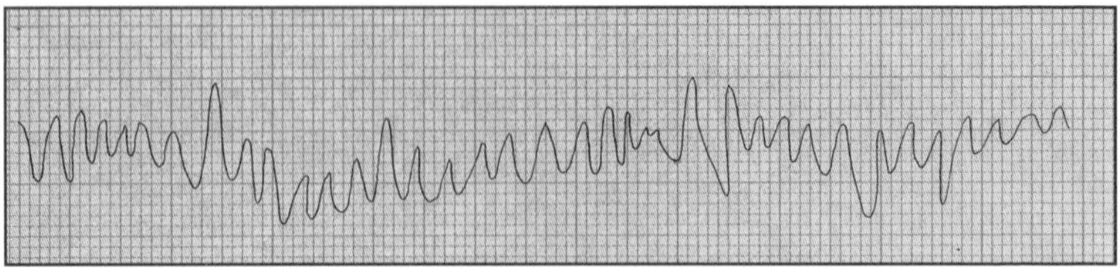

What is the rhythm?

➥ answer on page 409

Case 3.22

FAECES CHART

NAME	A PATIENT	**HOSPITAL NUMBER**	123456
DATE OF BIRTH	1/1/1970	**WARD** Buttercup	

DATE	TIME	STOOL TYPE	CONSISTENCY	BLOOD	MUCUS	PUS	SIGN
10/06	0800	MODERATE	6 or 7	✓	✓		
	1000	"	7	✓			
	1230	"	6	✓			
	1425	"	6		✓		
	1615	"	7	✓			
	1845	"	7	✓			
	2105	LARGE	7	✓	✓		
	2330	"	6	✓			
11/06	0200	"	7	✓	✓		
	0530	MODERATE	6	✓			
	0720	"	6	✓			
	0930	"	7	✓	✓		
	1145	"	7	✓	✓		
	1355	LARGE	7	✓	✓		
	1605	MODERATE	7	✓			
	1830	"	6	✓			
	2010	"	6	✓			
	2235	"	7	✓			
	2355	"	7	✓			

Summarise the findings on the stool chart and list the potential causes.

➥ answer on page 410

Case 3.23 ++

A previously fit and well 28-year-old woman is admitted with chest pain. The pain is sharp in nature, has some relationship to respiration and is eased by sitting forward. Her ECG is shown:

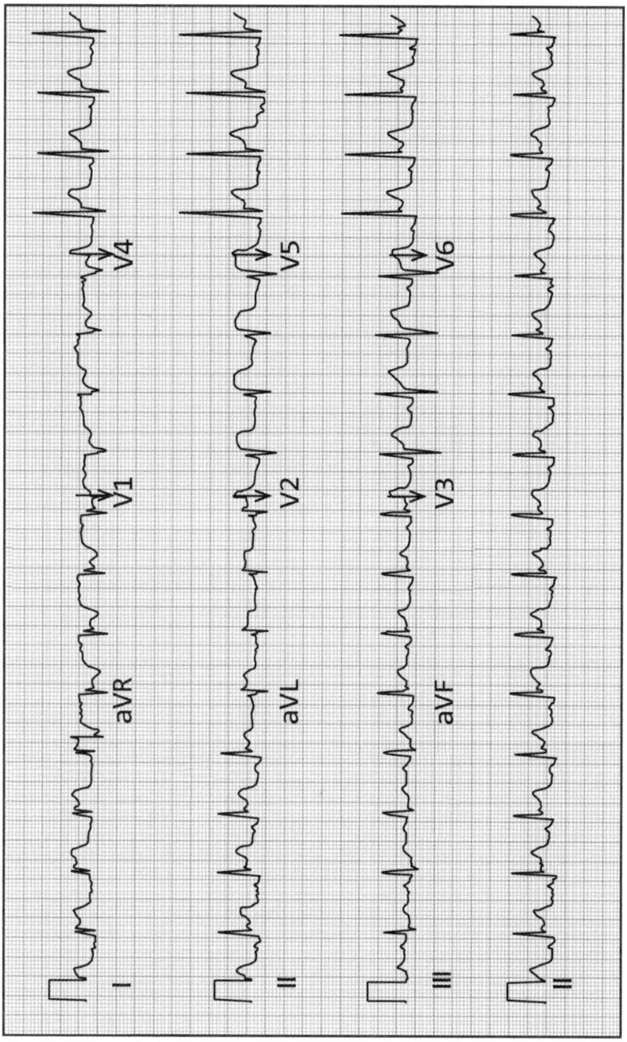

What is your interpretation?

➥ **answer on page 411**

Case 3.24 ++

A 70-year-old woman with a history of a myocardial infarction presents with palpitations that are of recent onset. Her ECG is shown.

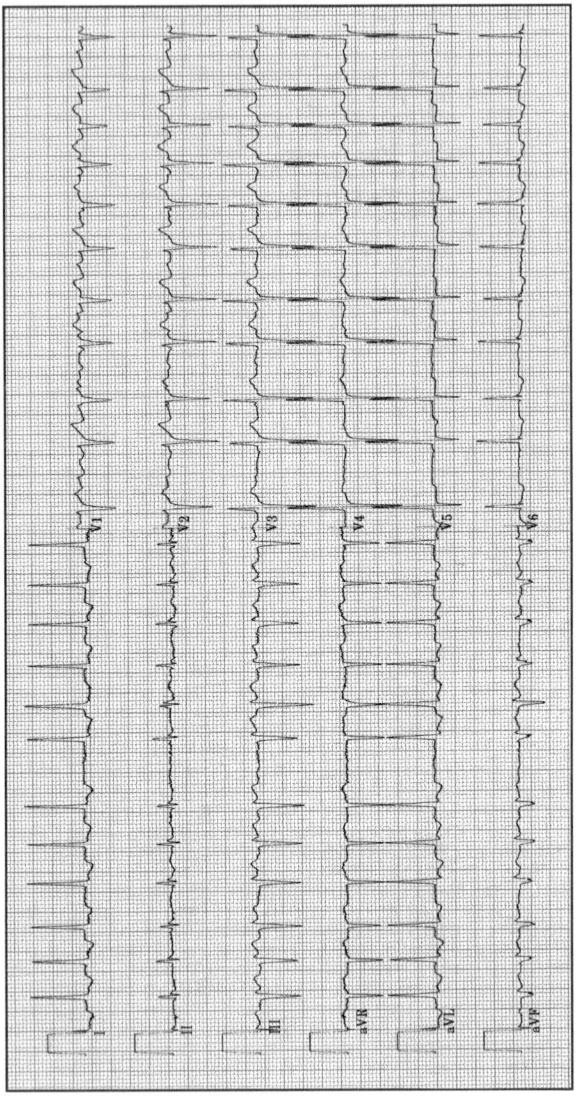

How would you interpret it?

➥ answer on page 413

Case 3.25 ++

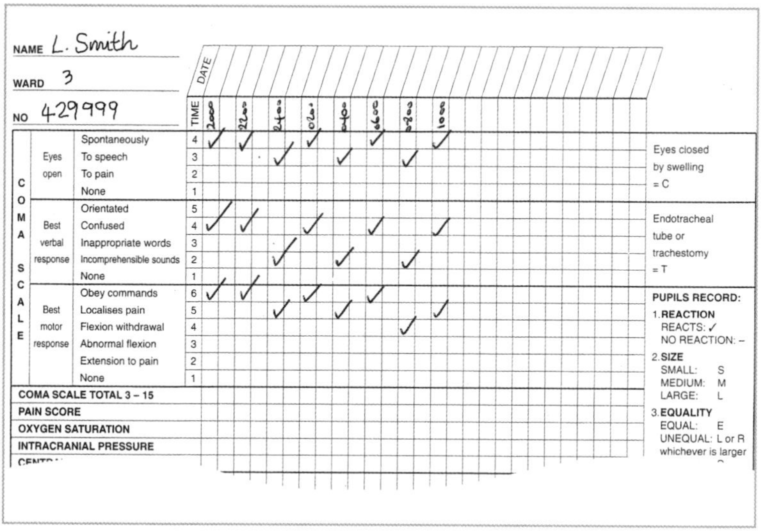

1. Explain the findings on the neuro-observation chart.
2. What are the potential causes?

➥ answer on page 415

Case 3.26 ++

A 74-year-old man is admitted complaining of dizziness. He has had several myocardial infarctions in the past. Clinical examination reveals a pulse rate of 30 beats/min, and a blood pressure of 62/46 mmHg. An ECG is performed.

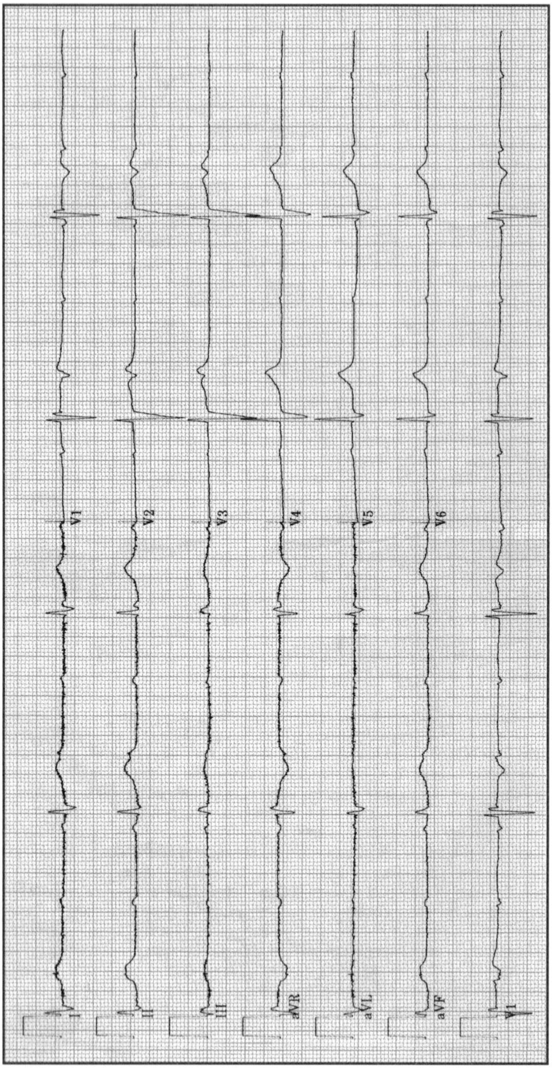

What does it show?

➥ **answer on page 416**

Case 3.27 ++

A patient's heart rate is monitored frequently after an admission with a suspected myocardial infarction.

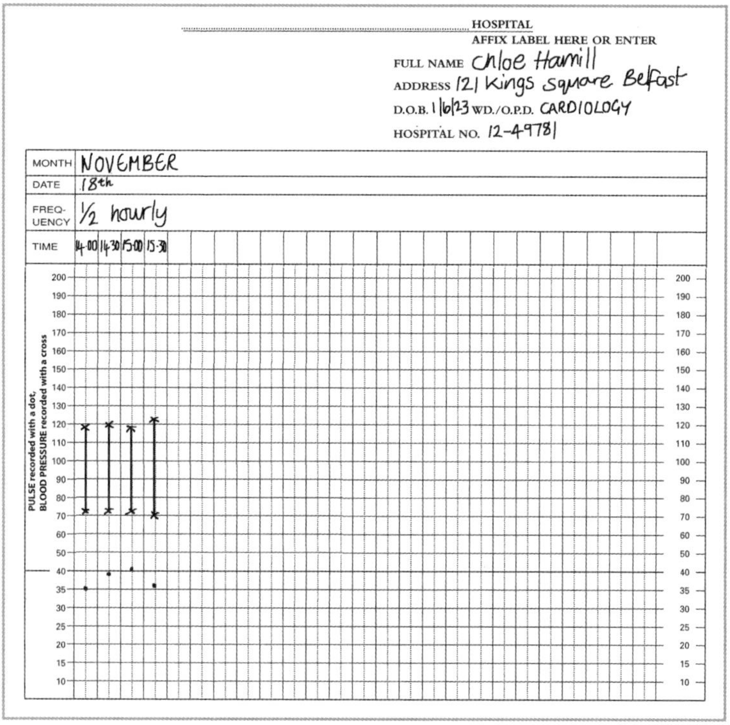

What is your interpretation, and what would you do for the patient?

➥ **answer on page 419**

Case 3.28 ++

A 68-year-old man who has been a life-long smoker is admitted with a lower respiratory tract infection. He was noted to be wheezy at the time of admission to hospital, and was treated with antibiotics and nebulised bronchodilators. His inflammatory markers settled, but he remained wheezy. Pulmonary function tests were performed 3 weeks later after resolution of his acute illness.

FEV_1	42% predicted
FVC	60% predicted
FEV_1/FVC	52%
*K*co	53% predicted

1. **Outline the abnormal findings in the results above.**
2. **What is the most likely cause for these abnormalities in this patient?**

➥ **answer on page 420**

Case 3.29 ++

A 36-year-old woman has been attending the respiratory outpatient department for 5 years because of sarcoidosis. Her disease has been well controlled recently, and her dose of oral steroids has been gradually reduced over a period of several months. On her most recent visit, she complains of increasing shortness of breath over the preceding 3 weeks. Her pulmonary function tests are shown alongside a set taken when she was feeling well.

	2 months before	**Present day**
FEV_1	69% predicted	63% predicted
FVC	52% predicted	49% predicted
FEV_1/FVC	68%	65% predicted
*K*co	90% predicted	61% predicted

What parameter has changed significantly between the two sets of readings, and how would you account for this?

➥ **answer on page 420**

Case 3.30 +++

A 65-year-old man is being investigated for hypertension. An ambulatory blood pressure monitor is fitted, and the following summary trace is provided.

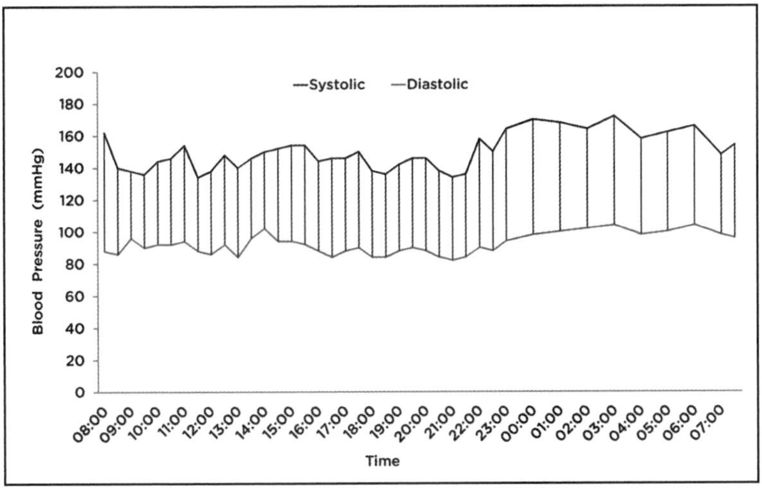

Image used with permission from Hamilton P, Corr M. Medical student quiz. *Ulster Medical Journal* 2016;**85**:55–6.

1. Interpret the trace.
2. What is the significance of this finding?

➥ **answer on page 420**

Case 3.31 +++

An elderly man is in the coronary care unit following a myocardial infarction. He is treated with primary angioplasty and is doing well until he develops further pain on day 2 post-procedure. His ECG is shown below:

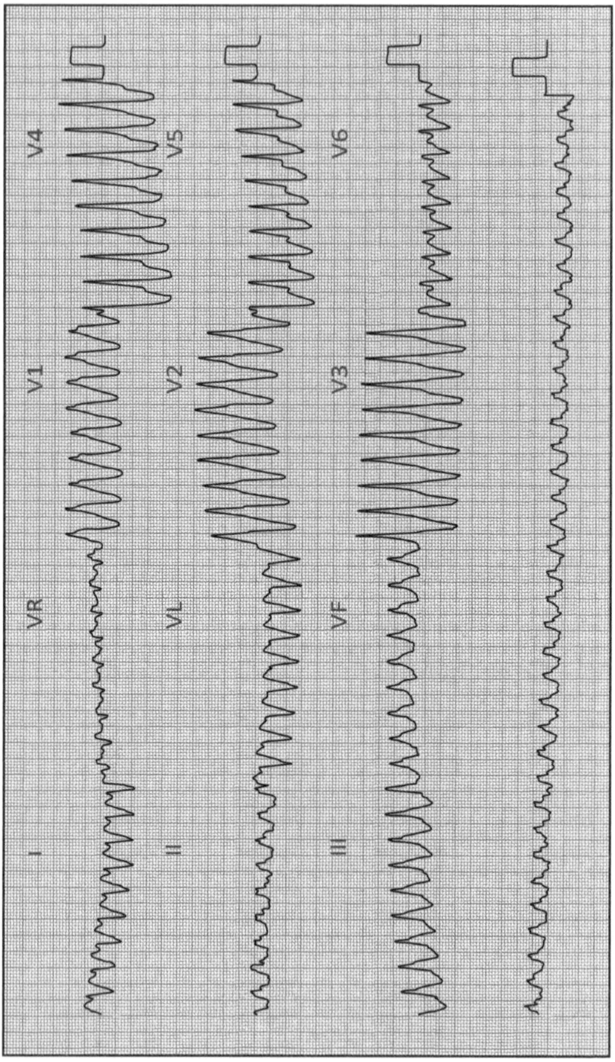

What is your interpretation?

➥ **answer on page 421**

Case 3.32 +++

A 64-year-old woman is admitted from A&E complaining of increasing shortness of breath. This has been worsening over a period of 2 months. There is little of note on examination. The admitting doctor arranges for pulmonary function tests to assess her symptom.

FEV_1	90% predicted
FVC	88% predicted
FEV_1/FVC	75%
*K*co	40% predicted

1. **Outline the abnormal findings in the results above.**
2. **What blood test would you order?**

→ **answer on page 422**

Case 3.33 +++

An 80-year-old female nursing home resident presents with acute confusion. No other history is available. On examination, she is tachypnoeic, with oxygen saturations of 83% on 85% oxygen. She is peripherally cyanosed. Blood pressure is 74/32 mmHg. On auscultating her lungs, she has medium inspiratory crepitations to her midzones.

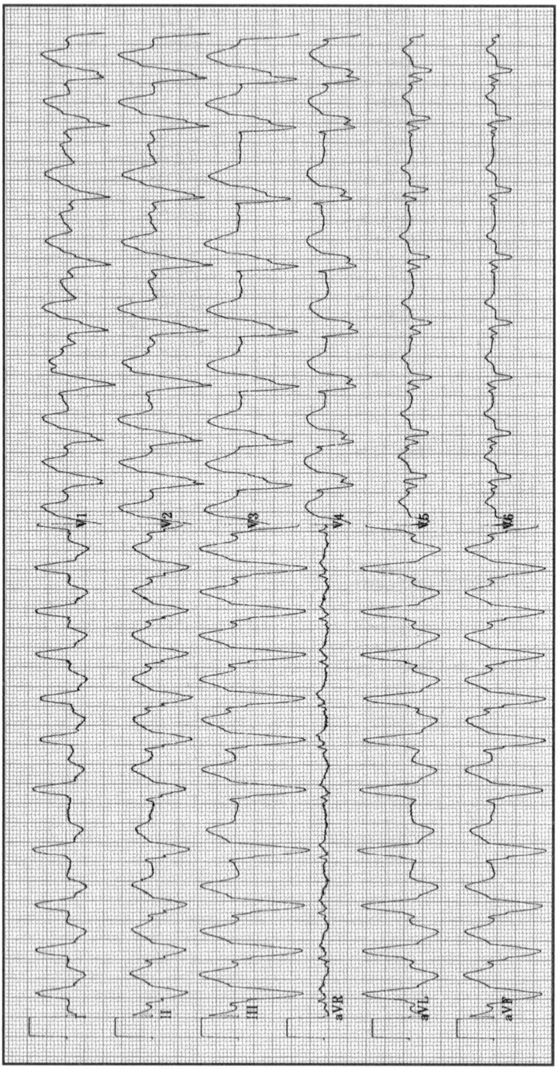

What is your interpretation?

➥ answer on page 423

AT THE BEDSIDE AND IN THE CLINIC: ANSWERS

3

Answer 3.1

➥ case on page 360

A CT angiogram can be used to investigate possible SAH in patients who have a normal cerebrospinal fluid examination. The problem with CT angiography (apart from the need to administer contrast, and the radiation dose) is that a percentage of the normal population have intracerebral aneurysms, and there is the possibly of incidentally finding such an abnormality in an individual who did not in fact have an SAH. The problem relates to the fact that the treatment of intracranial aneurysms is not without its potential complications. MRI of the brain may assist further in identifying small quantities of subarachnoid blood at this stage, due to its ability to identify blood of variable age on susceptibility-weighted sequences.

Answer 3.2

➥ case on page 360

The differential WCC reveals that lymphocytes are the predominant cell type here. The CSF:plasma glucose ratio is a little high, and the total protein is elevated - but only marginally. In summary, many of the parameters are abnormal, but not markedly so.

CAUSES OF LYMPHOCYTE-PREDOMINANT LEUKOCYTOSIS IN CSF	
Viral meningitis	Tuberculous meningitis
Mumps meningoencephalitis	Partially treated bacterial meningitis

The most common cause for these findings is viral meningitis - the virus itself may never be identified. Polymerase chain reaction analysis of CSF can be performed to test for a number of viruses, including herpes simplex. The treatment and outcome of viral meningitis are markedly different to those of partially treated bacterial meningitis, and if any diagnostic doubt exists, treatment should continue for bacterial meningitis.

Answer 3.3

➥ case on page 361

1. Leg ulcers can be the result of several underlying disease processes. Most commonly, ulcers can be due to venous insufficiency, arterial insufficiency or a combination of both. The patient's medical history puts her at risk of both venous (previous varicose vein surgery) and arterial (diabetes and ischaemic heart disease) ulcers. Findings on examination are, however, more in keeping with a venous ulcer.

   Management of venous ulceration is complex, but the mainstay relies on graduated pressure bandages. However, these bandages can exacerbate arterial insufficiency, and should not be routinely applied to all patients without first performing an ABPI measurement. The first step in the management of this patient's ulcer should therefore involve measurement of the ABPI.

2. The patient should be treated with graduated pressure bandages. Patients with an ABPI of less than 0.8 should not, in general, have compression bandages applied.

Answer 3.4

➥ case on page 361

DAILY WEIGHTS

DATE	TIME	WEIGHT	
10/06/05	0800 HRS	125 KG	
11/06/05	0800	124 KG	
12/06/05	0800	123.1 KG	
13/06/05	0800	122.2 KG	Steady weight loss until here
14/06/05	0800	115.4 KG	Dramatic weight loss
15/06/05	0800	115.9 KG	
16/06/05	0800	116.6 KG	
17/06/05	0800	118.1 KG	Gradual weight gain

1. Daily weight charts are an extension of the standard fluid balance ('input/output') chart. In the short term (hours and days) changes usually reflect a change in body fluid content. It is paramount (as seen from the chart)

that the recordings are taken at the same time each day. Dietitians keep weight records for those who are undernourished, receiving enteral or parenteral nutritional supplementation, or enrolled in dietary programmes. In such cases, changes in the longer term become more important. The common reasons for recording daily weight are conditions in which excess fluid is retained by the body - severe congestive cardiac failure, ascites or renal failure being prime examples.

A response to treatment, in particular diuretics and dietary sodium restriction, may be monitored using a weight chart in conjunction with a fluid balance chart.

This example documents a patient with significant ascites (excess fluid in the peritoneal cavity) over a period of several days after treatment. Over the initial 4 days a steady, albeit relatively small, daily reduction in weight is observed. This is in response to the introduction or increased dosing of diuretic therapy.

2. On 14/06/05 a more substantial reduction of 6.8 kg is observed. This is due to paracentesis with the removal of a substantial volume of fluid.

Answer 3.5

➥ case on page 362

1. The history is short and the symptoms significant. However, the only significant abnormality on the CSF sample is the elevated level of protein within the CSF. The plasma total protein is normal. The CSF protein is raised to a greater degree than one would usually expect for a viral or bacterial meningitis/encephalitis. Note that the WCC and the CSF:plasma glucose ratio are also not in keeping with an infective pathology. The differential diagnosis is therefore of diseases causing a high CSF protein.

   When interpreted in the context of the history of leg weakness after an episode of infectious diarrhoea, the diagnosis is most likely to be Guillain-Barré syndrome (an acute inflammatory polyneuropathy).

2. Nerve conduction studies (NCS) would help diagnosis (see Neurophysiological investigations on page 356 for further details).

Answer 3.6

➥ case on page 362

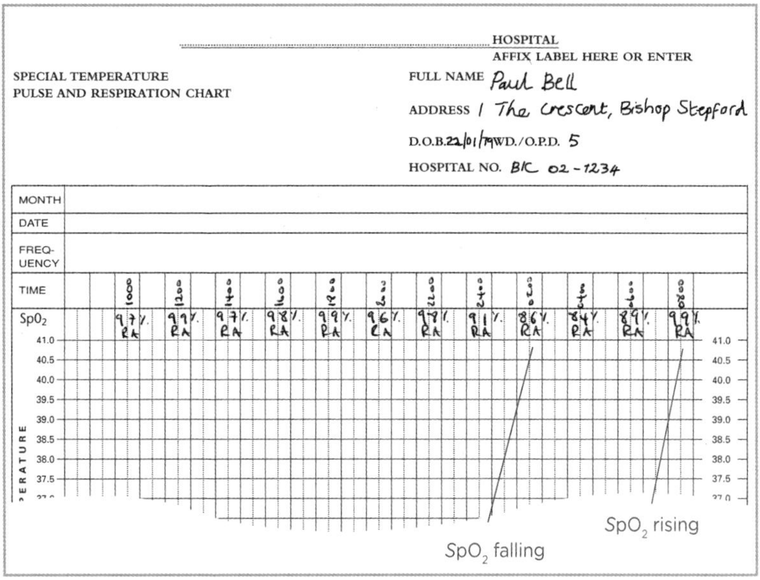

This chart outlines the blood oxygen saturations taken at 2-h intervals by pulse oximetry throughout a 24-h period. The vast majority are normal while breathing room air. If one was not to record the saturations during sleeping hours the patient may be deemed to be entirely normal. However, during the period 02:00–06:00 hours there is evidence of significant deoxygenation with a low of 84% at 04:00 hours.

A possible diagnosis here is obstructive sleep apnoea (OSA). If one were to waken the patient purposefully and then record the oxygen saturations they would probably return to normal. This diagnosis may be confirmed through formal sleep studies.

Answer 3.7

➥ case on page 363

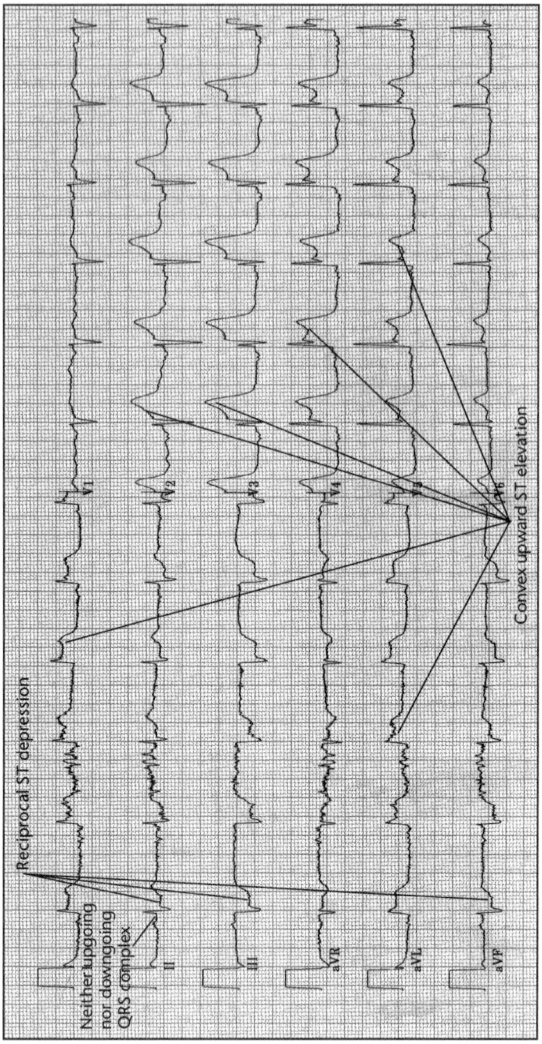

Heart rate

There are 4.2 big squares between consecutive R waves. The ventricular rate is therefore 300 ÷ 4.2 = 71 beats/min.

Heart rhythm

A P wave precedes each QRS complex. The P-R interval is normal (four small squares) and does not vary from beat to beat. The rhythm is sinus rhythm.

Cardiac axis

Lead I is upgoing. Lead III is downgoing. Lead II is neither upgoing nor downgoing. The axis is approaching that of left axis deviation.

P waves

P waves are of normal size and shape.

QRS complexes

There are no abnormal Q waves. The R and S waves are of normal height. The QRS complex is of normal duration (two small squares).

ST segment

The ST segment is elevated, in a convex shape, in leads I, aVL, V2, V3, V4 and V5. The ST segment is depressed and horizontal in leads II, III, aVR and aVF. When ST depression accompanies ST elevation, it is known as reciprocal ST depression.

Q-T interval

The Q-T interval is normal (1.5 large squares).

T waves

The T waves appear large, but are difficult to interpret on account of the ST-segment changes.

Conclusion: anterolateral ST elevation myocardial infarction or STEMI (ie affecting the anterior and lateral surfaces of the heart). Reciprocal ST depression in some of the limb leads.

Answer 3.8

➥ case on page 364

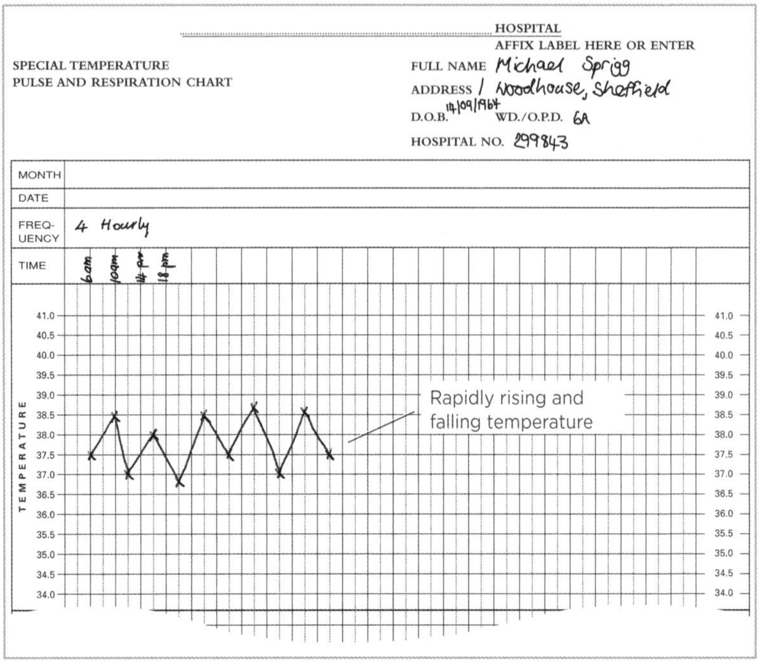

There is a simple but striking finding on the general observation chart over a period of several hours. The trend in temperature recordings is highly abnormal. It can be seen that the patient is apyrexic at times but has a significantly elevated temperature on other occasions. This is a swinging or spiking fever. Each temperature peak probably represents the shedding of bacterial toxins into the bloodstream. This finding may be due to any underlying infective source – although the pattern is characteristically seen in the setting of an abscess. A similar pattern can be seen in several rheumatological diseases, eg Still's disease.

Answer 3.9

➥ case on page 365

Start date 19/02/05

Drug Prescription and Administration Record (DPAR1)

Patient details	Drug allergies:
TIM SCOTT Patient details Affix label ADC 542219 DOB 11/03/69	ASPIRIN

Weight	Date	Signature
Weight	Date	Signature [illegible]

For the safety of the patient, please read the following instructions:

- Use generic names;
- Write in CAPITALS and BLACK ink;
- Do not alter existing instructions;
- Changes must be ordered by a new prescription;
- Discontinue a drug by drawing a line through it and signing.
- All drugs given must be initialled in the appropriate box.

REGULAR PRESCRIPTIONS

Date, month and year →

Drug	Frequency	Dose	Route	Start date	Stop date	Signature	Stop signature	Additional information	Times
CLOPIDOGREL	OD	75 MG	PO	19/02		[illegible]			08
AMLODIPINE	OD	10 MG	PO	19/02		[illegible]			08
WARFARIN								SEE INR CHART	
PARACETAMOL	QDS	1G	PO	19/02	21/02	[illegible]	[illegible]		08, 12, 16, 22
ERYTHROMYCIN	QDS	250 MG	PO	19/02		[illegible]			08, 12, 16, 22

Likely drug interaction (WARFARIN – ERYTHROMYCIN)

Tim Scott
ADC 542219 DOB 11/03/69

Date	INR result	Warfarin dose	Prescribed by	Given by	Time
19/02	2.35	4 mg	[illegible]	CM	2200
20/02	—	4 mg	[illegible]	CM	2200
21/02	2.98	3 mg	PKH	EFF	2200
22/02	—	3 mg	[illegible]	KRT	2200
23/02	3.99	2 mg	PKH	NHY	2200

Date	INR result	Warfarin dose	Prescribed by	Given by	Time

Rising INR

This scenario is based upon both a patient's drug chart and his warfarin chart. Those patients on warfarin while in hospital should be placed on a dedicated warfarin chart. This generally outlines the indication for its prescription, the desired target INR range and the daily warfarin dose and INR if taken. It is easy, but also dangerous, to view this chart in isolation. Following admission this patient is started on erythromycin and the warfarin dose remains at the usual level. The INR was recorded before the first inpatient dose and was 2.35, perfectly placed in the desired range for the indication, atrial fibrillation. On day 3 it is checked again and found to be 2.98. The dose is decreased by 1 mg, but again 2 days later the INR has continued to rise to 3.99. This is not in the highly dangerous range, but is enough to warrant consideration. The drug erythromycin is the cause. A macrolide antibiotic, it is known to enhance the anticoagulant effect of warfarin through its effect as an enzyme inhibitor in the liver.

Answer 3.10

➥ case on page 366

The important points to take away from the echocardiographic report are as follows:

Size of heart chambers (atria and ventricles)	Normal
Ventricular septal thickness	Normal
Left ventricular function	Severe left ventricular wall hypokinesis. Markedly reduced left ventricular ejection fraction
Details about each valve	Only a trace of aortic and mitral regurgitation
Vegetations or tumours	None seen
Estimated pulmonary artery pressure	Normal
Pericardial effusion	None

This woman has symptoms (dyspnoea and orthopnoea) of left ventricular failure. Her echocardiogram demonstrates the poor residual function of her left ventricle following her myocardial infarction.

Answer 3.11

➥ case on page 367

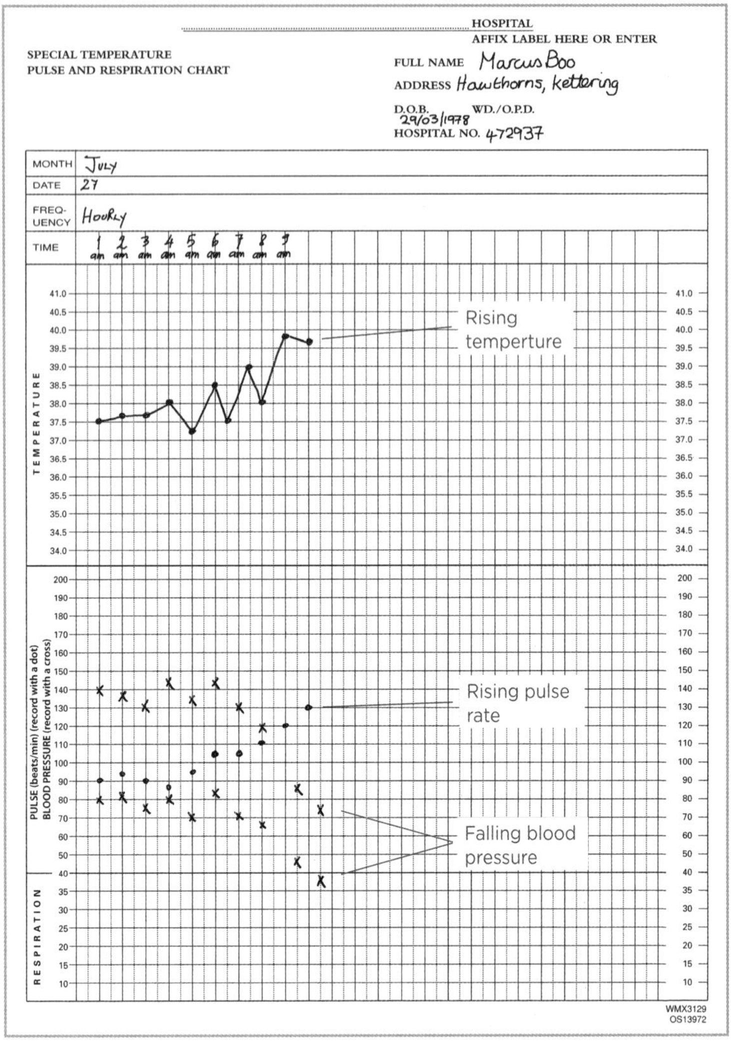

1. The diagnosis of sepsis requires a full patient assessment. However, the bedside chart may provide the first evidence of impending sepsis. Taking an assessment of the chart over several hours, rather than a snapshot, aids in the diagnosis as one views the alteration of three key parameters - blood pressure, pulse rate and temperature. A persistent pyrexia or swinging fever is seen in the context of haemodynamic instability (hypotension and tachycardia).

This example clearly shows a rising and sustained pyrexia with a maximum temperature of 39.9°C. A falling blood pressure, to a low of 78/38 mmHg, with an accompanying tachycardia of 130 beats/min, demonstrates a haemodynamically unstable state.

2. If this patient fails to respond to initial treatment with fluids and antibiotics he should be transferred to an HDU/ICU environment where inotropic support (eg noradrenaline) may be administered to support the cardiovascular system until the underlying infection has been identified and treated.

Answer 3.12

➥ case on page 368

This CSF sample shows essentially normal values for all the common indices. Additional analyses have been performed, including oligoclonal bands which are present.

These bands represent immunoglobulin G (IgG). The presence of this has been noted in a number of conditions - it is therefore of poor specificity in isolation. However, it is found in over 80% of patients with multiple sclerosis (MS). MS is the most common cause for its presence on CSF analysis. It is a supportive feature rather than a diagnostic feature of the disease. MS is the most likely diagnosis here.

CAUSES OF OLIGOCLONAL BANDS IN CSF
Multiple sclerosis
Subacute sclerosing panencephalitis
Guillain-Barré syndrome
Neurosyphilis
Lyme disease
Neurosarcoidosis

Answer 3.13

➥ case on page 369

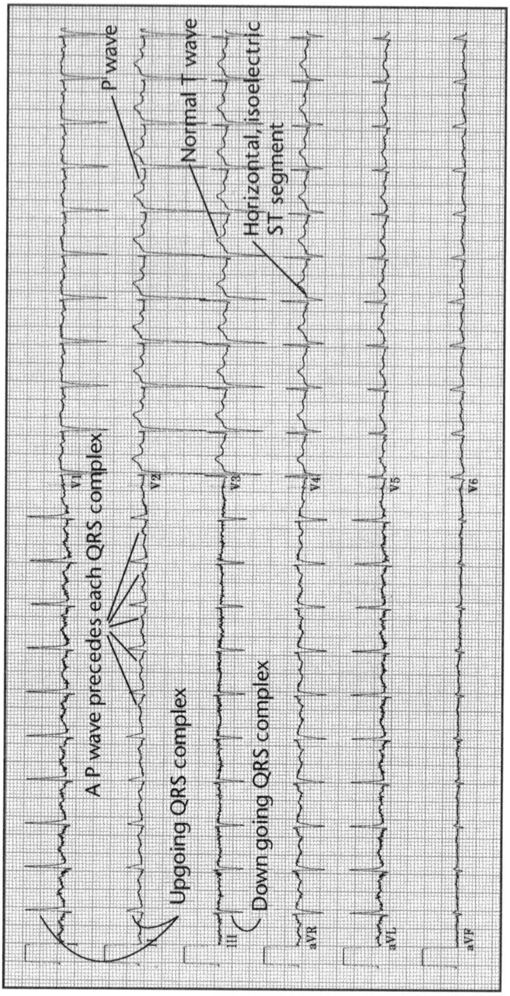

Heart rate

There are 12 small squares between consecutive R waves. The ventricular rate is therefore 1500 ÷ 12 = 125 beats/min.

Heart rhythm

A P wave precedes each QRS complex. The P–R interval is normal (four small squares) and does not vary from beat to beat. The rhythm is sinus rhythm.

Cardiac axis
Leads I and II are upgoing. Lead III is downgoing. The axis is normal.

P waves
P waves are of normal size and shape.

QRS complexes
There are no abnormal Q waves. The R and S waves are of normal height. The QRS complex is of normal duration (two small squares).

ST segment
The ST segment is horizontal and isoelectric.

Q-T interval
The Q-T interval is normal (1.5 large squares).

T waves
T waves are normal in size and shape.

Conclusion: sinus tachycardia. The most likely cause of this is anxiety. Sinus tachycardia is the most common ECG finding in patients with a pulmonary embolism, so this diagnosis should be considered. However, in this case, history and examination point to the true cause of this man's chest pain – muscular strain.

Answer 3.14

➥ case on page 370

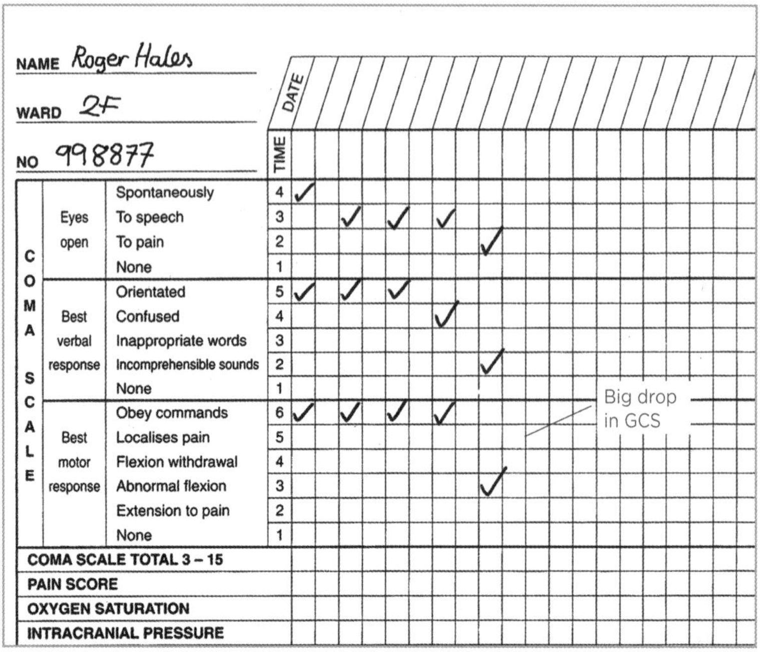

COMA SCALE				1	2	3	4	5
Eyes open	Spontaneously	4		✓				
	To speech	3			✓	✓	✓	
	To pain	2						✓
	None	1						
Best verbal response	Orientated	5		✓	✓	✓		
	Confused	4					✓	
	Inappropriate words	3						
	Incomprehensible sounds	2						✓
	None	1						
Best motor response	Obey commands	6		✓	✓	✓	✓	
	Localises pain	5						
	Flexion withdrawal	4						
	Abnormal flexion	3						✓
	Extension to pain	2						
	None	1						
COMA SCALE TOTAL 3 – 15								
PAIN SCORE								
OXYGEN SATURATION								
INTRACRANIAL PRESSURE								

Changes in conscious level may be sudden and permanent as well as fluctuant. A significant drop in the GCS should be acted upon without delay. This bedside chart records a large drop from 13 to 7. This sudden change requires both a fast answer to establish the cause, and action to be taken to ensure the welfare of the patient. A GCS of less than 8/15 is an indication for consideration of intubation as the patient's airway is likely to become compromised.

CAUSES OF LARGE SUDDEN DROP IN GCS	
Intracerebral bleed (including subarachnoid haemorrhage)	Trauma – diffuse axonal injury
Cerebral oedema	Seizure
Drugs and alcohol	Metabolic causes (such as hypoglycaemia)

Answer 3.15

➥ case on page 370

1. This man has a restrictive defect on spirometry as shown by the raised FEV_1/FVC.
2. The most likely cause would be pulmonary fibrosis, either secondary to his rheumatoid disease or as a side effect of its treatment with methotrexate.
3. An high-resolution CT scan of the chest would best aid diagnosis and management. This would identify any pulmonary changes associated with fibrosis.

Answer 3.16

➥ case on page 371

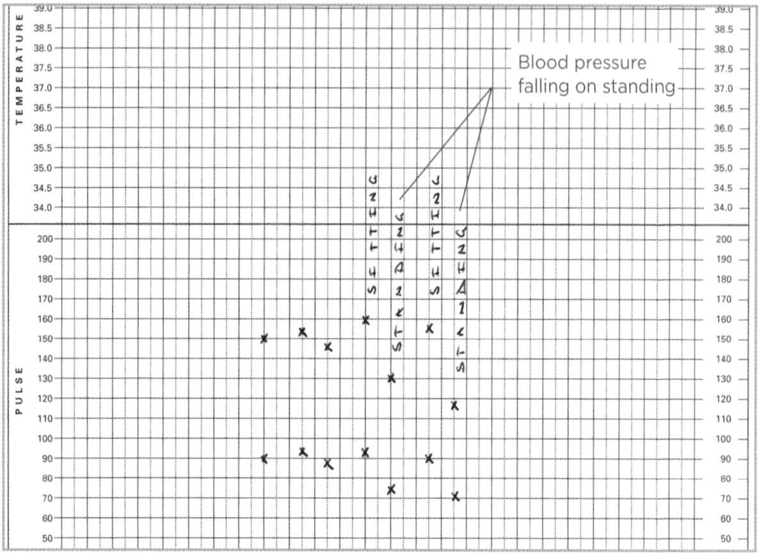

1. This basic chart demonstrates a series of blood pressure measurements. Unlike a conventional recording it indicates that some have been taken in different positions of posture. The likely indication for this is a patient with a history of falls, especially an elderly patient. For changes to be deemed significant, there must be a change in systolic blood pressure of greater than 20 mmHg when the patient changes from lying to standing. This patient has postural (orthostatic) hypotension.
2. Potential diagnoses are listed below:

CAUSES OF POSTURAL HYPOTENSION
Idiopathic
Dehydration (hypovolaemia)
Drug induced (eg diuretics, vasodilators, anti-parkinsonian medication)
Hypoadrenalism
Autonomic neuropathy
Multisystem atrophy
Idiopathic

Answer 3.17

➥ case on page 372

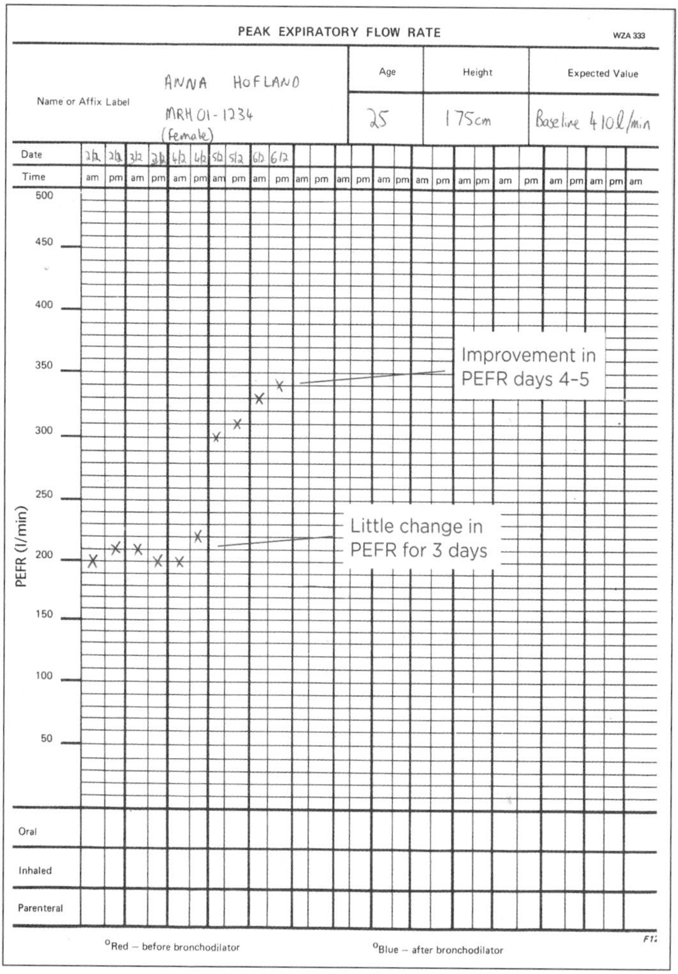

In this bedside chart, the patient's known baseline PEFR of 410 l/min has been documented. Using the patient details at the top of the chart, one can look up the predicted PEFR, which is 505 l/min. Thus, even when at 'her best' she has a reduction in expiratory flow compared with a 'normal' adult of the same build. At the time of admission her PEFR is only 200 l/min - less than half of her baseline. Over the course of the next 2 days there is little change in her PEFR. Her condition has stabilised. Days 4 and 5 of her stay show a significant and sustained increase in her readings. A steady rise to 340 l/min is seen. Either there has been a natural resolution of her asthma attack or the instigation of effective treatment has caused this change.

Answer 3.18

➥ case on page 373

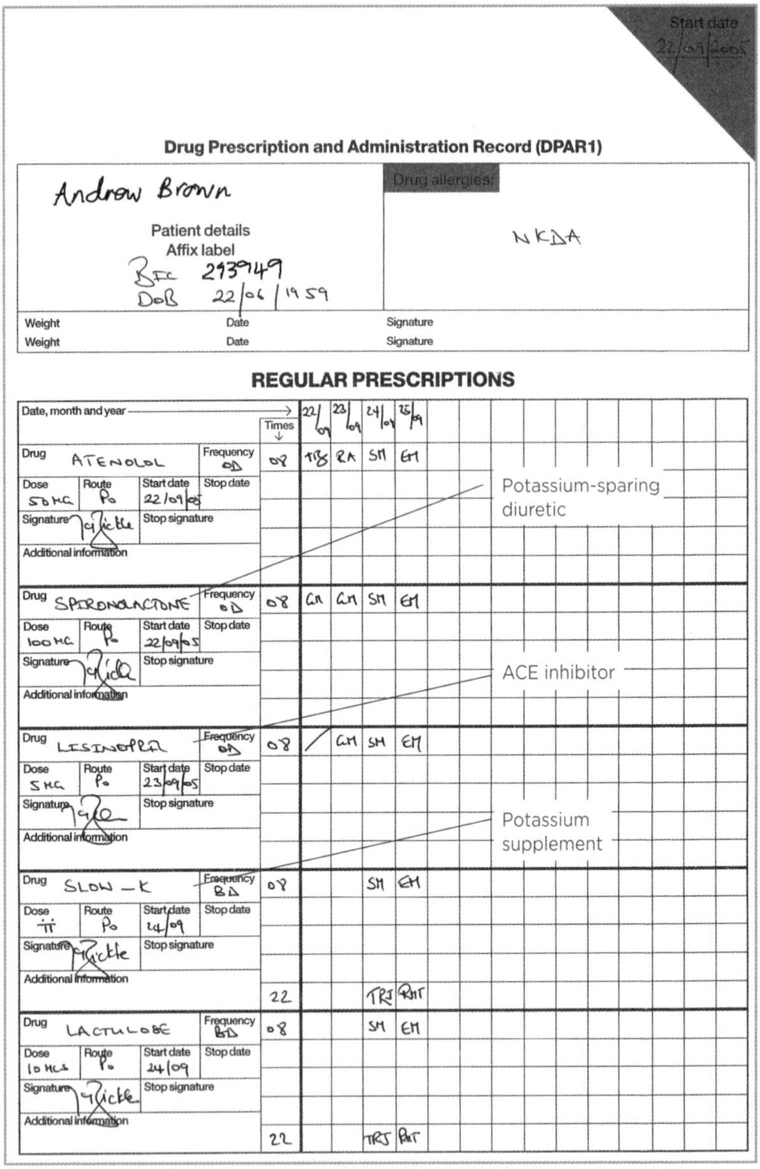
Start date 22/09/2005

Drug Prescription and Administration Record (DPAR1)

Andrew Brown
Patient details
Affix label
BFC 293949
DoB 22/06/1959

Drug allergies: NKDA

Weight | Date | Signature
Weight | Date | Signature

REGULAR PRESCRIPTIONS

Date, month and year	Times	22/09	23/09	24/09	25/09
Drug ATENOLOL; Frequency OD; Dose 50 MG; Route PO; Start date 22/09/05; Stop date; Signature; Stop signature; Additional information	08	TBS	RA	SM	EM
Drug SPIRONOLACTONE; Frequency OD; Dose 100 MG; Route PO; Start date 22/09/05; Stop date; Signature; Stop signature; Additional information	08	GM	GM	SM	EM
Drug LISINOPRIL; Frequency OD; Dose 5 MG; Route PO; Start date 23/09/05; Stop date; Signature; Stop signature; Additional information	08	/	GM	SM	EM
Drug SLOW-K; Frequency BD; Dose ii; Route PO; Start date 24/09; Stop date; Signature; Stop signature; Additional information	08			SM	EM
	22			TRJ	RMT
Drug LACTULOSE; Frequency BD; Dose 10 MLS; Route PO; Start date 24/09; Stop date; Signature; Stop signature; Additional information	08			SM	EM
	22			TRJ	RMT

This relatively simple drug chart illustrates the importance of appreciating the actions of common medications and the problems that can arise. On admission, the patient is on a K⁺-sparing diuretic (spironolactone) at a dose that suggests an indication for liver disease rather than heart failure. On day 1 of his admission, an angiotensin-converting enzyme (ACE) inhibitor is introduced. The combination of an ACE inhibitor (lisinopril) and spironolactone, although acceptable, should be appreciated and initially the serum potassium should be checked to ensure that it does not rise to a dangerous level. Therefore, when supplemental potassium is started the following day - perhaps by a busy doctor who does not usually cover this patient and who has limited understanding of the patient's overall case - we have a potential disaster. If left unchecked the K^+ may increase to a level causing cardiac dysrhythmias or, worse, cardiac arrest.

Answer 3.19

➥ case on page 374

Several features in the history should set off alarm bells for bacterial meningitis. The patient is young and in an institutional environment, and has an acute headache with photophobia. In addition, the CSF is cloudy with a raised WCC and a low CSF:plasma glucose ratio.

Three important points can be learned from this case:

1. If the leukocyte count is raised, analysis of the differential leukocyte count will help in distinguishing the cause.
2. A patient may have bacterial meningitis without any organisms being seen on microscopy. Don't be put off by this.
3. In bacterial meningitis, CT of the brain can be normal even when the CSF is highly abnormal.

This patient has bacterial meningitis and requires immediate treatment with intravenous antibiotics.

THE CLASSIC CSF FINDINGS IN BACTERIAL MENINGITIS	
A cloudy appearance Organisms seen in CSF Raised WCC (with >95% neutrophils) Red cell count (RCC) normal	Raised (but only mild-moderate) total protein Significantly reduced CSF glucose Reduced CSF:plasma glucose ratio (to less than two-thirds)

Answer 3.20

➡ case on page 375

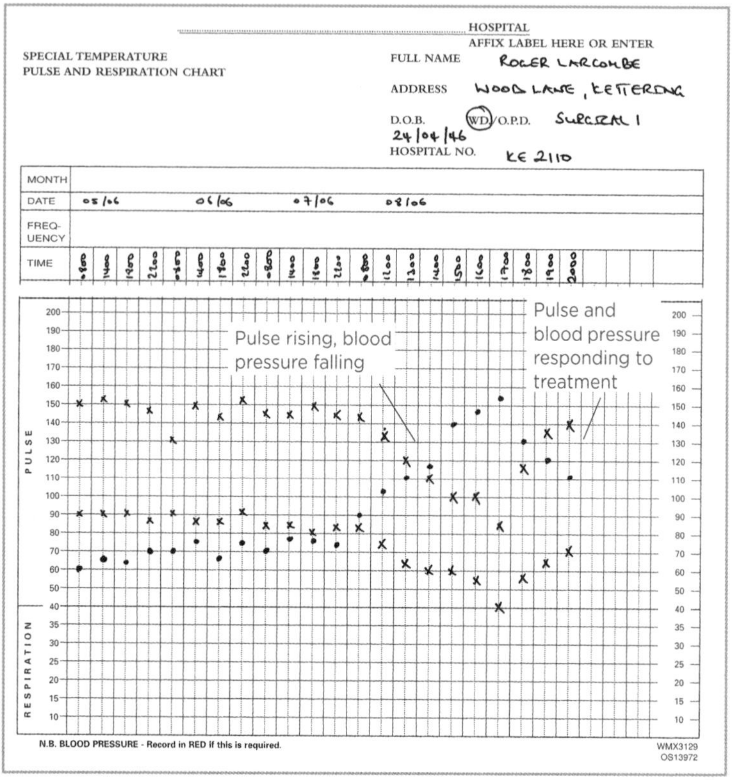

NAME	ROGER LARCOMBE	HOSPITAL NUMBER	KE2110
DATE OF BIRTH	24/04/1946	WARD	SURGICAL 1

DATE	TIME	AMOUNT	CONSISTENCY	BLOOD	MUCUS	PUS	SIGN
5/6	08 00	SMALL	4				[illegible]
	16 00	MODERATE	5				[illegible]
6/6	10 00	SMALL	5	DARK			[illegible]
	20 00	SMALL	4	DARK			[illegible]
7/6	0900	MODERATE	5	DARK			[illegible]
	1300	SMALL	4				[illegible]
	21 00	MODERATE	4	DARK			[illegible]
8/6	06 00	LARGE	5	BLACK+FOUL			[illegible]
	07 00	MODERATE	5	"			[illegible]
	09 00	LARGE	5	"			[illegible]
	13 00	MODERATE	5	"			[illegible]
	1700	MODERATE	5	"			[illegible]

Most patients will have several observation charts at the end of the bed. These should all be viewed in a systematic fashion to maximise the information obtained. In this scenario, both the vital signs chart and the bowel habit chart reveal the likely diagnosis.

An inpatient for several days following admission with dark stools and rectal bleeding, this patient has remained stable, albeit with persistently abnormal bowel motions. It can be seen that on occasion the motion is both loose and dark in nature, but is always relatively small in volume and the patient's general observations initially remain normal.

Fluid resuscitation, possibly with blood products, has occurred. Note on day 4 (08/06) that the patient becomes progressively more tachycardic and with this the blood pressure falls. This corresponds to an increase in the frequency of the motions, which are noted to be black and foul smelling in nature - this patient has melaena.

The melaena has been present to an extent since admission; however, on this occasion the patient has become haemodynamically unstable. There has been a significant upper gastrointestinal tract bleed. The patient should now undergo emergency endoscopy to locate and if possible treat the cause. In the meantime, intravenous fluids and possible red packed cells should be administered. Any coagulopathy should be corrected. One can see the blood pressure and tachycardia respond to fluid replacement (from 18:00 hours onwards).

Answer 3.21

➥ case on page 376

This rhythm as with all the ECGs above. However, for practical purposes, this rhythm should be instantly recognised as ventricular fibrillation (VF) by its erratic nature, and appropriate treatment given. This involves cardiac defibrillation.

After delivering three shocks, the rhythm on the monitor changes to that shown below. A pulse is still not present. What is the rhythm now?

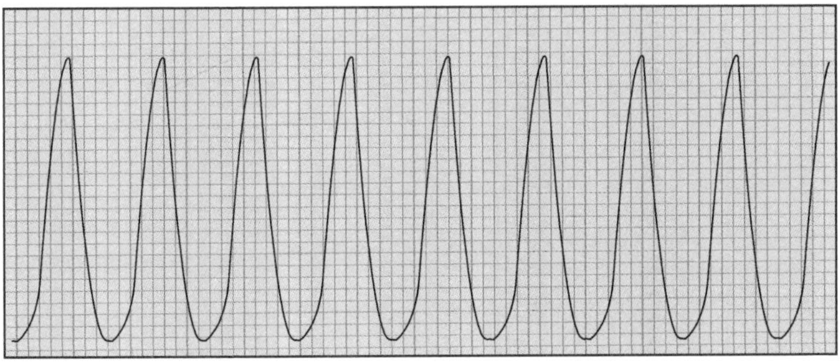

Again, this strip can be analysed in detail, but it should be instantly recognised by its shape as ventricular tachycardia (VT). The ECG shows a tachycardia with wide QRS complexes. This rhythm can be associated with a cardiac output, so it would be imperative to check for the presence of a pulse. Cardiac arrest associated with VT is treated with defibrillation.

Answer 3.22

➥ case on page 376

This patient is having bowel motion activity recorded formally using a faeces chart. At least eight motions each day have been passed. The consistency has been Bristol type 6 and 7 indicating very soft, watery motions. Furthermore it is mucoid and bloody. It would be important clinically for the fluid balance sheet to be assessed in conjunction with the stool chart to assess for adequate hydration. Possible causes for this pattern of bowel activity are listed in the box below.

Inflammatory bowel disease
Infective diarrhoea (eg *Shigella*, *Salmonella*)
Colorectal malignancy
Ischaemic colitis

Answer 3.23

➥ case on page 377

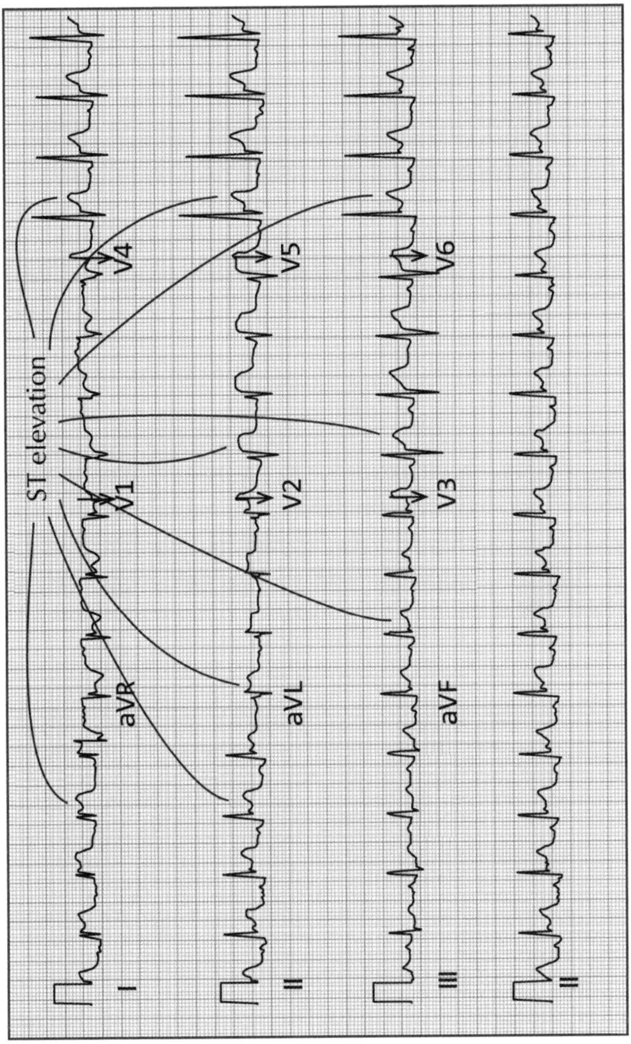

Heart rate

There are three big squares between consecutive R waves. The ventricular rate is therefore 300/3 = 100 beats/min.

Heart rhythm

A P wave precedes each QRS complex. The P-R interval is normal (four small squares) and does not vary from beat to beat. The rhythm is sinus rhythm.

Cardiac axis
Leads I, II and III are all upgoing. The axis is normal.

P waves
P waves are of normal size and shape.

QRS complexes
There appears to be a Q wave in aVR. The R and S waves are of normal height. The QRS complex is of normal duration (two small squares).

ST segment
There is ST-segment elevation in nearly all the leads. This is generally concave. There is no reciprocal ST depression.

Q–T interval
The Q–T interval is normal (1.6 large squares).

T waves
It is difficult to appreciate the T waves fully because of the distortion of the ST segments. They appear grossly normal.

Conclusion: acute pericarditis. Putting together the history (does not sound typical for myocardial ischaemia) and the ST-segment changes, this is the most likely diagnosis.

Answer 3.24

➥ case on page 378

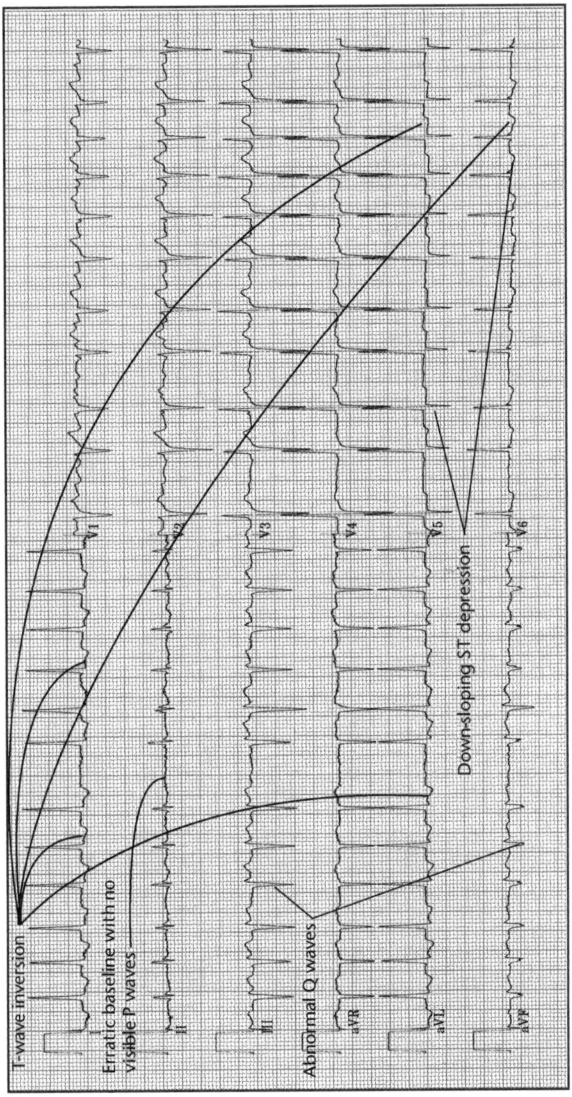

Heart rate

There are nine small squares between the first two consecutive R waves in lead I. The ventricular rate is therefore 1500 ÷ 9 = 167 beats/min. However, since the rhythm is clearly irregular, a more accurate assessment of heart rate can be made by measuring the distance between the first and eleventh R waves and dividing this distance by 10 to find the average R–R interval.

By this method, there are approximately 20.5 large squares between the first and eleventh R waves. The average R–R interval is therefore 2.05 large squares. The heart rate is 300 ÷ 2.05 = 146 beats/min.

Heart rhythm

No P waves are visible. The baseline is erratic. QRS complexes occur irregularly. The rhythm is atrial fibrillation.

Cardiac axis

Leads I and II are upgoing. Lead III is downgoing. The axis is normal.

P waves

No P waves are visible.

QRS complexes

There are abnormal Q waves in leads III and aVF, indicating a previous inferior myocardial infarction. The R and S waves are of normal height. The QRS complex is of normal duration (two small squares).

ST segment

The ST segment is horizontal and isoelectric in leads II, III, aVR, aVF, V1, V2 and V3. There is slight downsloping ST depression in the other leads, most marked in I and V6.

Q–T interval

The Q–T interval is normal (seven small squares).

T waves

T waves are normal in size. There is T-wave inversion in leads I, aVL, V5 and V6.

Conclusion: atrial fibrillation with a ventricular rate of 146 beats/min. Inferior Q waves. There is downsloping ST elevation and T-wave inversion in the leads looking at the lateral aspect of the heart. The patient may be on digoxin, but the T-wave changes probably indicate ischaemia. This may be related to the rapid heart rate, and may disappear if the rate is slowed. This woman's palpitations are due to a sudden onset of atrial fibrillation.

Answer 3.25

➥ case on page 379

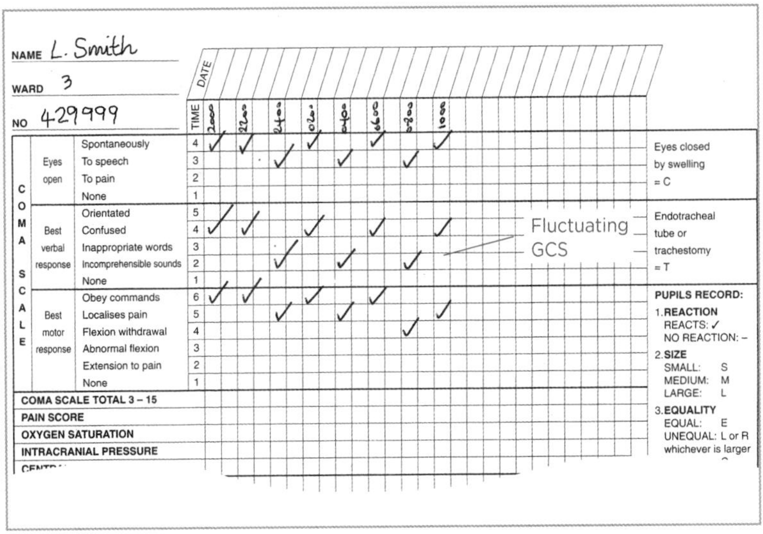

1. The GCS is a routinely used method of accurately and objectively recording a patient's level of consciousness. It is an easy-to-use scoring system which may be recorded in a reproducible fashion by nursing or medical staff. It comprises three independent categories - EYE OPENING, VERBAL RESPONSE and MOTOR RESPONSE. It is scored out of 15. The GCS must be measured in patients with head injury and after any neurosurgical intervention. This bedside chart illustrates its use in a patient after a fall.

   On admission the GCS is 14/15 on the basis of the patient being confused. At midnight the conscious level takes a drop from 14/15 to 10/15. Two hours later one can observe that the GCS has returned to its admission level of 14/15. Further frequent monitoring throughout the morning shows a repeat of this pattern - the GCS IS FLUCTUANT. An intracranial cause should be sought with urgent imaging.

2. This pattern is typically seen in subdural haematoma. Following a fall, the patient is lucid at times but the conscious level is variable. Extracranial causes, eg sepsis or hypoglycaemia, may also account for such patterns.

Answer 3.26

➥ case on page 380

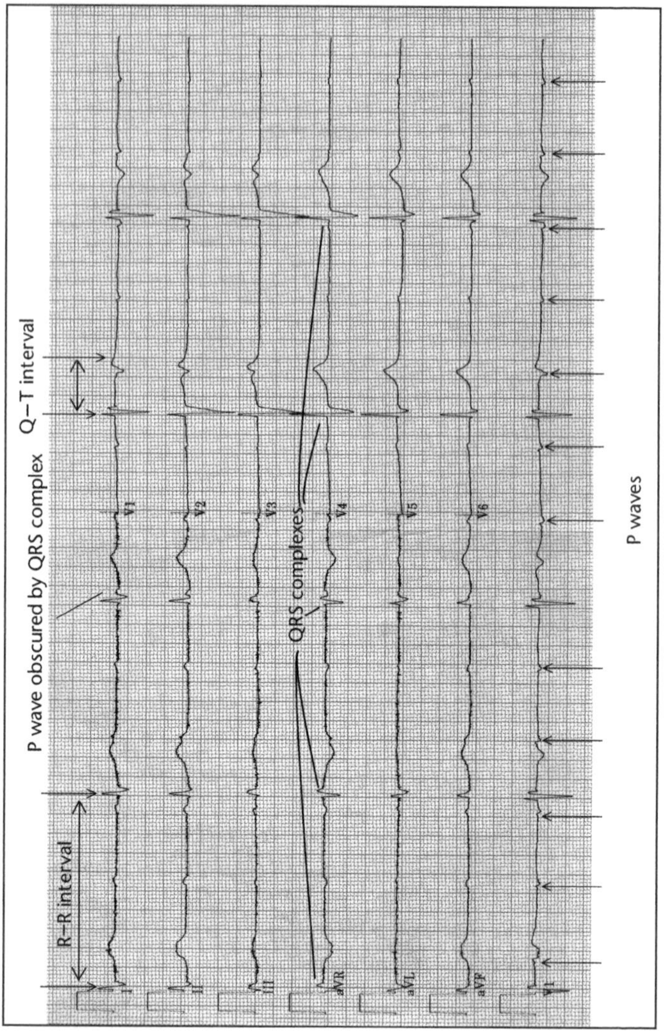

Heart rate

There are 10 big squares between consecutive R waves. The ventricular rate is therefore 300 ÷ 10 = 30 beats/min.

Heart rhythm

P waves are seen, but these show no consistent relationship with the QRS complexes. The P waves and QRS complexes are completely dissociated. The rhythm is third-degree heart block.

Cardiac axis
Leads I, II and III are all upgoing. The axis is normal.

P waves
P waves are of normal size and shape. One P wave is difficult to see because it is obscured by a simultaneous QRS complex.

QRS complexes
There are no abnormal Q waves. The QRS complexes are narrow (two small squares). This indicates that the electrical signal to the ventricles is originating in specialised conducting tissue. The R and S waves are of normal height.

ST segment
The ST segment is horizontal and isoelectric.

Q-T interval
The Q-T interval is prolonged (three large squares). The Bazett correction is therefore required. Three large squares= 3 x 0.2 second = 0.6 second. The R-R interval is 10 large squares = 10 x 0.2 second = 2 seconds. The Q-Tc is therefore:

$$\frac{0.6}{\sqrt{2}} = 0.42 \text{ second}$$

T waves
T waves are normal in size and shape.

Conclusion: third-degree heart block with a ventricular rate of 30 beats/min. This rhythm is resulting in symptomatic hypotension. Consideration should be given to an emergency pacing procedure, followed by the placement of a permanent pacemaker.

The patient eventually had a permanent pacemaker inserted. An ECG was performed to check its function, and is shown overleaf. Note the presence of pacing spikes, which indicate that the pacemaker is discharging. When a pacemaker stimulates the ventricles directly, the QRS complexes will be wide and bizarre. It is impossible to interpret anything else from the ECG in such circumstances, other than that an artificial pacemaker is present.

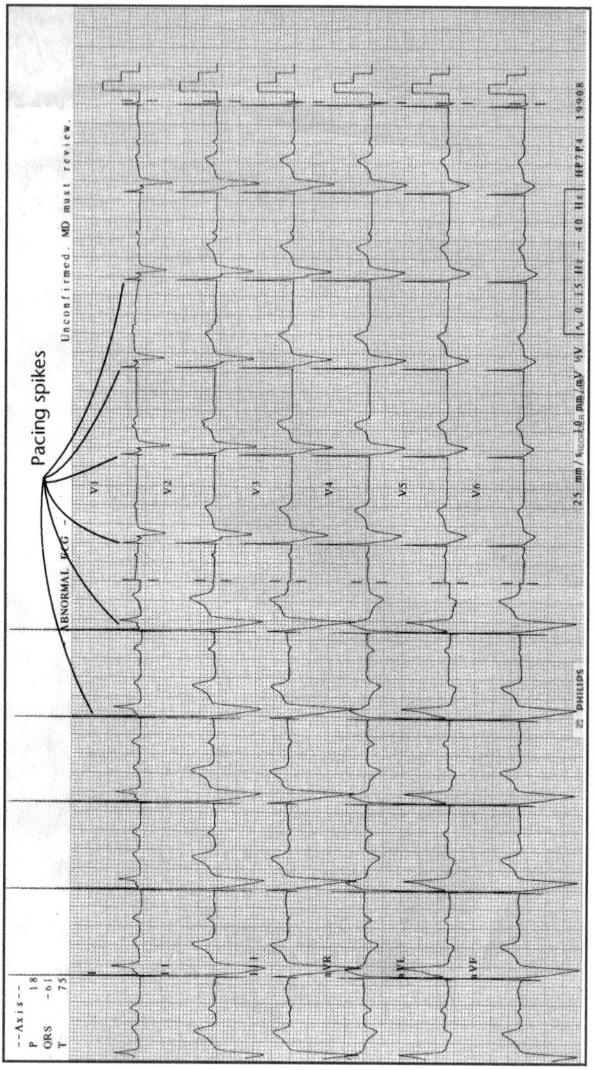
Pacing spikes
--Axis--
P 18
QRS -61
T 75
ABNORMAL ECG -
Unconfirmed. MD must review.
I
II
III
aVR
aVL
aVF
V1
V2
V3
V4
V5
V6
25 mm/s
10 mm/mV
0.15 Hz - 40 Hz
HP7R4 19908
PHILIPS

Answer 3.27

➥ case on page 381

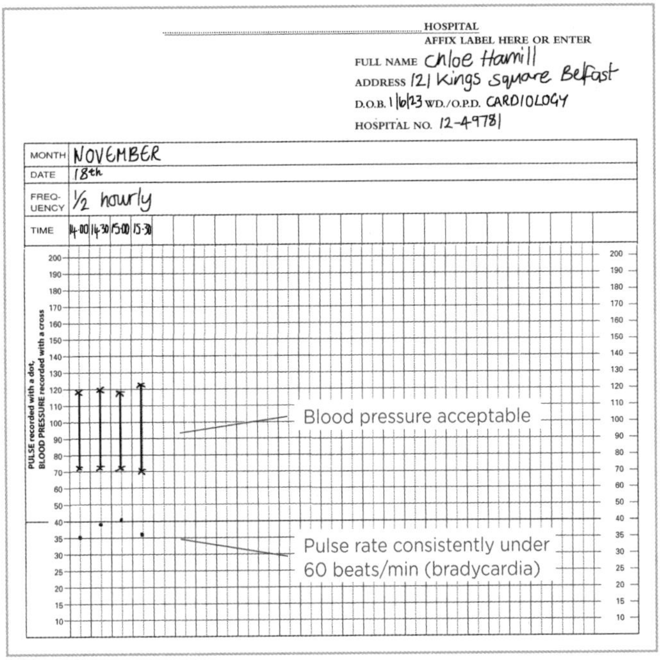

The patient has a marked bradycardia. The blood pressure seems acceptable, so gathering more information seems most appropriate at this stage. You should record a 12-lead ECG and attach the patient to a cardiac monitor.

After a short time, you are called to interpret the cardiac monitor. You see the following on the screen:

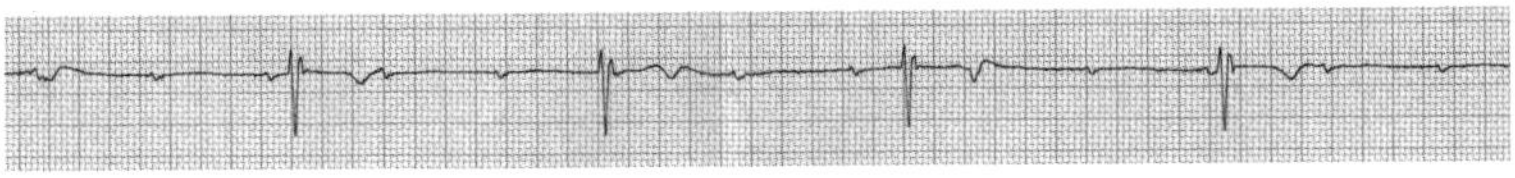

What is your interpretation of the heart rhythm?

The rhythm is complete heart block (or third-degree heart block) (see page 323 for further details). The patient requires drug treatment to speed the heart up, and will probably require the insertion of a pacemaker.

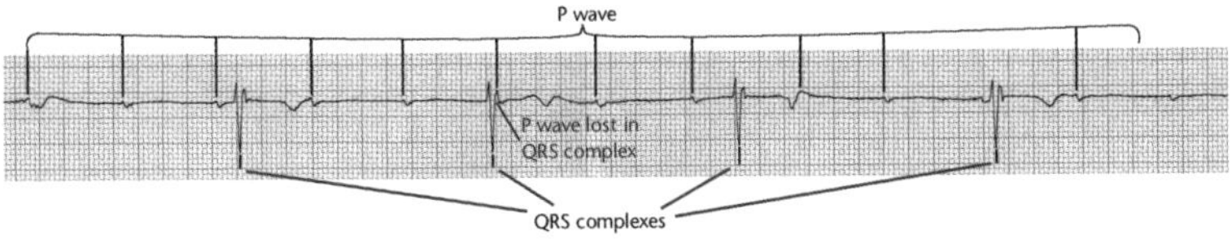

ANSWERS

Answer 3.28

➥ case on page 382

1. This patient's spirometry shows an obstructive pattern. His *K*co is low, indicating that something is interfering with gas transfer in the lungs. In this case, it is a reflection of his airway disease.
2. Given that this patient is a life-long smoker, it is likely that he has COPD. Consideration should be given to optimising inhaled bronchodilator therapy before discharge.

Answer 3.29

➥ case on page 382

The FEV_1 and FVC remain fairly similar between both sets of readings, indicating a restrictive lung defect. The major deterioration lies with the *K*co, which has taken a marked turn for the worse. This is most likely due to a deterioration in the underlying disease process because of the reducing dose of steroids. Consideration should be given to increasing the steroid dose.

Answer 3.30

➥ case on page 383

The average daytime BP is around 140/90 mmHg (an accurate mean result would be provided with such a report). Overnight, the BP is higher than during the day. This pattern is known as reverse nocturnal dipping.

Reverse nocturnal dipping is an abnormal finding, because BP should fall during sleep. Before pursuing this finding further, it would be important to enquire about the patient's activities when the monitor was fitted. Perhaps he works night shifts and is awake all night. Diurnal variation notwithstanding, the patient does have abnormally high BP and should be thoroughly investigated and adequately treated.

Answer 3.31

➥ case on page 384

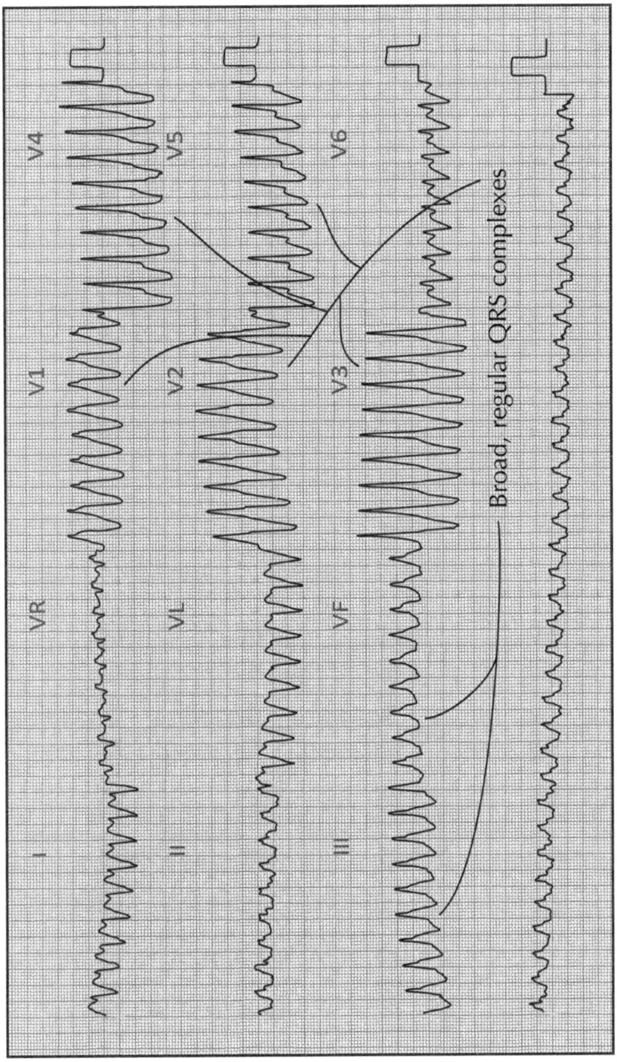

Heart rate

There are eight small squares between consecutive R waves. The ventricular rate is therefore 1500/8 = 188 beats/min.

Heart rhythm

P waves cannot be seen. Ventricular activity appears regular, however.

Cardiac axis

Leads I is downgoing and leads II and III are upgoing. There is right axis deviation.

P waves

P waves cannot be clearly seen.

QRS complexes

The QRS complexes are broad.

ST segment

It is difficult to appreciate any ST segments in this tracing.

Q-T interval

This cannot be clearly seen in this tracing.

T waves

The T waves are not well visualised.

Conclusion: this is a broad QRS complex tachycardia, which in this instance is due to ventricular tachycardia. This is a medical emergency requiring urgent management.

Answer 3.32

➥ case on page 385

1. FEV_1 and FVC are generally normal unless they are less than 80% of the predicted value. Spirometry is essentially normal in this example. The only abnormality shown is a low *K*co.
2. A classic cause of reduced *K*co with normal spirometry is anaemia. This patient should have a full blood picture analysed as a first-line measure.

Answer 3.33

➥ case on page 386

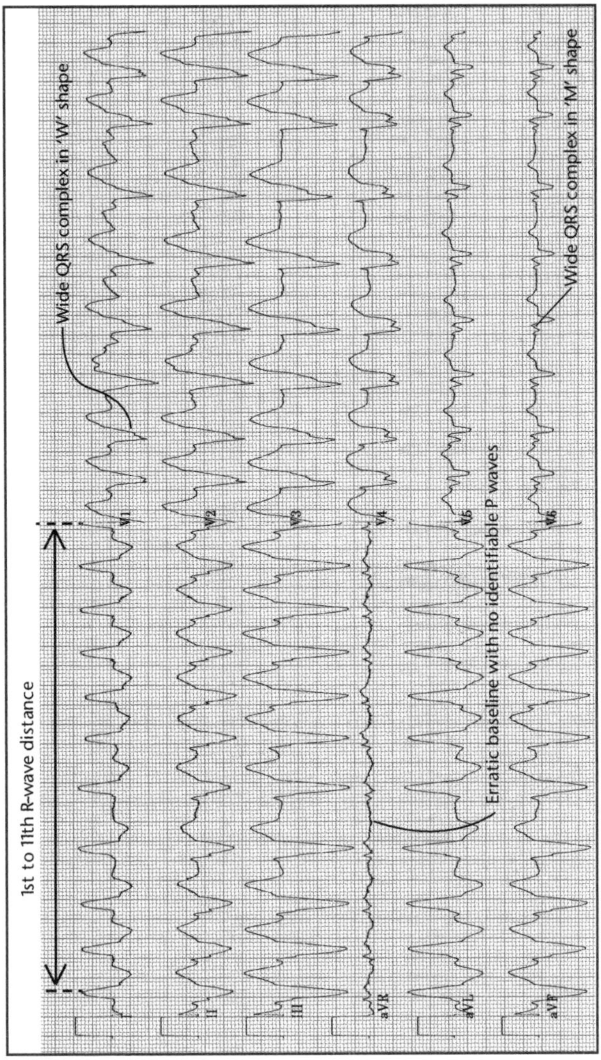

Heart rate

There are 11 small squares between the first two consecutive R waves in lead I. The ventricular rate is therefore 1500 ÷ 11 = 136 beats/min. However, since the rhythm is irregular, a more accurate assessment of heart rate can be made by measuring the distance between the first and eleventh R waves and dividing this distance by 10 to find the average R–R interval.

By this method, there are 24 large squares between the first and eleventh R waves. The average R–R interval is therefore 2.4 large squares. The heart rate is 300 ÷ 2.4 = 125 beats/min.

Heart rhythm

No P waves are visible. The baseline is erratic. QRS complexes occur irregularly. The rhythm is atrial fibrillation.

Cardiac axis

Lead I is upgoing. Leads II and III are downgoing. There is left axis deviation.

P waves

No P waves are visible.

QRS complexes

The QRS complexes are abnormally wide. The complex in V1 has a 'W' shape, and that in V6 is 'M' shaped. This is left bundle-branch block.

ST segment

The ST segment is difficult to visualise.

Q–T interval

The Q–T interval is difficult to measure.

T waves

T waves appear grossly abnormal in size and shape.

Conclusion: atrial fibrillation at 125 beats/min with left bundle-branch block. When this pattern is present, it is impossible to make any further comments about an ECG (ie ST-segment changes or T-wave abnormalities). Left bundle-branch block that is of new onset would be in keeping with an acute myocardial infarction. Old ECGs should be reviewed to determine whether this ECG finding is new.

4 COMPLETE CLINICAL CASES

Use your understanding and interpretative skills from the rest of the book to approach these complete cases. The cases represent full patient pathways in which data from a multitude of investigations are available for interpretation. These holistic cases will test your skills in real-life scenarios.

Bedside chart	4.1, 4.4, 4.11, 4.10, 4.13, 4.14
Biochemistry	4.2, 4.3, 4.4, 4.5, 4.6, 4.7, 4.10, 4.12, 4.13, 4.14, 4.15
Cardiology	4.4, 4.10, 4.12, 4.15
Endocrinology	4.6, 4.15
Genetics	4.2, 4.7
Haematology	4.2, 4.3, 4.5, 4.7, 4.8, 4.9, 4.10, 4.11, 4.13, 4.14
Imaging	4.1, 4.4, 4.5, 4.10, 4.11, 4.13, 4.15
Immunology	4.3
Microbiology	4.5, 4.7, 4.13
Neurology	4.1
Pathology	4.8, 4.9
Peritoneal fluid analysis	4.2, 4.5
Respiratory	4.4, 4.5, 4.12, 4.13, 4.14
Toxicology blood levels	4.12, 4.13
Urinalysis	4.14

Case 4.1

A 38-year-old teacher is brought to hospital by her concerned husband due to her unusual behaviour and sleepiness over the past 48 h. She has recently returned from supervising a school trip.

Her observation chart from the initial 6 h of her admission is shown.

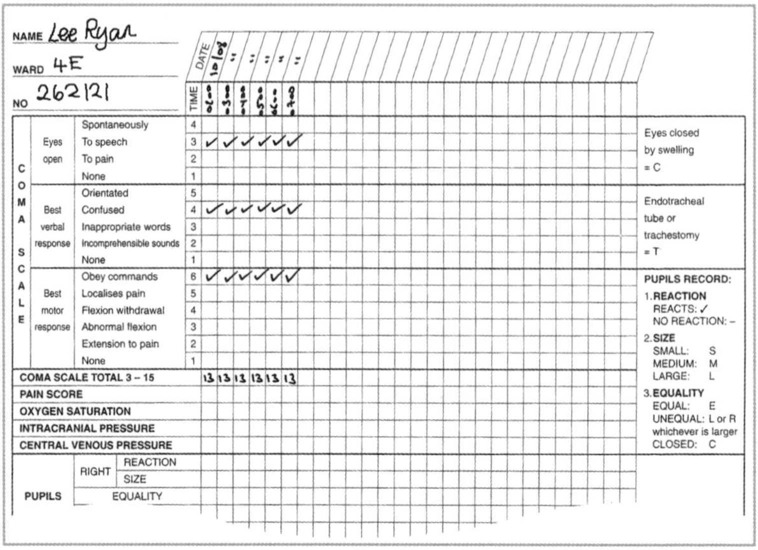

CT of the brain is arranged and the following report is telephoned to her doctor.

> **Neuroradiology department**
> Routine unenhanced images of the brain performed. No mass lesion seen. There is the suggestion of mild oedema within the temporal lobes bilaterally. MRI recommended.

Clinical examination revealed no signs of raised intracranial pressure. After discussion with the patient's consultant, lumbar puncture is performed. The details are below.

Opening pressure	16 cmCSF	
Appearance	Clear	
	No organisms seen on microscopy	
WCC	121 /mm^3 (>95% lymphocytes)	(<5/mm^3)
RCC	3 /mm^3	(0/mm^3)
Glucose	2.8 mmol/l (plasma glucose 5.6 mmol/l)	(Approx. 40–60% of plasma glucose)
Total protein	72 g/l (plasma total protein 0.44 g/l)	(0.15–0.45 g/l)

1. **Summarise the findings from the CSF analysis and suggest one further specific test that might be performed on the CSF given the clinical history.**

In the meantime an electroencephalogram is also performed. The report is sent back with the patient.

> **EEG department**
> There is evidence of slow wave changes.
> Periodic complexes are seen

2. **Given the result of the EEG, CSF analysis and CT brain imaging what is the likely diagnosis?**

➥ **answer on page 456**

Case 4.2

A 34 year-old oil-rig engineer is required to attend a medical before a secondment to his company's overseas operation in Brunei. He has been fortunate with his health with no previous problems. He admits to smoking 20 cigarettes a day and drinking approximately 38 units of alcohol a week. His conscientious doctor sends several tests. The following results were of some concern.

Iron	99 μmol/l	(11–32 μmol/l)
Ferritin	878 μg/l	(12–200 μg/l)
TIBC	12 μmol/l	(42–80 μmol/l)
Transferrin saturation	65%	

1. **What can one infer from this iron profile?**
2. **Ferritin is an acute phase reactant. Name some other acute phase reactants.**

His liver function tests are recalled on the computer and are shown below.

Bilirubin	11 μmol/l	(3-17 μmol/l)
AST	25 U/l	(5-35 U/l)
ALT	32 U/l	(5-35 U/l)
ALP	67 U/l	(30-150 U/l)
GGT	152 U/l	(7-33 U/l males)
Albumin	40 g/l	(35-50 g/l)

3. **What do the liver function tests show?**

The doctor is concerned about an underlying genetic disorder and a blood sample is sent to the genetics laboratory. The result below was obtained.

Genetics laboratory
Homozygous abnormality on chromosome 6p - *HFE* gene - missense mutation *C282Y*

The doctor tries to arrange treatment, but unfortunately the patient leaves his job and no further medical action is taken. Nothing is heard of him for several years, until he is admitted to a local hospital with a distended abdomen and fever.

Physical examination demonstrates the presence of ascites. Peritoneal aspiration is performed and shown below.

Neutrophil count (WCC)	312 cells/mm^3
Ascites albumin content	19 g/l
Serum albumin	32 g/l
Microscopy and Gram stain	Gram-negative rods
Culture	*E. coli*
Amylase	92 U/l

4. **What is the diagnosis?**

He is treated for the acute condition and further blood tests are performed to assess his liver function.

Bilirubin	84 μmol/l	(3-17 μmol/l)
AST	134 U/l	(5-35 U/l)
ALT	65 U/l	(5-35 U/l)
GGT	109 U/l	(11-58 U/l males)
ALP	122 U/l	(30-150 U/l)
Albumin	26 g/l	(35-50 g/l)
Prothrombin time	24.9 s	(12-16 s)
APTT	34.5 s	(24-38 s)
Fibrinogen	4.5 g/l	(2-4 g/l)

5. **What do these liver function tests suggest?**

➥ **answer on page 457**

Case 4.3

A 39-year-old secretary attends hospital with a painful and swollen right knee, pains in the fingers and fatigue. The finger pains have been with her for several weeks and are especially bad first thing in the morning, making her work difficult. The knee is a more recent complaint.

On examination there is active synovitis in the small joints of the hands and a large effusion of the right knee.

Among the initial blood tests from the A&E officer are those shown.

Hb	99 g/l	(120-160 g/l females)
MCV	89.9 fl	(76-96 fl)
WCC	11.2 x 10^9/l	(4.0-11.0 × 10^9/l)
Platelets	199 x 10^9/l	(150-400 × 10^9/l)
Adjusted Ca^{2+}	2.45 mmol/l	(2.10-2.65 mmol/l)
PO_4^{3-}	0.87 mmol/l	(0.8-1.45 mmol/l)
Albumin	36 g/l	(35-50 g/l)
Urate	0.34 mmol/l	(0.15-0.50 mmol/l)
CRP	312 mg/l	(<10 mg/l)

1. **Describe the findings.**

An enthusiastic junior doctor carries out knee aspiration, to exclude septic arthritis. The results are shown.

Specimen received	Synovial fluid from right knee
Appearance	Clear
Microscopy	<2 leukocytes per mm^3
Plane polarised light microscopy	No crystals seen
Synovial fluid culture	No growth

A few days later the result of her autoimmune screen becomes available.

Rheumatoid factor	199 IU/ml
Gastric parietal cell antibodies	1:280
Intrinsic factor antibodies	+ve
Anti-nuclear	-ve
Anti-nucleolar	-ve
Anti-nuclear (speckled)	-ve
Anti-mitochondrial	-ve
Anti-smooth muscle	-ve
Anti-gastric parietal cell	-ve
Anti-CCP	+ve

She is treated for her arthritis and attends regular review for many years with a variable course to her illness. On one occasion she complains of increasing shortness of breath and on auscultation of the chest there are inspiratory crepitations at the bases.

Spirometry is arranged. The results are shown.

FEV_1	68% predicted
FVC	50% predicted
FEV_1/FVC	85%
*K*co	51% predicted

The accompanying chest X-ray is shown.

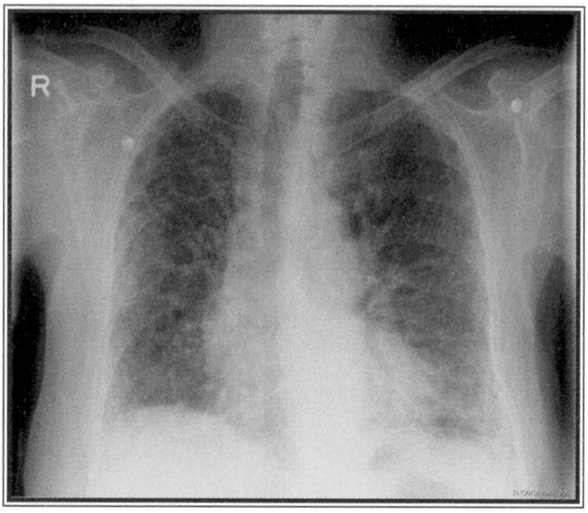

2. **What problem does this patient now have and how may it be related to her treatment?**
3. **What further radiological investigation would be of benefit?**

Six months later the patient sustains a forearm fracture. She is referred for a DXA scan. The results can be seen below.

Region (age matched)	BMD (g/cm²)	T score	Z score
Neck of femur	0.526	-3.0	-2.7
L1	0.812	-2.7	-2.8
L4	0.846	-3.0	-2.9

4. **Outline the significance of these results.**

➥ **answer on page 460**

Case 4.4

A 74-year-old man is admitted with a painful abdomen. He has a history of hypertension and atrial fibrillation. He had a laparotomy as a younger man for a gastric ulcer. He has not passed a motion in several days. On examination his abdomen is tender with rebound.

An abdominal X-ray is taken and shown below.

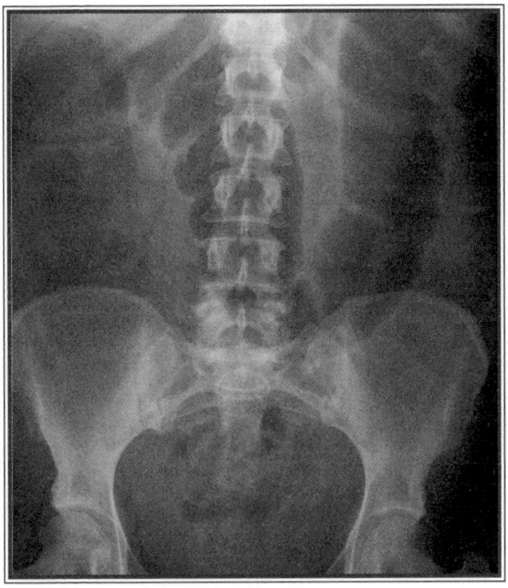

1. **Interpret this abdominal X-ray.**

The patient's condition rapidly deteriorates. An arterial blood gas is analysed.

FiO_2	0.21	
pH	7.26	(7.35-7.45)
PaO_2	11.5 kPa	(11-13 kPa)
$PaCO_2$	2.9 kPa	(4.7-6.0 kPa)
HCO_3^-	12.6 mmol/l	(24-30 mmol/l)
BE	-15.8 mmol/l	(-2 to +2 mmol/l)
Lactate	8.3 mmol/l	(0.5-2.0 mmol/l)

2. **Interpret this ABG.**

The patient has emergency surgery. After a short stay in the high dependency unit (HDU) he returns to the ward. Several days later he complains of further abdominal discomfort after his patient-controlled analgesia (PCA) device is stopped. On examination he is tender in the suprapubic space and this area is dull to percussion. A urinary catheter has been *in situ* since surgery.

His fluid (input/output) chart is observed.

.... HOSPITAL

DAILY FLUID CHART

AFFIX LABEL HERE OR ENTER
FULL NAME John Dickens
ADDRESS 2 Ford Street, Belfast
D.O.B. 16/04/1931 WD./O.P.D. 5
HOSPITAL NO. 264567

24 Hours Beginning 26/01/2005

TIME	INTAKE: BY MOUTH Amount ml.	Type	INTRAVENOUS OR OTHER ROUTES Amount ml.	Type	Add.	OUTPUT: Urine ml.	Faeces	Vomit ml.	Gast. Asp. ml.	Drain ml.	REMARKS
							/	/	/	/	
0800			50			30					
0900			50			34					
1000			50			45					
1100			50			10					
1200			50			10					
1300			50			5					
1400			50			5					
1500			50			0					
1600			50			0					
1700			50			0					
1800			50			0					
1900											
2000											
2100											
2200											
2300											
2400											
0100											
0200											
0300											
0400											
0500											
0600											
0700											

DATE:- INTAKE Name ....

TOTAL	By Mouth	Intravenous or Other Routes	Urine	Faeces	Vomit	Gast. Asp.	Drain
Day Total	ML	ML	ML	ML	ML	ML	ML
Night Total	ML	ML	ML	ML	ML	ML	ML
Total for 24 hours	ML	ML	ML	ML	ML	ML	ML

TOTAL INTAKE [ ] TOTAL OUTPUT [ ]

WCA 229/OS 10280

3. Describe the findings.

Blood and urine are sent for analysis

Na^+	134 mmol/l	(135–145 mmol/l)
K^+	6.6 mmol/l	(3.5–5.0 mmol/l)
Urea	19.7 mmol/l	(2.5–6.7 mmol/l)
Creatinine	403 μmol/l	(79–118 μmol/l)
Cl^-	98 mmol/l	(95–105 mmol/l)
HCO_3^-	12.6 mmol/l	(24–30 mmol/l)
Mg^{2+}	0.72 mmol/l	(0.7–1.0 mmol/l)
PO_4^{3-}	0.89 mmol/l	(0.8–1.45 mmol/l)

4. What problem has occurred?

Immediate treatment is given for hyperkalaemia.

5. An ECG was done just before treatment. Describe the findings on the ECG seen below.

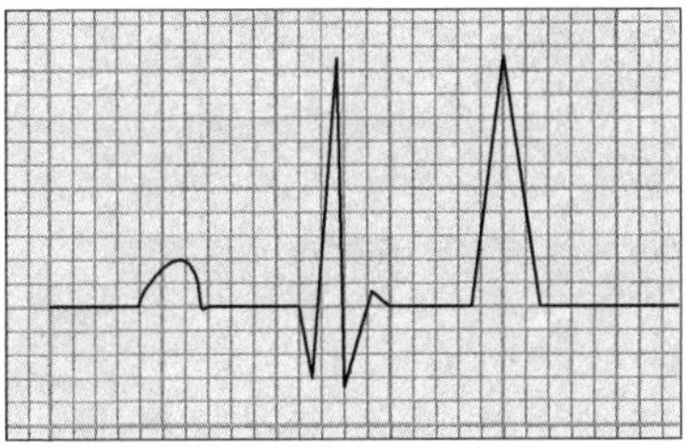

6. Which imaging study would you request to review the abdomen?

➥ answer on page 463

Case 4.5

A 54-year-old pilot is admitted to the local hospital with a complaint of increasing shortness of breath. She has noted this especially while flying recently. She has been seen by her occupational health doctor and prohibited from flying until investigations have been undertaken. She also complains of a cough and intermittent fever.

On examination the trachea is sited centrally. The left lung base is dull to percussion, vocal resonance is decreased and breath sounds are decreased.

Included in your initial investigations are a chest X-ray, FBP, U+E, CRP and ABG.

All are shown below for interpretation.

Hb	145 g/l	(120–160 g/l females)
MCV	98.7 fl	(76–96 fl)
Platelets	293 x 10^9/l	(150–400 × 10^9/l)
WCC	14.4 x 10^9/l	(4.0–11.0 × 10^9/l)
Neutrophils	11.3 x 10^9/l	(2.0–7.5 × 10^9/l)
Lymphocytes	2.2 x 10^9/l	(1.5–4.0 × 10^9/l)
Monocytes	0.5 x 10^9/l	(0.2–0.8 × 10^9/l)
Eosinophils	0.2 x 10^9/l	(0.04–0.4 × 10^9/l)
Basophils	0.09 x 10^9/l	(0.0–0.1 × 10^9/l)
Na^+	137 mmol/l	(135–145 mmol/l)
K^+	3.8 mmol/l	(3.5–5.0 mmol/l)
Urea	8.6 mmol/l	(2.5–6.7 mmol/l)
Creatinine	101 μmol/l	(79–118 μmol/l)
Cl^-	107 mmol/l	(95–105 mmol/l)
CRP	176 mmol/l	(<10 mg/l)

1. **What abnormalities are seen?**

FiO_2	0.21	
pH	7.50	(7.35–7.45)
PaO_2	7.8 kPa	(11–13 kPa)
$PaCO_2$	3.1 kPa	(4.7–6.0 kPa)
HCO_3^-	25.8 mmol/l	(24–30 mmol/l)
BE	+ 6.2 mmol/l	(-2 to +2 mmol/l)

2. **Describe the findings on this ABG.**

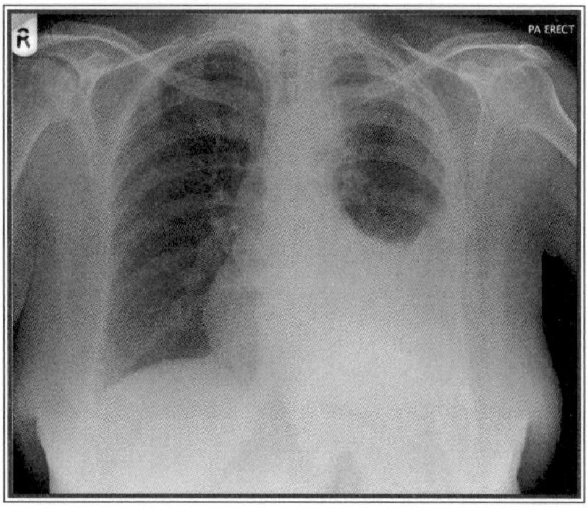

3. **Comment on this chest X-ray.**

A decision is made to perform a pleural tap for diagnostic purposes based on the findings from the initial investigations. The results are shown.

Total protein	38 g/l
LDH	246 U/l
pH	7.37
Microscopy	Nil seen

4. **How would you interpret these results?**

She is treated with a cephalosporin antibiotic based on known sensitivities. Three days into this treatment she develops diarrhoea. Stool samples are sent by her nurse. The result is shown below.

Clostridium difficile toxin positive

5. **What is the best course of action based on these findings?**

➥ **answer on page 467**

Case 4.6

A 62-year-old male patient with inoperable lung cancer is admitted on the general medical take-in with acute confusion. Physical examination is unremarkable. Routine blood tests are sent, and the following results are obtained.

Na^+	115 mmol/l	(135–145 mmol/l)
K^+	4.4 mmol/l	(3.5–5.0 mmol/l)
Urea	3.5 mmol/l	(2.5–6.7 mmol/l)
Creatinine	65 μmol/l	(79–118 μmol/l)
Cl^-	97 mmol/l	(95–105 mmol/l)
HCO_3^-	24.1 mmol/l	(24–30 mmol/l)

1. **His weight is 61 kg. Estimate his glomerular filtration rate.**

On the basis of these tests, a host of other investigations are organised. The results of these are shown below.

Free thyroxine	18.1 pmol/l	(7.6–19.7 pmol/l)
TSH	2.2 mU/l	(0.4–4.5 mU/l)

2. **What is his thyroid status?**

Short Synacthen® test		
Time (min)	0	30
Cortisol (nmol/l)	140	822

3. **Interpret this test result.**
4. **His blood glucose is 4.6 mmol/l. Calculate his plasma osmolality.**

His measured serum osmolality is similar to the calculated value.

Urinary sodium	55 mmol/l
Urine osmolality	525 mosmol/kg

5. **What is the overall diagnosis?**

➥ **answer on page 469**

Case 4.7

A 28-year-old patient is admitted to hospital on account of weight loss. She has an inherited condition. Browsing through old medical notes, the admitting doctor noted the following results.

Sweat analysis
112 mg sweat collected

Cl^-	67 mmol/l	(95–105 mmol/l)
Na^+	101 mmol/l	(135–145 mmol/l)

Genetics laboratory
ΔF508 mutation on long arm of chromosome 7

1. **What genetic condition does this patient have, and what is the inheritance pattern?**

The medical team are concerned about pancreatic exocrine insufficiency and measure faecal elastase. The following result is returned.

Faecal elastase undetectable.

2. **Does the patient have pancreatic exocrine insufficiency?**

During the course of her inpatient stay, the patient develops a cough with a degree of haemoptysis. The doctor is concerned about the possibility of a pulmonary embolism, and requests the following test urgently.

D-dimer	0.25 mg/l	(<0.5 mg/l)

3. **How does the D-dimer result help in managing the patient?**

The patient then becomes pyrexic, and clinical signs suggest pneumonia. The medical team commence co-amoxiclav. Sputum is sent for culture. Two days later the following result is obtained.

Sputum culture
Significant growth of *Moraxella catarrhalis*
Sensitivities shown:

Co-amoxiclav	R
Ciprofloxacin	R
Cefotaxime	S
Piperacillin/tazobactam	S
Gentamicin	S

On the basis of these sensitivities, and a worsening clinical state, the patient's antibiotics are changed to gentamicin.

A short time later the patient complains of hearing loss. The following audiogram is obtained.

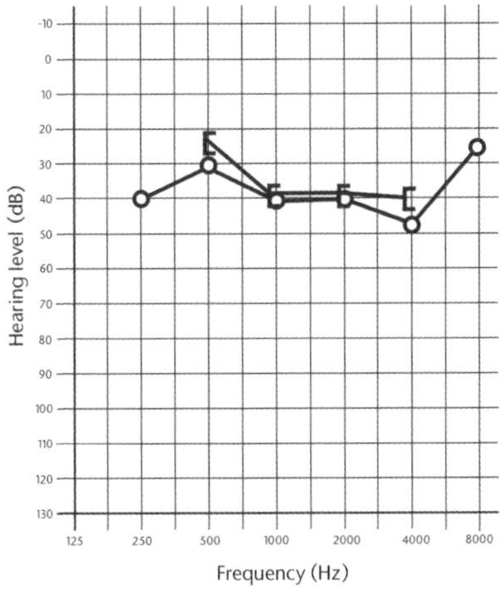

4. **What type of hearing loss has she developed, and how would you explain it?**

➥ **answer on page 470**

Case 4.8 ✚

A 72-year-old man presents with increasing epigastric discomfort. He has been troubled with heartburn for several years. He admits to drinking 'more than he should'. The admitting doctor noted pallor, and requested the following.

Hb	77 g/l	(130–180 g/l males)
MCV	69.5 fl	(76–96 fl)
Platelets	512 x 10^9/l	(150–400 × 10^9/l)
WCC	8.7 x 10^9/l	(4.0–11.0 × 10^9/l)
Iron	5 μmol/l	(11–32 μmol/l)
Ferritin	9 μg/l	(12–200 μg/l)
TIBC	95 μmol/l	(42–80 μmol/l)
Vitamin B_{12}	265 ng/l	(191–663 ng/l)
Folate	12.3 μg/l	(>2 μg/l)

1. **How would you interpret these results?**

A blood film is examined. The following report is obtained.

Hypochromic, microcytic cells
Poikilocytosis and anisochromia
Occasional pencil cells seen

2. **Is this result in keeping with your answer to question 1?**

He proceeds to have an oesophagogastroduodenoscopy (OGD). Two abnormalities are noted. First, he is noted to have an abnormal appearance of the lower oesophagus. Second, gastritis is observed. A biopsy is taken from the lower oesophagus and the stomach. A CLO test is performed. You note the following after 24 h.

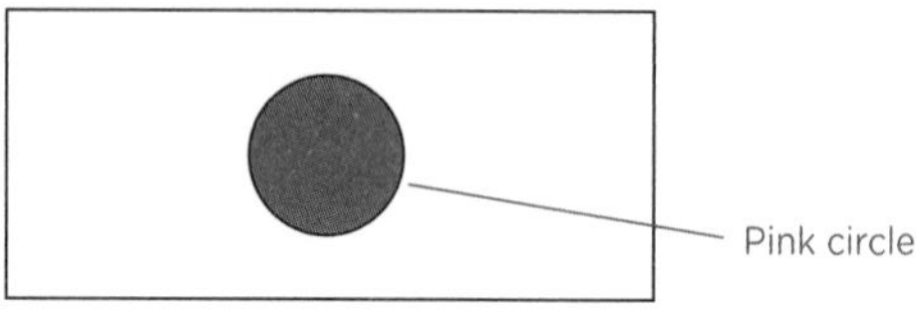

3. **What treatment should be commenced on the basis of this CLO result?**

One week later, the following result is phoned through from the pathology laboratory:

Pathology laboratory
Intestinal metaplasia in the lower oesophageal epithelium

4. **What is the condition affecting the oesophagus?**

➥ **answer on page 471**

Case 4.9

An 85-year-old man who is a smoker is admitted complaining of abdominal discomfort. No abnormalities are detected on clinical examination, but some basic blood tests are requested. Your colleague is concerned about the following test result, and asks for your help.

Hb	175 g/l	(130–180 g/l males)
PCV	0.55	(0.4–0.54 males)
MCV	86.4 fl	(76–96 fl)
Platelets	369 x 10^9/l	(150–400 × 10^9/l)
WCC	8.9 x 10^9/l	(4.0–11.0 × 10^9/l)

1. **What is this abnormality called, and how would you proceed?**

The result is repeated and confirmed. He proceeds to have an estimation of red cell mass.

Red cell mass estimation	
Red cell mass	137% predicted

2. **What does this result indicate?**

On the basis of this result, an arterial blood gas analysis was performed when the patient was breathing room air.

pH	7.37	(7.35–7.45)
PaO_2	12.6 kPa	(11–13 kPa)
$PaCO_2$	4.7 kPa	(4.7–6.0 kPa)
HCO_3^-	25.7 mmol/l	(24–30 mmol/l)
BE	+1.2 mmol/l	(-2 to +2 mmol/l)

3. **How would you interpret the blood gas?**

An ultrasound scan of the abdomen revealed a mass in keeping with a renal cell carcinoma.

The patient proceeded to surgery, and underwent a nephrectomy. He spent 2 days in the intensive care unit after the operation, but returned to the ward on day 3 after the operation. His urine output deteriorated on day 4, and a urine specimen was sent for analysis.

Urine sodium	<20 mmol/l

4. **What does this result tell you about the cause of the oliguria, and how would you treat the patient?**

The patient's urine output recovers. Several days later he complains of a burning pain on passing urine, and of having to pass urine more often than normal. The following result is obtained on urinalysis.

Protein	Nil
Blood	Nil
Nitrites	++
Leukocyte esterase	+++

5. **How would you interpret the urinalysis, and what further urine test would you request?**

↪ **answer on page 472**

Case 4.10 ++

A 72-year-old man with a history of hypertension and ischaemic heart disease was admitted 90 minutes after the witnessed onset of acute right-sided arm and leg weakness, and right-sided facial droop.

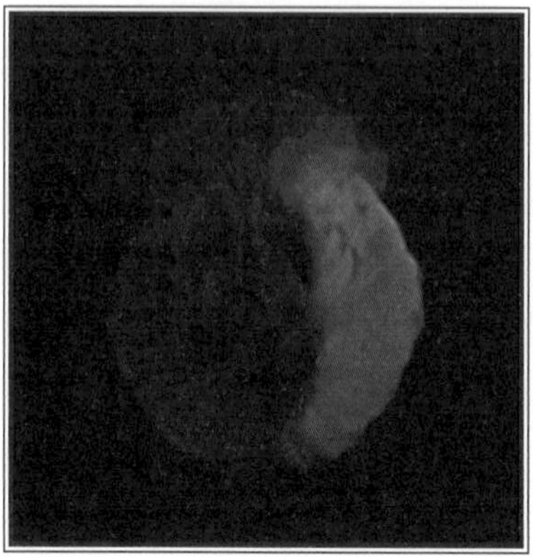

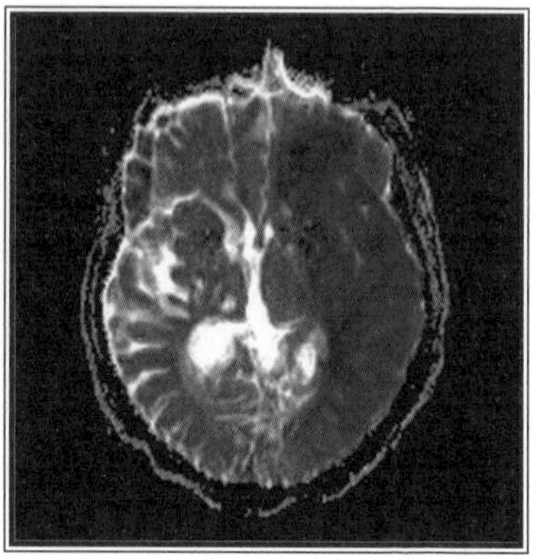

1. What is the diagnosis, and what treatment should be considered?

Treatment is administered and the patient makes a reasonable recovery in the first few hours. You are then called to assess him due to a deterioration in his condition. This is his neurological observations chart:

NAME J Adams
WARD Nightingale
NO 674

DATE 31st Oct

COMA SCALE		TIME	1800	1900	2000	2100	2200	2300
Eyes open	Spontaneously	4			✓	✓	✓	
	To speech	3	✓	✓				
	To pain	2						✓
	None	1						
Best verbal response	Orientated	5			✓	✓	✓	
	Confused	4	✓	✓				
	Inappropriate words	3						✓
	Incomprehensible sounds	2						
	None	1						
Best motor response	Obey commands	6	✓	✓	✓	✓	✓	
	Localises pain	5						
	Flexion withdrawal	4						
	Abnormal flexion	3						✓
	Extension to pain	2						
	None	1						
COMA SCALE TOTAL 3 – 15								
PAIN SCORE								
OXYGEN SATURATION								
INTRACRANIAL PRESSURE								

Eyes closed by swelling = C

Endotracheal tube or trachestomy = T

PUPILS RECORD:
1. **REACTION**
REACTS: ✓
NO REACTION: –
2. **SIZE**
SMALL: S
MEDIUM: M
LARGE: L
3. **EQUALITY**
EQUAL: E
UNEQUAL: L or R whichever is larger

2. What do you think has happened, and what are your priorities?

You arrange another CT scan which shows haemorrhagic transformation in the same region as the abnormality seen on the first scan.

3. **What are your priorities now?**

A blood test result comes back showing the following:

Hb	122 g/l	(130–180 g/l males)
MCV	86 fl	(76–96 fl)
WCC	7.6 x 10^9/l	(4.0–11.0 × 10^9/l)
Platelets	23 x 10^9/l	(150–400 × 10^9/l)

4. **How will this affect your management?**

The patient stabilises, and over the course of 2 weeks makes a reasonable improvement in conscious level. The limb weakness remains profound. You review him because he has developed anterior chest pain that reminds him of a previous myocardial infarction.

5. **How would you interpret his ECG?**

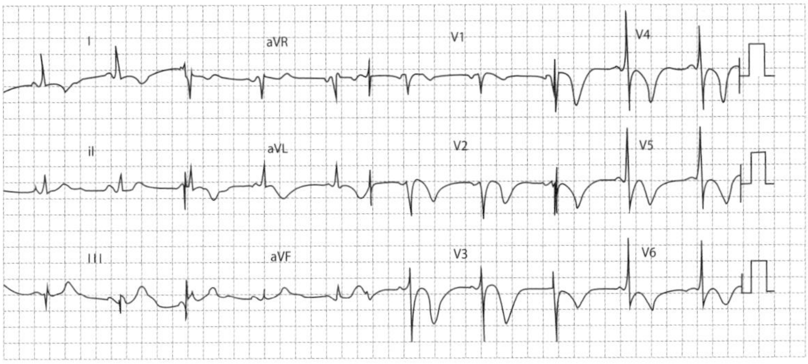

His chest pain settles after 1 hour; 12 hours later you request a blood test that shows the following:

High sensitivity troponin T	154 ng/l	(<14 ng/l)

6. **What has happened and what are the challenges in management?**

➥ **answer on page 473**

Case 4.11 ++

A 64-year-old man is admitted for investigation of generalised aches and pains, and lethargy. He is previously healthy and is on no prescribed medication. His fluid balance is monitored and, for the first day of hospitalisation, is as follows:

	Intake					Output				
Time	By mouth		IV or other			Urine	Faeces	Vomit (ml)	Gast. Asp. (ml)	Drain (ml)
	Amount (ml)	Type	Amount (ml)	Type	Add.					
08:00										
09:00	150					450				
10:00										
11:00	400									
12:00	100					400				
13:00										
14:00	300					350				
15:00										
16:00	250									
17:00	150					400				
18:00	300									
19:00										
20:00	150					400				
21:00	300									
22:00										
23:00						350				
24:00										
01:00										
02:00						500				
03:00										
04:00						350				
05:00										
06:00										
07:00						300				

Total	By Mouth	IV or other	Urine	Faeces	Vomit	Gast. Asp.	Drain
Day	1800 ml		2350 ml				
Night	300 ml		1150 ml				
Total	2100 ml		3500 ml				
Total Intake	2100 ml		Total Output	3500 ml			

1. **How would you interpret the fluid balance chart? What is your differential diagnosis?**

You request a panel of blood tests that come back (shown below). His kidney function had been found to be normal 4 months before.

Hb	86 g/l	(130–180 g/l males)
MCV	80 fl	(76–96 fl)
WCC	4.2 x 10^9/l	(4.0–11.0 × 10^9/l)
Platelets	173 x 10^9/l	(150–400 × 10^9/l)
ESR	96 mm/h	(0–15 mm/h males)
Na^+	144 mmol/l	(135–145 mmol/l)
K^+	4.8 mmol/l	(3.5–5.0 mmol/l)
Urea	14.2 mmol/l	(2.5–6.7 mmol/l)
Creatinine	246 μmol/l	(79–118 μmol/l)
Cl^-	95 mmol/l	(95–105 mmol/l)
HCO_3^-	24 mmol/l	(24–30 mmol/l)
Glucose	4.2 mmol/l	(4.0–8.0 mmol/l)
Total protein	96 g/l	(<0.45 g/l)
Albumin	30 g/l	(35–50 g/l)

2. **What are the abnormalities, and what is the likely diagnosis?**

A skeletal survey is performed. Here is the skull X-ray.

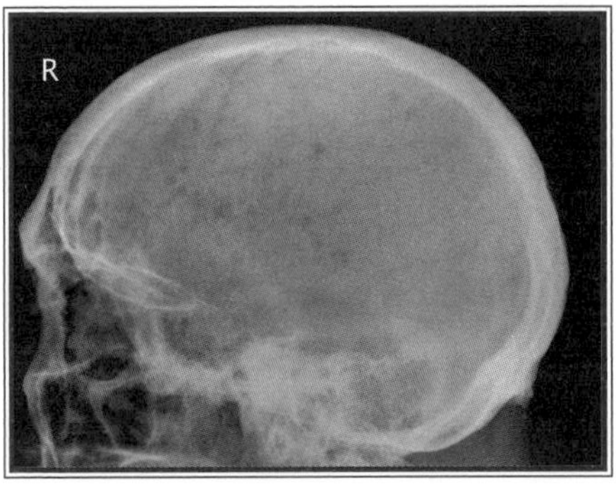

3. **How does the X-ray appearance relate to the likely diagnosis?**

After several days, the laboratory phones through the following results:

IgG	27.2 g/l	(0.8–4.0 g/l)
IgA	0.5 g/l	(7.0–14.5 g/l)
IgM	0.4 g/l	(0.45–2.0 g/l)
Plasma protein electrophoresis:		
IgG paraprotein band approximately 25 g/l in size		

You request a blood calcium level. It is returned as 2.59 mmol/l.

4. **What is the cause of the abnormality seen on the fluid balance chart at the start of the case?**

➥ **answer on page 474**

Case 4.12 ++

A 45-year-old woman with a history of depression is admitted at 1.30am after the ingestion of an unknown quantity of antidepressants (specific type unknown). She is fully conscious on arrival at the hospital and insists that she does not want to live, but is refusing to answer your questions.

You perform a blood gas analysis:

FiO_2	0.40	
pH	7.28	(7.35–7.45)
PaO_2	32.3 kPa	(11–13 kPa)
$PaCO_2$	3.4 kPa	(4.7–6.0 kPa)
HCO_3^-	14.7 mmol/l	(24–30 mmol/l)

1. How would you interpret this test? What else would you like to measure?

The biochemistry laboratory phones through her initial results to a member of the team:

Na^+	142 mmol/l	(135–145 mmol/l)
K^+	3.8 mmol/l	(3.5–5.0 mmol/l)
Urea	4.6 mmol/l	(2.5–6.7 mmol/l)
Creatinine	55 µmol/l	(79–118 µmol/l)
Cl^-	95 mmol/l	(95–105 mmol/l)
HCO_3^-	15 mmol/l	(24–30 mmol/l)
Glucose	5.2 mmol/l	(4.0–8.0 mmol/l)
Total bilirubin	10 µmol/l	(3–17 µmol/l)
ALP	62 U/l	(30–150 U/l)
AST	22 U/l	(5–35 U/l)
ALT	31 U/l	(5–35 U/l)
GGT	132 U/l	(7–33 U/l females)
Paracetamol	45 mg/l	(Nil)
Salicylate	<20 mmol/l	(Nil)
Alcohol	126 mmol/l	(Nil)

2. How would you interpret these tests, and how would your management change?

An ECG is performed and a rhythm strip printed.

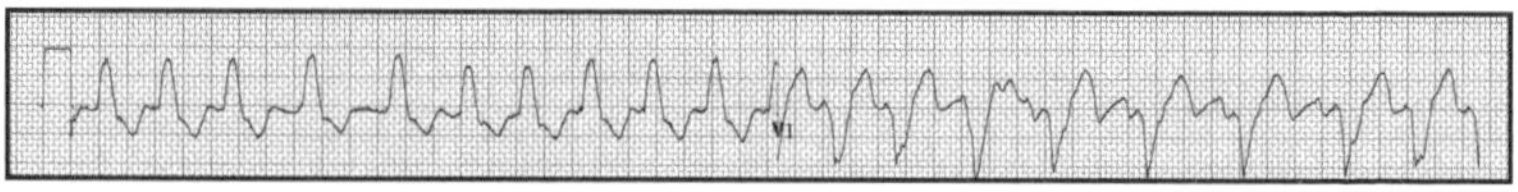

3. What substance has she taken an overdose of, and what is the priority in management?

While you are preparing to give her a drug, her monitor starts to alarm. There is no response from the patient and there is no pulse. Her bedside cardiac monitor shows the following rhythm:

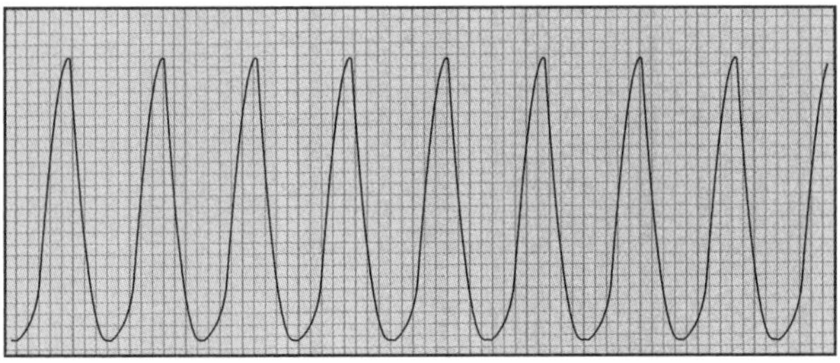

4. What is the rhythm and how will you manage the patient?

➥ answer on page 476

Case 4.13 ++

An 18-year-old student is found by her housemates. She is in a confused state on the floor and is surrounded by several packets of paracetamol. It is 22:00 hours and they are able to ascertain that she took the tablets around 15:30 hours that day. She smells of alcohol. She had been on medications for low mood but is otherwise healthy. On arrival at hospital half an hour later blood tests were taken which are shown.

Na^+	139 mmol/l	(135–145 mmol/l)
K^+	3.7 mmol/l	(3.5–5.0 mmol/l)
Urea	5.1 mmol/l	(2.5–6.7 mmol/l)
Creatinine	52 μmol/l	(79–118 μmol/l)
Cl^-	105 mmol/l	(95–105 mmol/l)
HCO_3^-	25 mmol/l	(24–30 mmol/l)
Paracetamol	160 mg/l	(Nil)
Alcohol	25 mmol/l	(Nil)
Salicylates	Nil	(Nil)
Bilirubin	12 μmol/l	(3–17 μmol/l)
AST	78 U/l	(5–35 U/l)
ALT	65 U/l	(5–35 U/l)
GGT	99 U/l	(7–33 U/l females)
ALP	67 U/l	(30–150 U/l)
Albumin	39 g/l	(35–50 g/l)
Prothrombin time (PT)	18.7 s	(12–16 s)
APTT	35.4 s	(24–38 s)
Fibrinogen	6.7 g/l	(2–4 g/l)

1. **With the above results in mind outline the treatment approach for this patient.**

Following the commencement of her treatment blood tests are taken on a regular basis and are shown below.

Time (hours)	Bilirubin (μmol/l)	AST (U/l)	ALT (U/l)	ALP (U/l)	GGT (U/l)	Albumin (g/l)	PT (s)
4	13	44	56	65	64	42	16.05
12	15	44	56	65	64	41	17.05
20	16	8001	7056	55	64	39	17.15
28	16	9977	10 230	75	54	38	18.55
36	19	12 333	11 156	65	61	34	19.05
44	23	12 993	12 333	64	62	32	21.05
52	27	13 144	12 456	75	73	28	21.44
56	29	13 111	12 346	77	74	24	24.05
60	36	13 244	12 153	85	77	22	30.05

2. **Outline the trend and significance of these results. What treatment should be considered now?**

She is transferred to a regional centre where she undergoes surgery. In the initial days postoperatively she progresses well, but on day 5 becomes short of breath and a chest X-ray is taken which is shown below.

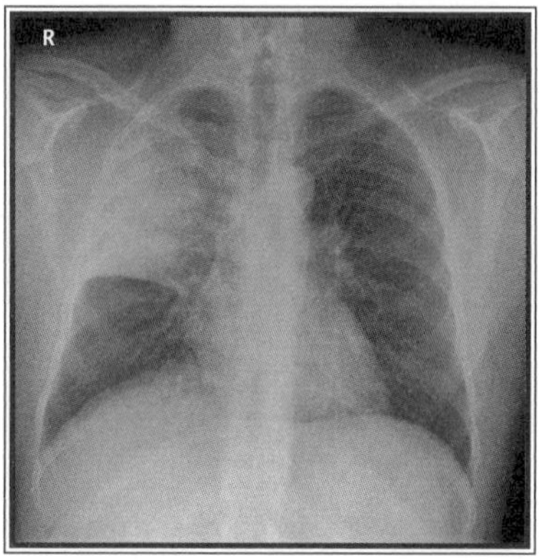

3. **Report the findings on this chest X-ray.**

At the same time a sample is sent for arterial blood gas analysis. The patient was breathing room air.

FiO_2	0.21	
pH	7.35	(7.35–7.45)
PaO_2	5.2 kPa	(11–13 kPa)
$PaCO_2$	4.3 kPa	(4.7–6.0 kPa)
HCO_3^-	24.8 mmol/l	(24–30 mmol/l)
BE	-4.2 mmol/l	(-2 to +2 mmol/l)

4. **What abnormality is observed on the arterial sample?**

She is commenced on antimicrobial therapy and sputum is sent for analysis. The following day the results of her sputum analysis are conveyed from microbiology.

> Gram-positive cocci in keeping with *Streptococcus pneumoniae*

During the middle of the night you are called by the nurse to see her as some of her vital signs are concerning. Her bedside chart is shown.

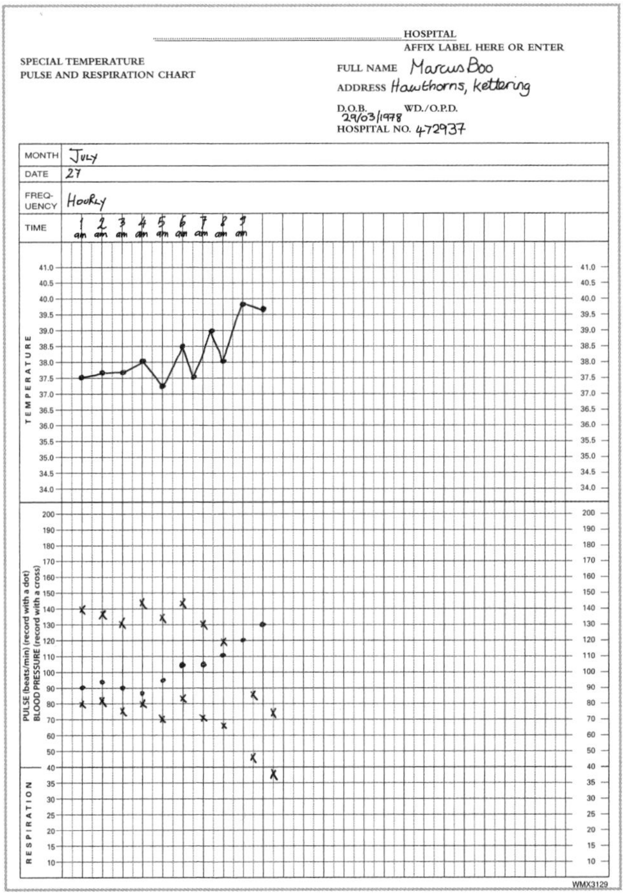

5. **Describe the findings on the chart and the underlying cause.**

➥ **answer on page 478**

Case 4.14 +++

An 18-year-old shop assistant is admitted with generalised abdominal pain that has been worsening for 36 hours. On examination, you find the abdomen to be generally tender, although there is no clinical evidence of peritonism. The nurse hands you her observations recording sheet.

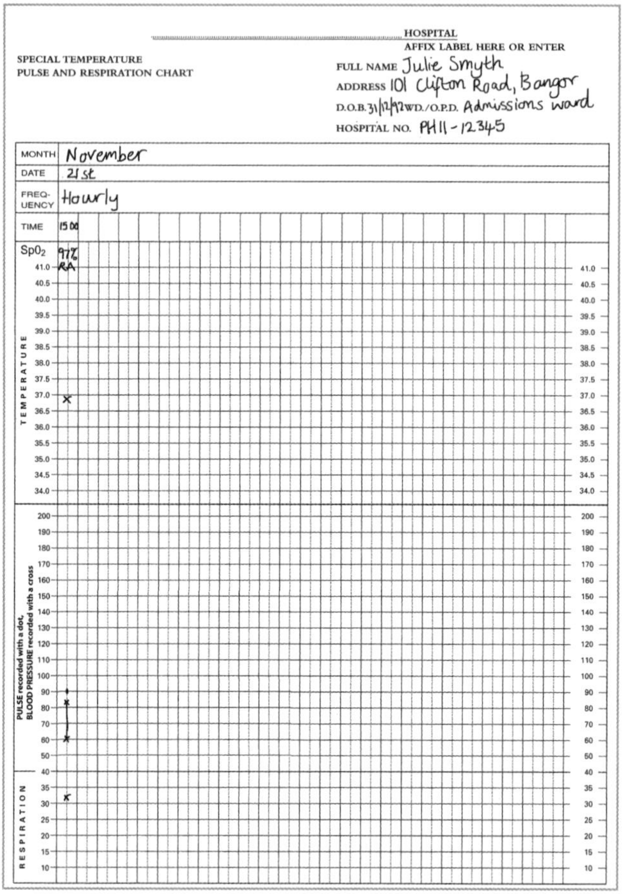

1. **What parameters are notably abnormal? Does this narrow your differential diagnosis?**

Shortly, you receive her initial blood results.

Hb	132 g/l	(120–160 g/l females)
MCV	84 fl	(76–96 fl)
WCC	7.6 x 10^9/l	(4.0–11.0 × 10^9/l)
Platelets	368 x 10^9/l	(150–400 × 10^9/l)
Na^+	142 mmol/l	(135–145 mmol/l)
K^+	3.9 mmol/l	(3.5–5.0 mmol/l)
Urea	6.2 mmol/l	(2.5–6.7 mmol/l)
Creatinine	46 μmol/l	(79–118 μmol/l)
Cl^-	94 mmol/l	(95–105 mmol/l)
HCO_3^-	8 mmol/l	(24–30 mmol/l)
Amylase	52 U/l	(25–125 U/l)

2. What is the major abnormality? Are any possible diagnoses less likely bearing in mind these results?

On account of the abnormalities seen, you perform a blood gas analysis. The results are shown. The patient is breathing room air.

FiO_2	0.21	
pH	7.21	(7.35–7.45)
PaO_2	12.5 kPa	(11–13 kPa)
$PaCO_2$	2.9 kPa	(4.7–6.0 kPa)
HCO_3^-	7.6 mmol/l	(24–30 mmol/l)

3. What are the causes of the acid-base abnormality demonstrated and what tests might you arrange to differentiate between them?

You request urinalysis. The results are shown.

Glucose	++++
Bilirubin	Neg
Ketones	++++
Specific gravity	1.005
Blood	Neg
Protein	Neg
Nitrite	Neg
Leukocytes	Neg

4. Based on all the results so far, what is the apparent cause of the abdominal pain?

Treatment is commenced, and the patient appears to improve. You are asked to review her in 4 hours. Her bedside charts on the opposite page show the trend of vital signs.

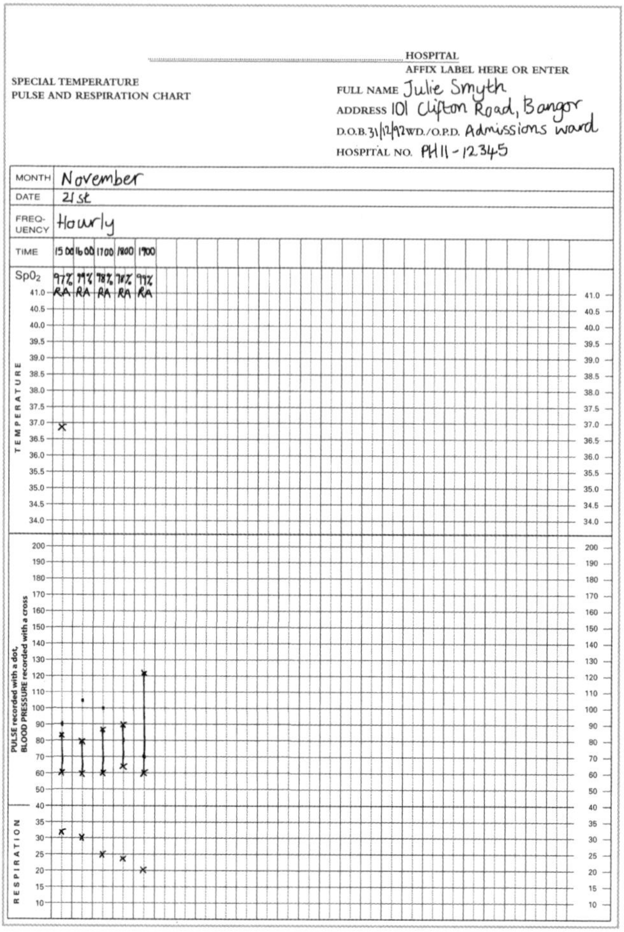

Time	Glucose (mmol/l)	Ketones (mmol/l)
1500	28.2	7.2
1600	26.3	6.1
1700	19.5	4.9
1800	12.7	4.1
1900	8.6	2.8

5. **Are you satisfied that the patient is improving?**

Repeat blood tests show the following:

Na^+	142 mmol/l	(135-145 mmol/l)
K^+	2.4 mmol/l	(3.5-5.0 mmol/l)
Urea	6.2 mmol/l	(2.5-6.7 mmol/l)
Creatinine	46 μmol/l	(79-118 μmol/l)
Cl^-	94 mmol/l	(95-105 mmol/l)
HCO^{3-}	12 mmol/l	(24-30 mmol/l)
FiO_2	0.21	
pH	7.30	(7.35-7.45)
PaO_2	12.7 kPa	(11-13 kPa)
$PaCO_2$	3.4 kPa	(4.7-6.0 kPa)
HCO_3^-	12.5 mmol/l	(24-30 mmol/l)

6. **What action would you take now?**

➥ **answer on page 482**

Case 4.15 +++

A 51-year-old male teacher is referred for investigation of high blood pressure. He has been started on an ACE inhibitor by his GP after two readings showing moderate hypertension. He does not smoke. You arrange ambulatory blood pressure monitoring.

Ambulatory Blood Pressure Monitor - Summary of Results

Name of patient: Mr Richard Eakin
Age: 51 years
Hospital Number: PH99-29283
Number of Attempted Readings: 50
Number of Successful Readings: 48 (96%)

	Minimum (mmHg)	Maximum (mmHg)	Mean (mmHg)
Wake period	136/72	212/108	162/88
Sleep period	122/80	216/108	174/92
Overall	122/80	216/108	164/89

1. **What is your interpretation of this recording?**

As a result of this investigation, you arrange a series of tests, the results of which are shown below.

Na^+	144 mmol/l	(135–145 mmol/l)
K^+	3.3 mmol/l	(3.5–5.0 mmol/l)
Urea	4.3 mmol/l	(2.5–6.7 mmol/l)
Creatinine	46 μmol/l	(79–118 μmol/l)
Cl^-	93 mmol/l	(95–105 mmol/l)
HCO_3^-	25 mmol/l	(24–30 mmol/l)
Glucose	7.2 mmol/l	(Random 4.0-8.0 mmol/l)
Total cholesterol	5.2 mmol/l	(<5.0 mmol/l)
HDL-cholesterol	0.9 mmol/l	(>1.0 mmol/l)
LDL-cholesterol	4.1 mmol/l	(<3.0 mmol/l)
Cholesterol:HDL ratio	5.78	
Urinary albumin:creatinine ratio	67	

Chest X-ray report
Heart size normal
Normal mediastinal contours
Lungs clear

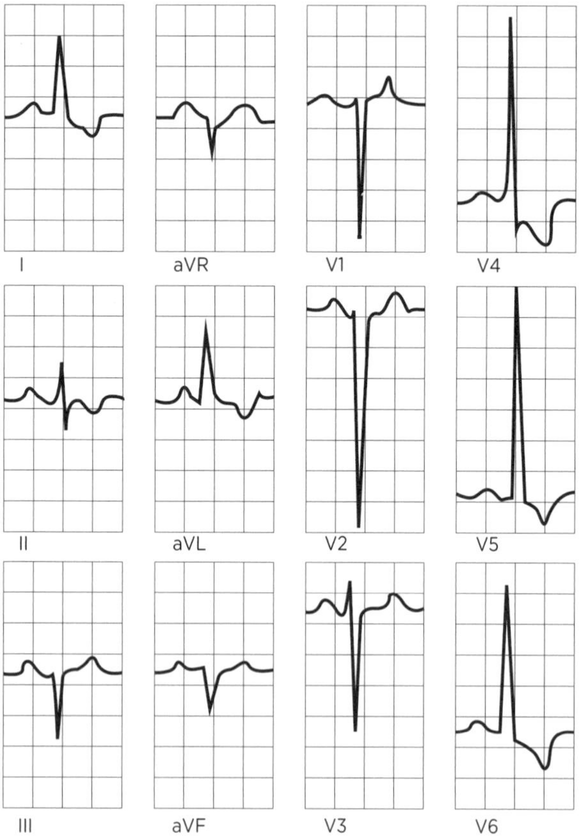

Transthoracic echocardiogram report
Moderate concentric left ventricular hypertrophy. Left ventricular function appears normal. No significant valvular disease. Other chambers appear normal.

Renal ultrasonography and Doppler ultrasonography: report of study of renal vessels
Both kidneys appear normal in size, shape and echogenicity. Normal Doppler waveform tracings were obtained from vessels on both sides.

2. **What are your conclusions based on these results? What further tests would be helpful?**
3. **How would you interpret the test, and how does this affect cardiovascular risk?**

You decide to stop treatment to allow a hormone test to be carried out.

Plasma renin activity	0.3 ng/ml per h
Aldosterone	24 ng/l
Aldosterone:renin ratio	80

4. **What are the implications of this test, and how might you investigate further?**

➥ **answer on page 486**

4 COMPLETE CLINICAL CASES: ANSWERS

Answer 4.1

➥ case on page 426

1. Given the finding of an altered conscious level, the patient is placed on a neuro-observation chart. The observation chart shows a stable Glasgow Coma Scale of 13/15. The patient is deemed to be confused and opens her eyes to speech.

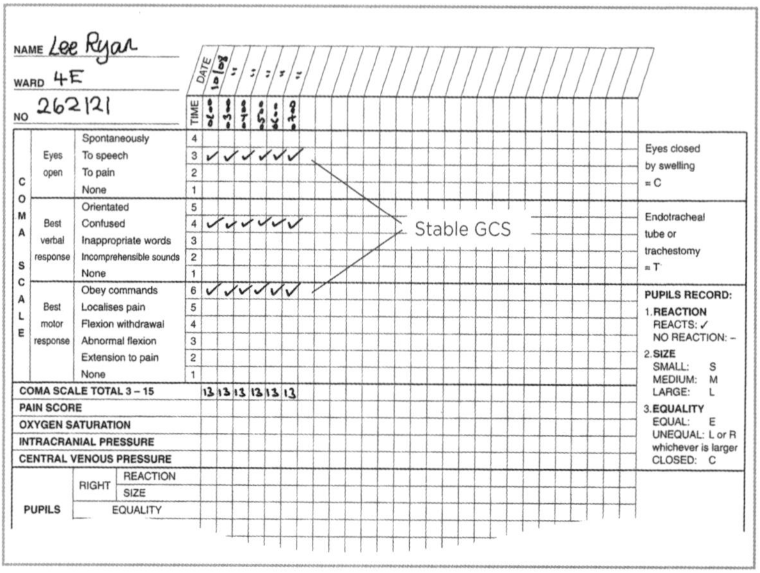

The CT brain imaging is abnormal. Lumbar puncture and an EEG are therefore performed to help come to a diagnosis.

Opening pressure	16 cmCSF	
Appearance	Clear	
	No organisms seen on microscopy	
WCC	121/mm³	Normal
RCC	3/mm³	
Glucose	2.8 mmol/l	Low
Total protein	72 g/l	Mild elevation

This collection of findings is termed a CSF pleocytosis.

CAUSES OF A CSF PLEOCYTOSIS
Viral meningitis
Encephalitis
Partially treated bacterial meningitis
TB or fungal meningitis
Intracranial abscess
Post-subarachnoid haemorrhage

One should have inferred from the clinical scenario so far that the cause of her symptoms and CSF findings is a viral meningitis/encephalitis. An additional test would be for PCR of the CSF to enable detection of viruses, especially herpes simplex virus (HSV).

2. The EEG findings demonstrate the characteristic neurophysiological findings of HSV encephalitis.

   Further tests in HSV encephalitis would include:

- **MRI of brain:**
  - Oedema within the temporal lobes bilaterally (better elucidated than on CT).
- **PCR of CSF:**
  - HSV-1: present.

CASE SUMMARY
A CSF pleocytosis
Herpes simplex encephalitis

Answer 4.2

➥ case on page 427

Iron	99 μmol/l	High
Ferritin	878 μg/l	High
TIBC	12 μmol/l	Low
Transferrin saturation	65%	High

1. These results suggest a state of iron overload. This may be due to hereditary haemochromatosis. Haemochromatosis may present with:

- Cardiomyopathy
- Liver disease

- Pituitary disease
- Diabetes mellitus
- Joint problems (pseudogout).

All manifestations are related to the deposition of iron within organs.

2. Other acute phase reactants include:

- CRP
- ESR
- Ceruloplasmin.

Note that albumin acts as a 'negative acute phase reactant' - its levels decreasing with inflammation.

Bilirubin	11 μmol/l	
AST	25 U/l	
ALT	32 U/l	
ALP	67 U/l	
GGT	152 U/l	High
Albumin	40 g/l	

3. As is commonly the case, both at diagnosis and in established disease, the LFTs are essentially normal. The only abnormal LFT is the GGT which is mildly elevated. Given his clinical history this is likely to reflect heavy alcohol consumption rather than haemochromatosis.

Idiopathic haemochromatosis is an autosomal recessive condition. Only homozygotes develop clinically overt disease. There is now a gene test for haemochromatosis and screening of first-degree relatives of patients is offered. The most common genetic defect is homozygosity of the *C282Y* missense mutation of the *HFE* gene on chromosome 6p. In addition, a different mutation - *H63D* - can play a role in some cases.

With appropriate early management, patients with haemochromatosis should, in large part, not develop liver failure.

Neutrophil count (WCC)	312 cells/mm^3	High
Ascites albumin content	19 g/l	
Serum albumin	32 g/l	
Microscopy and Gram stain	Gram-negative rods	Abnormal finding
Culture	*E. coli*	Abnormal finding
Amylase	92 U/l	

4. The presentation with ascites implies the development of liver cirrhosis with portal hypertension. The peritoneal aspiration performed tells us three things:

- The serum-ascites albumin gradient (SAAG) is 32 - 19 = 13 g/l. This tells us that the patient probably has portal hypertension.
- The ascitic fluid is infected with the Gram-negative microorganism *E. coli*.
- There is a high neutrophil count.

This all implies spontaneous bacterial peritonitis. In the acute setting, the most important result to note would be the WCC. An elevated WCC should be taken as evidence for peritonitis and appropriate therapy instituted before culture results are obtained. If the WCC had been normal, one should consider ascites secondary to the development of hepatocellular carcinoma. Haemochromatosis patients with cirrhosis are susceptible to this primary liver malignancy.

5. The accompanying LFTs show:

- Poor synthetic function (prothrombin time UP and albumin DOWN)
- Mildly deranged liver function
- The patient has developed liver failure as a result of the combined hepatotoxic insults of iron and alcohol.

Bilirubin	84 μmol/l	High
AST	134 U/l	High
ALT	65 U/l	High
GGT	109 U/l	High
ALP	122 U/l	High
Albumin	26 g/l	Low
Prothrombin time	24.9 s	High
APTT	34.5 s	
Fibrinogen	4.5 g/l	

CASE SUMMARY

Haemochromatosis
Spontaneous bacterial peritonitis
Liver failure

Answer 4.3

➥ case on page 429

Hb	99 g/l	Low
MCV	89.9 fl	
WCC	11.2×10^9/l	Slightly high
Platelets	199×10^9/l	
Adjusted Ca^{2+}	2.45 mmol/l	
PO_4^{3-}	0.87 mmol/l	
Albumin	36 g/l	
Urate	0.34 mmol/l	
CRP	312 mg/l	High

1. The important findings from the FBP, bone profile and other biochemistry tests are:

- A normocytic anaemia (low haemoglobin and normal MCV)
- A substantially raised CRP
- A normal urate
- A normal bone profile.

Sometimes normal blood results are as important as positive ones. In this case, gout is on the list of differential diagnoses for an acute-onset, painful, swollen joint so the urate level is important to measure. However, remember that the urate level can be normal in acute gout.

Specimen received	Synovial fluid from right knee
Appearance	Clear
Microscopy	<2 leukocytes per mm^3
Plane polarised light microscopy	No crystals seen
Synovial fluid culture	No growth

The knee aspirate sample is normal. No white cells or organisms were identified, and culture was negative, excluding septic arthritis. Similarly, no crystals were seen to suggest a crystalline arthritis.

Rheumatoid factor	199 IU/ml	High
Gastric parietal cell antibodies	1:280	High
Intrinsic factor antibodies	+ve	Abnormal
Anti-nuclear	-ve	
Anti-nucleolar	-ve	
Anti-nuclear (speckled)	-ve	
Anti-mitochondrial	-ve	
Anti-smooth muscle	-ve	
Anti-gastric parietal cell	-ve	
Anti-CCP	+ve	Abnormal

The result of the autoimmune screen is important. The rheumatoid factor is highly elevated, which in the context of the clinical symptoms and earlier finding of a raised CRP and normochromic anaemia implies a diagnosis of rheumatoid disease. There are three important points to remember about rheumatoid factor:

- Its level does not necessarily reflect disease activity.
- It can be raised in a number of states other than rheumatoid disease (ie poor specificity).
- It does not need to be positive for the diagnosis of rheumatoid disease to be made (20% of patients are rheumatoid factor negative).
- More highly specific is the newer RA autoantibody anti-CCP (anti-cyclic citrullinated peptide), which is normal in this case.

Interestingly, the screen also has antibodies to gastric parietal cells and intrinsic factor in keeping with a diagnosis of pernicious anaemia. It is common for patients to suffer from several coexisting autoimmune diseases.

FEV_1	68% predicted	Low
FVC	50% predicted	Low
FEV_1/FVC	85%	High
*K*co	51% predicted	Low

2. The positive findings from spirometry with transfer factor are:

- A reduced FEV_1
- A reduced FVC
- A high FEV_1:FVC ratio
- A reduced transfer factor.

This demonstrates a restrictive pattern wholly in keeping with interstitial lung fibrosis.

Chest X-ray report
This is a PA chest X-ray of Mrs B taken on 2 January 2006. She is 39 years of age. The technical quality of the film is satisfactory. There is evidence of increased interstitial lung markings throughout both bases. The lung volumes appear reduced overall. These findings are typical of interstitial lung fibrosis. High-resolution CT of the chest is advised.

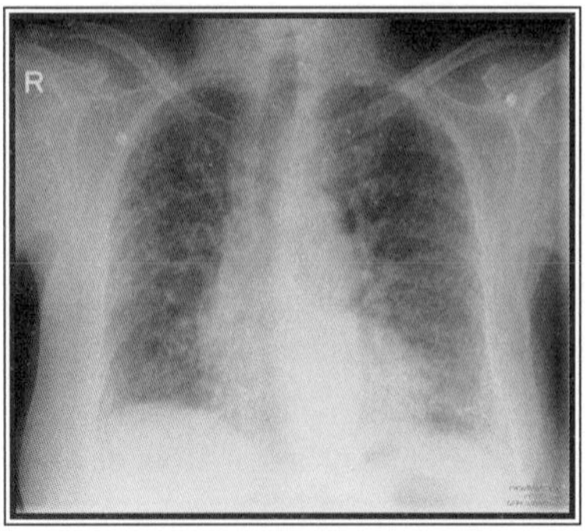

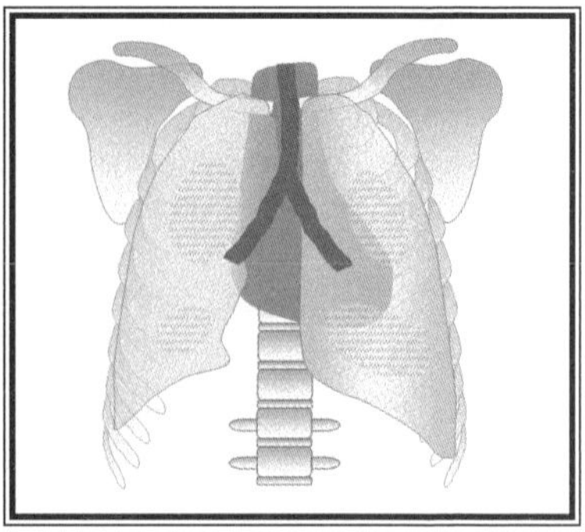

The presence of fibrosis may be due to:

- The disease itself – pulmonary fibrosis is one of the pulmonary manifestations of rheumatoid disease
- A side effect of treatment with methotrexate (first-line disease-modifying anti-rheumatic drug treatment for this condition).

3. As seen in the report above, high resolution CT is advisable as this will help clarify in greater detail the nature and extent of the disease.

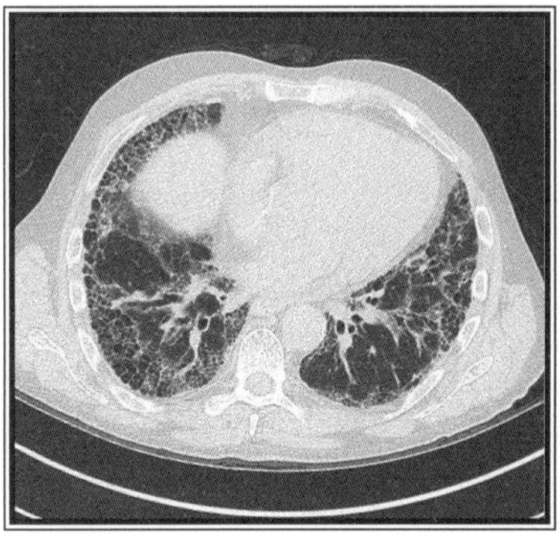

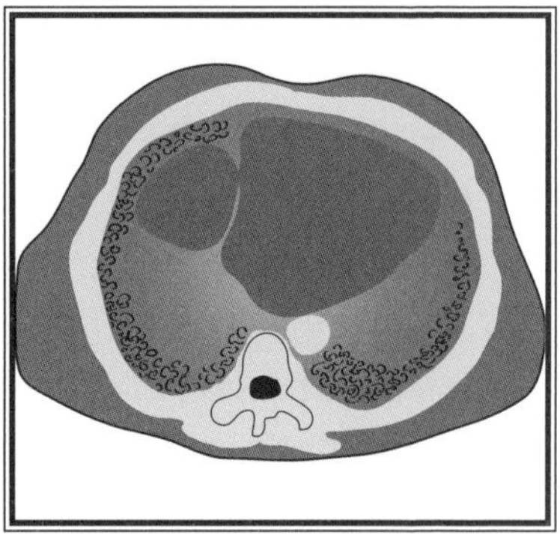

Region (age matched)	BMD (g/cm^2)	T score	Z score	
Neck of femur	0.526	-3.0	-2.7	Low
L1	0.812	-2.7	-2.8	Low
L4	0.846	-3.0	-2.9	Low

4. Patients with rheumatoid disease often have exacerbations ('flares') of their disease requiring treatment with either intravenous or oral steroids. Both the disease itself and steroid treatment put such patients at risk of developing osteoporosis which is diagnosed by dual energy X-ray

absorptiometry (DXA) scanning. A *T* score of less than −2.5 indicates osteoporosis. A score of −1.5 to −2.5 implies the presence of osteopenia.

CASE SUMMARY
Knee effusion (due to rheumatoid disease) Interstitial lung fibrosis (rheumatoid lung) Steroid-induced osteoporosis

Answer 4.4

➥ case on page 431

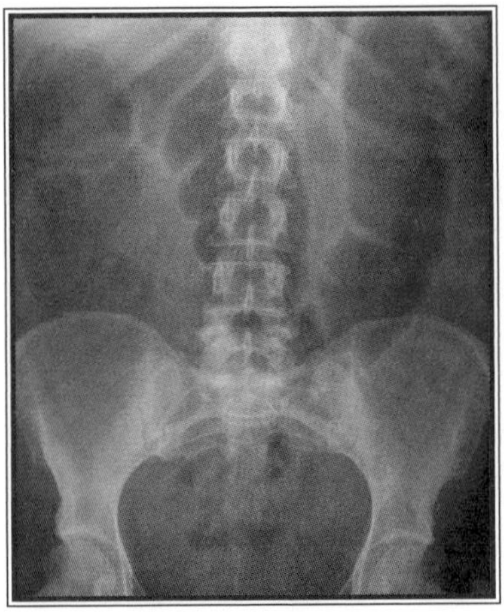

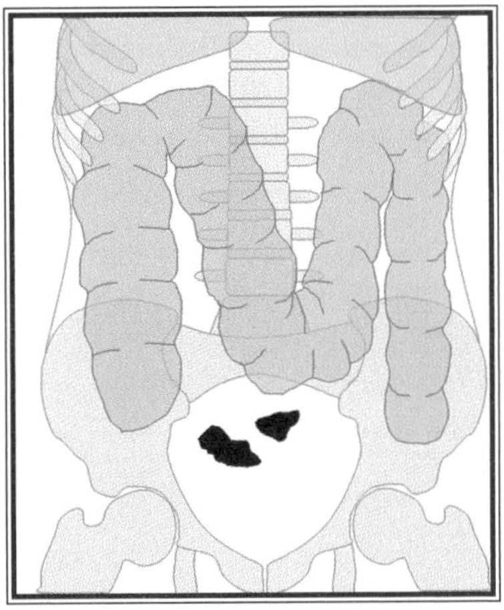

Abdominal X-ray report
This is a supine abdominal X-ray. The patient is 74 years of age. The technical quality is adequate.
The distribution of gas within the large bowel is abnormal. The luminal diameter is 7 cm at the splenic flexure. Haustral markings can be seen. There is a paucity of gas beyond this point. No extraluminal gas is seen. Appearances in keeping with large bowel obstruction.

2. Interpretation of the ABG.

FiO_2	0.21	
pH	7.26	Low
PaO_2	11.5 kPa	
PaCO_2	2.9 kPa	Low
HCO_3^-	12.6 mmol/l	Low
BE	-15.8 mmol/l	High
Lactate	8.3 mmol/l	High

The findings on arterial blood analysis are:

- Oxygenation is adequate.
- A low pH. This patient is profoundly acidotic.
- A low *Pa*CO_2. Respiratory compensation is occurring.
- A low HCO_3^-. The origin of excess acid is metabolic in nature.
- A high lactate. This is a 'rogue' acid being produced in large quantities. In this case ischaemia of the large bowel is the cause.

The anion gap can be calculated:

$$\text{Anion gap} = (Na^+ + K^+) - (Cl^- + HCO_3^-) = 23.6\ \text{mmol/l}$$

3. This patient has a high anion gap metabolic acidosis, most likely due to lactic acidosis, secondary to an ischaemic bowel.

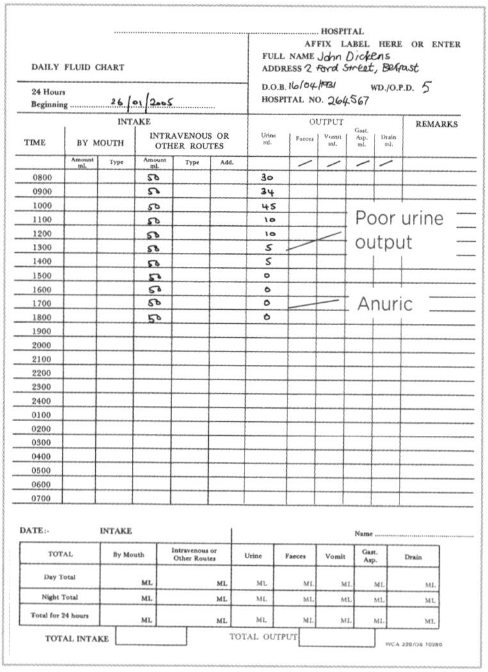

.... HOSPITAL

DAILY FLUID CHART

24 Hours Beginning 26/01/2005

AFFIX LABEL HERE OR ENTER
FULL NAME John Dickens
ADDRESS 2 Ford Street, Belfast
D.O.B. 16/04/1931 WD./O.P.D. 5
HOSPITAL NO. 264567

TIME	INTAKE: BY MOUTH Amount ml.	Type	INTRAVENOUS OR OTHER ROUTES Amount ml.	Type	Add.	OUTPUT: Urine ml.	Faeces	Vomit ml.	Gast. Asp. ml.	Drain ml.	REMARKS
							/	/	/	/	
0800			50			30					
0900			50			34					
1000			50			45					
1100			50			10					
1200			50			10					
1300			50			5					
1400			50			5					
1500			50			0					
1600			50			0					
1700			50			0					
1800			50			0					
1900											
2000											
2100											
2200											
2300											
2400											
0100											
0200											
0300											
0400											
0500											
0600											
0700											

DATE:- INTAKE Name ....

TOTAL	By Mouth	Intravenous or Other Routes	Urine	Faeces	Vomit	Gast. Asp.	Drain
Day Total	ML	ML	ML	ML	ML	ML	ML
Night Total	ML	ML	ML	ML	ML	ML	ML
Total for 24 hours	ML	ML	ML	ML	ML	ML	ML

TOTAL INTAKE TOTAL OUTPUT

WCA 329/06 10280

One should infer from the bedside chart that:

- there is a significant positive balance
- the urine output has tailed off in the last 4 hours
- before becoming anuric the urine output was poor.

Na^+	134 mmol/l	
K^+	6.6 mmol/l	High
Urea	19.7 mmol/l	High
Creatinine	403 μmol/l	High
Cl^-	98 mmol/l	
HCO_3^-	12.6 mmol/l	Low
Mg^{2+}	0.72 mmol/l	Low
PO_4^{3-}	0.89 mmol/l	

4. This patient has anuria which was preceded by a period of oliguria. In the first instance the urinary catheter should be checked and flushed to ensure that there is no blockage.

   The blood results show that this patient has developed acute renal failure. From the clinical history it appears that this is at least being contributed to by obstruction of the renal tract.

   The patient has life-threatening hyperkalaemia. A potassium of greater than 6.5 mmol/l (in the context of acute renal failure) requires immediate treatment.

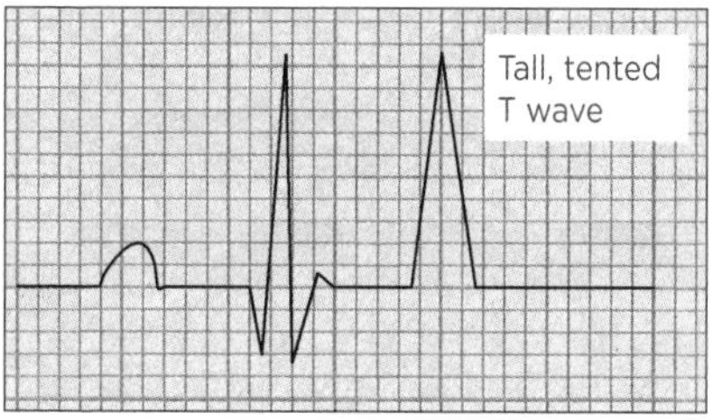

5. The ECG shows classic changes related to hyperkalaemia. The T waves are tall and peaked.

6. CT of the abdomen

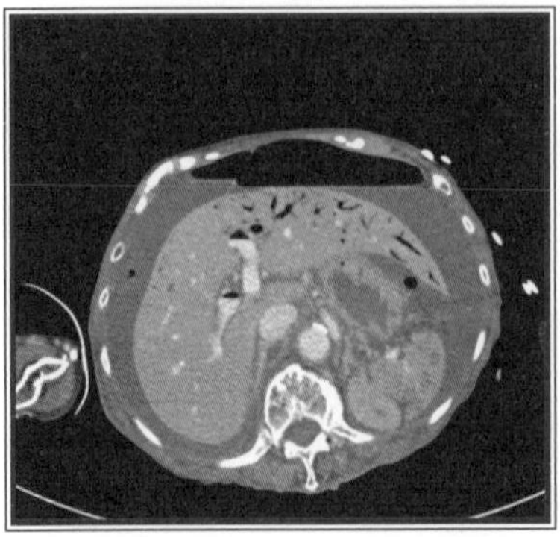

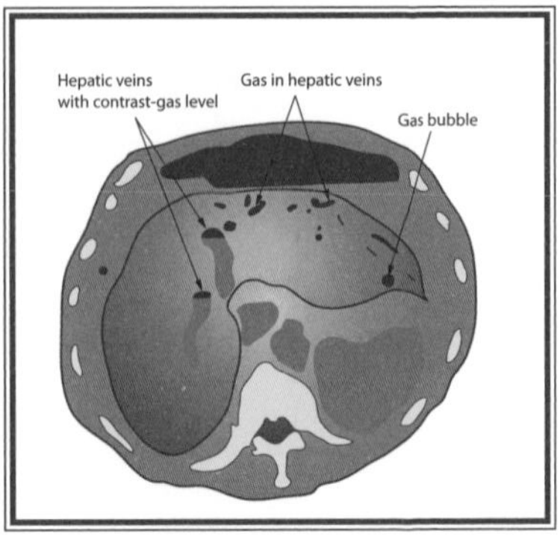

CT with IV contrast may often identify ischaemic bowel. Features include:

- Non-enhancing bowel wall
- Intramural ± free gas
- Visceral vessel thrombus.

CASE SUMMARY

Large bowel obstruction
Bowel ischaemia with metabolic acidosis
Acute renal impairment (due to bladder outlet obstruction)
ECG abnormality (due to hyperkalaemia)

Answer 4.5

➥ case on page 433

Hb	145 g/l	
MCV	98.7 fl	
Platelets	293 x 10^9/l	
WCC	14.4 x 10^9/l	High
Neutrophils	11.3 x 10^9/l	High
Lymphocytes	2.2 x 10^9/l	
Monocytes	0.5 x 10^9/l	
Eosinophils	0.2 x 10^9/l	
Basophils	0.09 x 10^9/l	
Na^+	137 mmol/l	
K^+	3.8 mmol/l	
Urea	8.6 mmol/l	High
Creatinine	101 μmol/l	
Cl^-	107 mmol/l	
CRP	176 mmol/l	High

1. From the initial investigations one should have identified the following:

- There is a raised WCC (predominantly comprising neutrophils), along with a raised CRP. The possibility of infection should be entertained.
- In addition, you will note a mildly raised urea, reflective of a mild degree of dehydration.

FiO_2	0.21	
pH	7.50	High
PaO_2	7.8 kPa	Low
$PaCO_2$	3.1 kPa	Low
HCO_3^-	25.8 mmol/l	
BE	+ 6.2 mmol/l	High

2. The ABG features two findings:

- A low PaO_2. The patient is hypoxic. She has type 1 respiratory failure.
- A low $PaCO_2$. The patient is short of breath and hyperventilating, causing a low CO_2. This has led to a respiratory alkalosis.

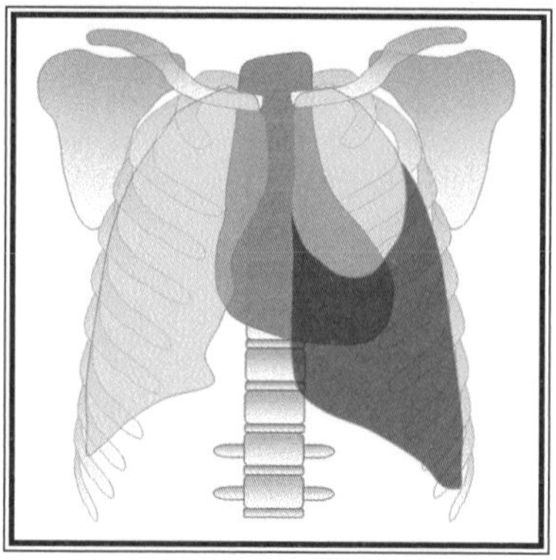

3. The chest X-ray indicates the likely cause for the findings.

Radiology report
This is a PA chest X-ray of Captain Janice Boeing taken on 19 December 2005. She is a 54-year-old woman. The technical quality of the film is satisfactory. The most striking finding is an area of radio-opacity on the left side of the chest from the lower zone extending to the midzone. The left hemidiaphragm silhouette and the left costophrenic angle are not identified. The remainder of the film is normal in appearance. These findings are in keeping with a moderate left-sided pleural effusion.

Total protein	38 g/l	High
LDH	246 U/l	High
pH	7.37	
Microscopy	Nil seen	

4. From the pleural fluid analysis one can see:

- This is an exudate with an elevated total protein and LDH level.

5. Putting all this information together and correlating it with the patient's clinical features, the likely cause for this pleural effusion is an underlying pneumonia. This is termed a 'parapneumonic pleural effusion'.

   The patient goes on to develop diarrhoea. The most likely cause is simple diarrhoea secondary to the commencement of antibiotics. However, one must be suspicious of *Clostridium difficile* as a causative organism for the diarrhoea, particularly since this patient has received a cephalosporin antibiotic.

   The stool sample indicates the presence of *C. difficile* toxin. Ideally the causative antibiotic should be stopped if possible. Specific treatment should also be commenced to treat the *C. difficile* if appropriate.

CASE SUMMARY

Pneumonia
Exudate pleural effusion (parapneumonic)
Type 1 respiratory failure with hyperventilation
Clostridium difficile infection (secondary to antibiotic treatment)

Answer 4.6

➥ case on page 435

1. From the information given, the eGFR could be calculated (see page 9 for details). Alternatively, the following formula could be used to give an approximation of the GFR:

$$\text{Creatinine clearance (ml/min)} = \frac{(140 - 62) \times 61}{(0.81 \times 65) \div 88.4} = 89.87 \text{ ml/min}$$

Free thyroxine	18.1 pmol/l
TSH	2.2 mU/l

2. His thyroid status is normal.

Short Synacthen® test		
Time (min)	0	30
Cortisol (nmol/l)	140	822

Rise to >600 following Synacthen® (822)

3. This is a normal short Synacthen® test indicating normal adrenal gland function.
4. Plasma osmolality is calculated as:

   Plasma osmolality = 2 × (115 + 4.4) + 3.5 + 4.6 = 246.9 mosmol/kg

5. This patient fits the diagnostic criteria for SIADH, which is most likely secondary to his lung cancer, most commonly with the small cell subtype. His confusion may be due to hyponatraemia.

CASE SUMMARY

Hyponatraemia
SIADH

Answer 4.7

➥ case on page 436

1. This patient has cystic fibrosis, which is inherited in an autosomal recessive manner.

Faecal elastase undetectable. — Abnormal

2. Yes. Pancreatic insufficiency is common in cystic fibrosis. Low faecal elastase supports this diagnosis.
3. The D-dimer is normal. This indicates a very low probability of a thromboembolic event such as a pulmonary embolism. Other causes of haemoptysis should be sought. In very rare situations, the D-dimer can be normal in the presence of thrombosis, so clinical judgement is always essential when interpreting this result.
4. The audiogram shows sensorineural deafness. This is a rare but characteristic side effect of aminoglycoside antimicrobials such as gentamicin.

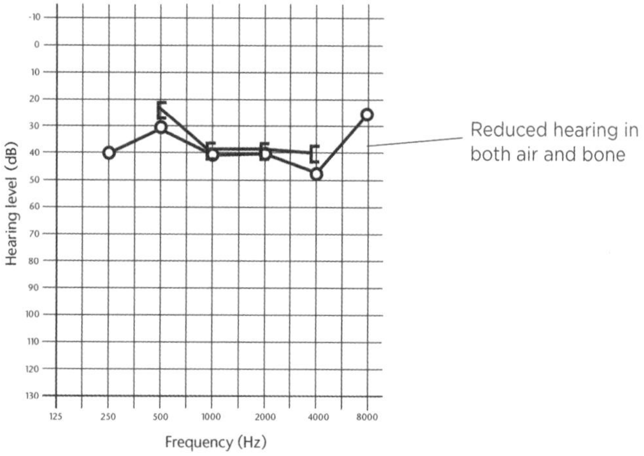

CASE SUMMARY

Cystic fibrosis
Pancreatic exocrine insufficiency
Pneumonia
Gentamicin-induced hearing loss

Answer 4.8

➥ case on page 437

Hb	77 g/l	Low
MCV	69.5 fl	Low
Platelets	512 x 10^9/l	High
WCC	8.7 x 10^9/l	
Iron	5 µmol/l	Low
Ferritin	9 µg/l	Low
TIBC	95 µmol/l	High
Vitamin B_{12}	265 ng/l	
Folate	12.3 µg/l	

1. This patient has a microcytic anaemia. The mild thrombocytosis may be due to active bleeding. The haematinics show iron deficiency.
2. Yes. The abnormal blood cells described can all be found with iron deficiency.
3. The result is CLO positive, indicating gastric infection with *Helicobacter pylori*. The patient should be commenced on a course of antibiotics with a proton pump inhibitor, in an attempt to eradicate the infection.
4. The patient has Barrett's oesophagus, and will require surveillance OGDs for monitoring the disease.

CASE SUMMARY

Iron deficiency anaemia
Helicobacter pylori-positive gastritis
Barrett's oesophagus

Answer 4.9

➥ case on page 438

Hb	175 g/l	
PCV	0.55	>0.5
MCV	86.4 fl	
Platelets	369 x 10^9/l	
WCC	8.9 x 10^9/l	

1. The PCV is elevated, indicating polycythaemia. A measurement of the red cell mass is required to distinguish true polycythaemia from apparent polycythaemia.

Red cell mass estimation		
Red cell mass	137% predicted	>125% predicted

2. The red cell mass result indicates true polycythaemia, and a cause should be sought.

pH	7.37	All normal
PaO_2	12.6 kPa	
$PaCO_2$	4.7 kPa	
HCO_3^-	25.7 mmol/l	
BE	+1.2 mmol/l	

3. The arterial blood gas analysis is entirely normal.

Urine sodium	<20 mmol/l	Low

4. The urinary sodium concentration is low, suggesting that the oliguria is due to prerenal causes, ie hypovolaemia. The patient requires intravenous fluid resuscitation.

Protein	Nil	
Blood	Nil	
Nitrites	++	Abnormal
Leukocyte esterase	+++	Abnormal

5. The urine contains nitrites and leukocyte esterase. In keeping with the clinical history, these changes are most commonly caused by a urinary tract infection. The most useful next investigation would be a urine culture.

CASE SUMMARY

Renal cell carcinoma
Postoperative prerenal uraemia
Urinary tract infection

Answer 4.10

➥ case on page 440

1. The patient has had a stroke caused by infarction in the territory of the left middle cerebral artery. All patients presenting with cerebral infarcts in the appropriate time period should be considered for thrombolytic therapy. It is important to ensure that there are no contraindications for thrombolysis. These include, but are not limited to, recent trauma or surgery, bleeding disposition and uncontrolled hypertension. Thrombolysis must be administered relatively soon after symptom onset (current evidence suggests within 4.5 hours).

2. The patient's level of consciousness has dramatically worsened. The integrity of the patient's airway should be assessed and the airway protected if necessary. Breathing and circulation should be assessed next. A sudden drop in blood pressure might be indicative of a large amount of bleeding somewhere in the body, precipitated by the thrombolytic agent. A bedside blood glucose reading should be taken because hypoglycaemia could present in this manner. Assuming that all these parameters are satisfactory, you should then rapidly consider the intracranial status. Options include extension of the infarction or intracerebral haemorrhage. A repeat CT scan of the brain should be performed without delay.

3. The CT scan confirms that the patient's infarct has undergone haemorrhagic transformation. The priorities always start with ensuring that the 'ABCs' are stable. The patient may require airway protection if the level of consciousness means that it is not secure. The next priority would be to correct any problem that might increase bleeding propensity and increase blood loss into the brain. Blood tests of coagulation and a platelet count should be arranged urgently. A haematologist should be contacted about blood product replacement. A neurosurgeon should also be contacted for an opinion as to whether surgical intervention with evacuation of the haemorrhage might be helpful.

Hb	122 g/l	
MCV	86 fl	
WCC	7.6 x 10^9/l	
Platelets	23 x 10^9/l	Very low

4. A patient with intracranial bleeding in the setting of thrombocytopenia should receive an infusion of platelets with the intention of increasing the platelet count to a safe level. In the longer term, the patient should be investigated to find out why the platelet count was so low.

5. This ECG shows horizontal ST depression in the anterior and lateral leads. This might simply represent myocardial ischaemia (angina) but the possibility of a non-ST-elevation myocardial infarction (NSTEMI) should be borne in mind. Biochemical testing for cardiac troponin will be necessary to distinguish between these two possibilities.

High sensitivity troponin T	154 ng/l	High

6. The elevated blood troponin level would suggest that the patient has had a myocardial infarction. Given the ECG noted earlier, the most likely diagnosis is an NSTEMI. In 'normal circumstances' the patient would receive anti-platelet therapy and heparin. The complicating factor in this case is that the patient is recovering from a recent intracerebral haemorrhage and any treatment given for the heart might result in further bleeding in the brain. Difficult decisions will have to be made by senior clinicians.

CASE SUMMARY

Stroke (infarction)
Haemorrhagic transformation of ischaemic stroke post-thrombolysis
Thrombocytopenia
NSTEMI

Answer 4.11

➥ case on page 442

1. The patient's urinary output seems excessive when compared with the amount of fluid consumed. The most common cause for this pattern is treatment with diuretics (eg for oedema in heart failure). We are told, however, that the patient is on no treatment, so this is not the cause. Other causes of polyuria include diabetes mellitus, diabetes insipidus, hypercalaemia and following the relief of urinary tract obstruction.

Hb	86 g/l	Low
MCV	80 fl	Normal
WCC	4.2 x 10^9/l	
Platelets	173 x 10^9/l	
ESR	96 mm/h	Markedly Elevated
Na^+	144 mmol/l	
K^+	4.8 mmol/l	
Urea	14.2 mmol/l	High
Creatinine	246 μmol/l	High
Cl^-	95 mmol/l	
HCO_3^-	24 mmol/l	
Glucose	4.2 mmol/l	Normal
Total protein	96 g/l	High
Albumin	30 g/l	Low

2. Several abnormalities are demonstrated, and the key to making the diagnosis is thinking of a condition that could explain all the results. It is possible that several disease processes coexist in the patient, but a single unifying diagnosis would be much more likely. The abnormalities are: normocytic anaemia, elevated ESR, acute kidney injury, high total protein and low albumin. The glucose level is normal making diabetes mellitus less likely. The normal sodium concentration makes diabetes insipidus less likely, but does not exclude it.

   The key to suspecting the correct diagnosis here lies with correct interpretation of the protein and albumin results. Total protein is a measure of albumin plus globulins. As this patient's albumin level is low and the total protein level is high, one can extrapolate that the globulin (IgG, IgA and IgM) level must be high. The disease most likely to give an elevated globulin level along with all the other abnormalities documented is multiple myeloma.

3. Lytic bone lesions are a recognised feature of multiple myeloma. Patients would routinely undergo a 'skeletal survey' to identify bony pathology in this condition. The appearance is of a 'pepperpot' skull, with the main differentials being metastases and hyperparathyroidism.

IgG	27.2 g/l	High
IgA	0.5 g/l	Low
IgM	0.4 g/l	Low
Plasma protein electrophoresis: IgG paraprotein band approximately 25 g/l in size		Abnormal

4. The IgG level is highly elevated, and the levels of other immunoglobulins are suppressed. The particular type of myeloma in this patient is one in which abnormal plasma cells are producing massive quantities of IgG. This test confirms myeloma as the diagnosis.

   Although the blood calcium level is apparently normal, the cause of the polyuria documented is hypercalcaemia. Don't forget to correct calcium levels for abnormalities with serum albumin. As this patient's albumin level is 30 g/l, the 'corrected calcium' level is 2.84 mmol/l which is high (see page 13 for details).

CASE SUMMARY

Multiple myeloma
Hypercalcaemia

Answer 4.12

➥ case on page 444

FiO_2	0.40	Note that she is receiving supplemental oxygen
pH	7.28	Low
PaO_2	32.3 kPa	This would be expected given the FiO_2
$PaCO_2$	3.4 kPa	Low
HCO_3^-	14.7 mmol/l	Low

1. Oxygenation is adequate given that the patient is breathing 40% oxygen. The pH is low in keeping with an acidosis. The bicarbonate and carbon dioxide levels are also low, so the patient has a metabolic acidosis with respiratory compensation. It would be helpful to perform a U+E profile, so that the anion gap can be calculated. Given the clinical scenario, however, a raised anion gap acidosis would be expected. You should also measure paracetamol concentrations, because, although the patient denies taking paracetamol, its level should generally be measured in all patients presenting after an overdose (as the treatment of paracetamol toxicity is simple, and not treating could have catastrophic consequences).

Na^+	142 mmol/l	
K^+	3.8 mmol/l	
Urea	4.6 mmol/l	
Creatinine	55 μmol/l	
Cl^-	95 mmol/l	
HCO_3^-	15 mmol/l	Low
Glucose	5.2 mmol/l	
Total bilirubin	10 μmol/l	
ALP	62 U/l	
AST	22 U/l	
ALT	31 U/l	
GGT	132 U/l	High
Paracetamol	45 mg/l	High
Salicylate	<20 mmol/l	
Alcohol	126 mmol/l	High

2. The bicarbonate is low in keeping with the known metabolic acidosis. The anion gap is 35.8 mmol/l which is raised. Please note that the list of causes for acid-base abnormalities listed in Chapter 1 is not exhaustive. The GGT is high, and this is often the case in patients who have consumed alcohol recently. The patient has taken some paracetamol as the blood level was 45. It would be important to consult the paracetamol overdose

nomogram to check if treatment is required. Given that the blood sample was drawn at 5 hours post-ingestion, we can be confident that treatment for paracetamol poisoning is not required in this case. Her blood alcohol level is reasonably high, indicating that she has recently consumed alcohol.

3. The major abnormality with the ECG is the broadening of the QRS complexes. Taken in the context of a patient who has ingested an antidepressant and has a metabolic acidosis, we can be fairly certain that she has taken a tricyclic antidepressant. Given the ECG abnormalities, she is at high risk of cardiac arrhythmia and/or seizures. She should be placed on a cardiac monitor and intravenous sodium bicarbonate administered to correct the cardiac arrhythmia and the acidosis.

4. You should instantly recognise this rhythm tracing as ventricular tachycardia. On occasion, this rhythm can generate sufficient cardiac output such that a pulse is felt. In this case, no pulse can be felt and the patient is in cardiac arrest. The cardiac arrest treatment algorithm should be started without delay (treatment details outside the scope of this text). As this rhythm often responds to defibrillation, this should be a treatment priority. Sodium bicarbonate should also be administered to the patient.

CASE SUMMARY
Tricyclic antidepressant overdose Ventricular tachycardia

Answer 4.13

➥ case on page 445

Na^+	139 mmol/l	
K^+	3.7 mmol/l	
Urea	5.1 mmol/l	
Creatinine	52 µmol/l	
Cl^-	105 mmol/l	
HCO_3^-	25 mmol/l	
Paracetamol	160 mg/l	Abnormal
Alcohol	25 mmol/l	Abnormal
Salicylates	Nil	
Bilirubin	12 µmol/l	
AST	78 U/l	High
ALT	65 U/l	High
GGT	99 U/l	High
ALP	67 U/l	
Albumin	39 g/l	
Prothrombin time (PT)	18.7 s	
APTT	35.4 s	Prolonged
Fibrinogen	6.7 g/l	

1. The following should have been interpreted from the data provided in this scenario.

   This woman has probably taken a substantial overdose of paracetamol in combination with alcohol.

   The level of 160 mg/l is 6.5 hours after ingestion. The significance of this is seen overleaf on the paracetamol nomogram. 160 mg/l is well above this line.

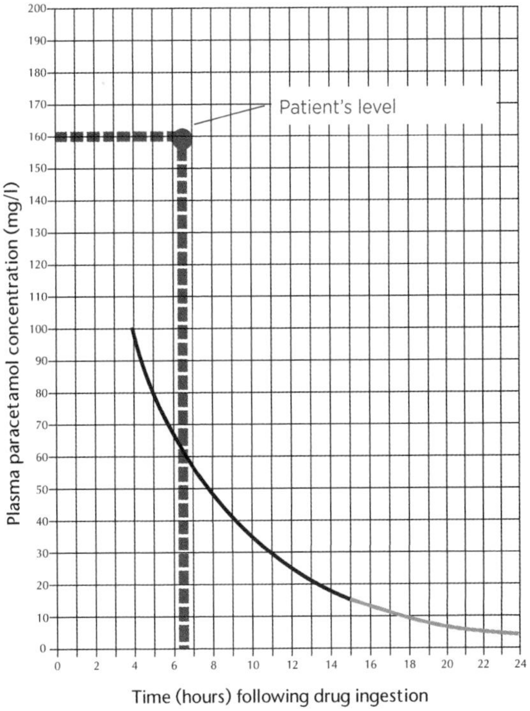

2. The patient should be treated with an intravenous infusion of *N*-acetylcysteine. The exact dose depends on the weight of the patient.

Falling trend

Time (hours)	Bilirubin (μmol/l)	AST (U/l)	ALT (U/l)	ALP (U/l)	GGT (U/l)	Albumin (g/l)	PT (s)
4	13	44	56	65	64	42	16.05
12	15	44	56	65	64	41	17.05
20	16	8001	7056	55	64	39	17.15
28	16	9977	10 230	75	54	38	18.55
36	19	12 333	11 156	65	61	34	19.05
44	23	12 993	12 333	64	62	32	21.05
52	27	13 144	12 456	75	73	28	21.44
56	29	13 111	12 346	77	74	24	24.05
60	36	13 244	12 153	85	77	22	30.05

Rising trend

This chart shows the changes in liver function over the 2–3 days following overdose. A huge surge in transaminases is seen from 20 hours indicating substantial hepatocellular damage from the toxic effects of paracetamol. Hepatic necrosis is taking place and the liver is failing. This can be seen because the prothrombin time is rising and the albumin is falling, as the ability of the liver to synthesise protein is diminishing. A liver transplantation should be considered.

3. Her transfer to a regional centre was to facilitate liver transplantation. Five days after her operation her chest X-ray, sputum analysis and ABG indicate that she had developed a postoperative pneumonia.

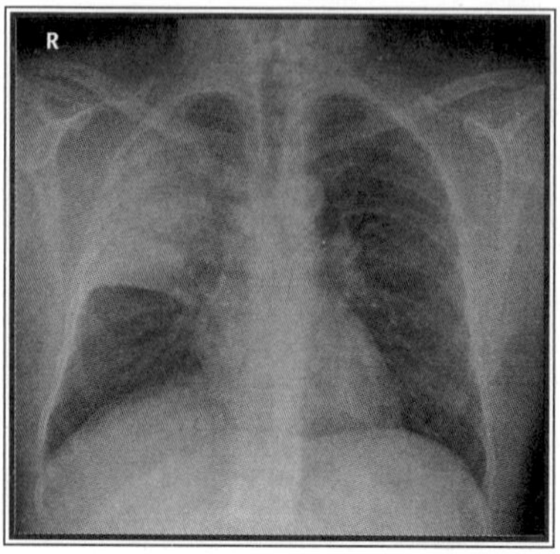

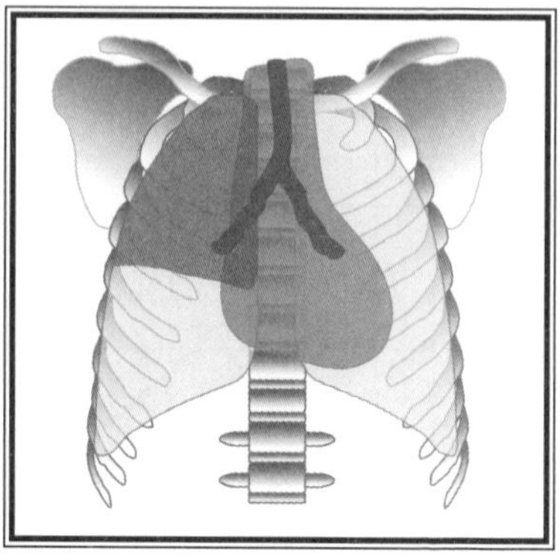

Chest X-ray report

This is a PA chest radiograph. It is the second in a series of postoperative films on this patient. The patient is 18 years of age and is an inpatient on the liver unit. The technical quality of the film is sound. The most obvious abnormality on this film is an area of increased radio-opacity in the right upper lobe. These findings are in keeping with consolidation. The remainder of the film is normal. These findings are in keeping with a right upper lobe pneumonia.

FiO_2	0.21	
pH	7.35	
PaO_2	5.2 kPa	Low
$PaCO_2$	4.3 kPa	
HCO_3^-	24.8 mmol/l	
BE	-4.2 mmol/l	

4. The arterial blood gas shows a marked hypoxia with a normal pH.

   She has type 1 respiratory failure, caused by pneumonia.

   From the sputum analysis a specific causative organism has been identified - *Streptococcus pneumoniae*. It must be emphasised that culturing takes time. Treatment should be instigated with empirical therapy, and altered later, if necessary, on the basis of the growth and sensitivities.

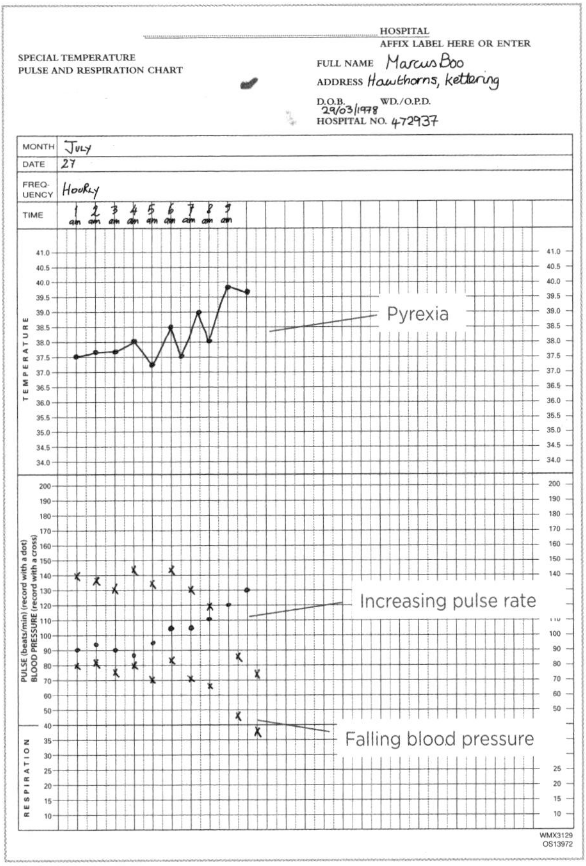

5. The bedside chart shows three key findings:

   1. Pyrexia
   2. Hypotension
   3. Tachycardia.

   In the context of an established pneumonia this may be in keeping with septic shock.

CASE SUMMARY

Paracetamol overdose requiring treatment
Development of hepatic failure requiring liver transplantation
Postoperative type 1 respiratory failure due to pneumonia
Development of septic shock

Answer 4.14

➥ case on page 448

1. The patient's respiratory rate is increased. Your first thought might be that the patient has a primary problem with breathing, and indeed this could be the case. A basal pneumonia, for example, can present with abdominal discomfort. However, there are many reasons for tachypnoea outside the chest, eg patients breathe faster when they are in pain or if they have a metabolic acidosis (to facilitate respiratory compensation). As a result of the wide range of problems that can manifest with an increased respiratory rate, this sign is often regarded as the most sensitive parameter that something serious is wrong with a patient.

   The patient's blood pressure is low. Again this could be due to a wide variety of reasons. Commonly, blood pressure falls with blood loss, sepsis and dehydration. Bearing in mind the abdominal pain, sensible suggestions would include a bleeding peptic ulcer, appendicitis, ischaemic bowel and colitis.

   Taking abdominal pain in context with tachypnoea and hypotension, the range of possible diagnoses remains wide and further tests are required.

Hb	132 g/l	
MCV	84 fl	
WCC	7.6 x 10^9/l	
Platelets	368 x 10^9/l	
Na^+	142 mmol/l	
K^+	3.9 mmol/l	
Urea	6.2 mmol/l	
Creatinine	46 μmol/l	
Cl^-	94 mmol/l	
HCO_3^-	8 mmol/l	Low
Amylase	52 U/l	

2. The major abnormality is the very low bicarbonate level. This is highly suggestive of a metabolic acidosis, although a measure of pH and $PaCO_2$ would be required to be certain.

   The normal haemoglobin is reassuring in terms of the fact that major blood loss would seem less likely. It should be borne in mind, however, that, after an acute bleed, it takes some time before the haemoglobin concentration falls - bleeding cannot therefore be ruled out using this test alone. The normal white cell count makes an infective cause less likely. The normal amylase level makes acute pancreatitis less likely, although sometimes the level can rise after a few hours, so if there is suspicion of pancreatitis, the level should be repeated.

FiO_2	0.21	
pH	7.21	Low
PaO_2	12.5 kPa	
$PaCO_2$	2.9 kPa	Low
HCO_3^-	7.6 mmol/l	Low

3. The blood gas analysis shows first that oxygenation is adequate. There is a metabolic acidosis present with respiratory compensation. You should then proceed to calculate the anion gap based on information presented earlier in the case. This is calculated as (142 + 3.9) - (94 + 7.6) = 44.3 mmol/l, and is therefore markedly raised. Note that it would also be reasonable to use the bicarbonate level from the initial set of blood tests for your calculation, although it is good practice always to use the most up-to-date results when making impressions about a patient's current state. Please refer to page 27 for a list of causes of this pH abnormality. Tests that would be useful at this stage could include; blood glucose, urinary glucose, blood ketones, urinary ketones, blood lactate and blood salicylate level if there is any suggestion of poisoning.

Glucose	++++	Abnormal
Bilirubin	Neg	
Ketones	++++	Abnormal
Specific gravity	1.005	
Blood	Neg	
Protein	Neg	
Nitrite	Neg	
Leukocytes	Neg	

4. The presence of significant quantities of glucose and ketones on urinalysis, taken in the context of an increased anion gap metabolic acidosis, is highly suggestive of diabetic ketoacidosis (DKA). This is recognised as an uncommon cause of abdominal pain and should always be borne in mind because it can be easily missed. The diagnosis should be confirmed by measuring blood glucose and ketone levels.

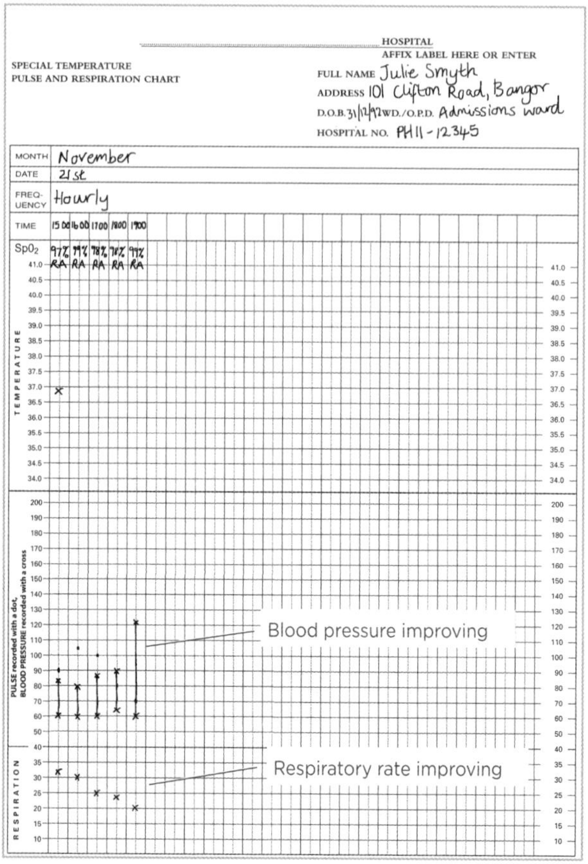

Time	Glucose (mmol/l)	Ketones (mmol/l)
1500	28.2	7.2
1600	26.3	6.1
1700	19.5	4.9
1800	12.7	4.1
1900	8.6	2.8

Glucose and ketone levels falling

5. The upper chart shows an improving respiratory rate and blood pressure. This is good evidence that the patient is improving. The administration of fluid and insulin to a patient with DKA is life saving and can result in a dramatic improvement in condition. The falling blood ketone level is more important than the normalisation of glucose levels. It would be important to see that the patient's acid-base status is normalising as a result of the treatment that you are giving.

An important point to note is that there is often a precipitating factor for DKA. Sometimes, as in this case, DKA can represent the first presentation of type 1 diabetes. More commonly, in patients with known diabetes, DKA results from missing insulin doses or an infection. In a case such as this one, you should be very vigilant not to miss an underlying intra-abdominal precipitant for the DKA (eg appendicitis).

Repeat blood tests show the following:

Na^+	142 mmol/l	
K^+	2.4 mmol/l	Low
Urea	6.2 mmol/l	
Creatinine	46 μmol/l	
Cl^-	94 mmol/l	
HCO^{3-}	12 mmol/l	
FiO_2	0.21	
pH	7.30	Low, but improved from before
PaO_2	12.7 kPa	
$PaCO_2$	3.4 kPa	Low, but normalising
HCO_3^-	12.5 mmol/l	Low, but mormalisiing

6. The patient's potassium level has fallen to an extremely low level due to the insulin given to treat the DKA. This could result in a cardiac arrhythmia. The patient should have a 12-lead ECG recorded to look for evidence of hypokalaemia, and should be connected to a bedside cardiac monitor. The patient should then receive an intravenous infusion of potassium.

   The patient still has a high anion gap metabolic acidosis, but this is improving as the DKA is treated. This would be expected to normalise entirely when the ketone level is back to normal and the patient has received sufficient fluid replacement. If it does not, another concomitant cause for the acidosis should be sought.

CASE SUMMARY

Wide anion gap metabolic acidosis due to diabetic ketoacidosis
Hypokalaemia due to insulin treatment

Answer 4.15

➥ case on page 451

1. Ninety-six per cent of blood pressure readings were successful, meaning that the study is valid and its results meaningful. The average daytime pressure was 162/88 mmHg, which is in keeping with significant hypertension. The other major finding on the report is that the patient's blood pressure rises at night. This is abnormal. Assuming that the patient had a good night's sleep on the night of the study and that he does not have obstructive sleep apnoea, this is a worrying finding. 'Reverse dipping' of blood pressure at night increases the chances of finding a secondary cause for the hypertension.

Na^+	144 mmol/l	
K^+	3.3 mmol/l	Low
Urea	4.3 mmol/l	
Creatinine	46 µmol/l	
Cl^-	93 mmol/l	
HCO_3^-	25 mmol/l	
Glucose	7.2 mmol/l	Not normal, but unsure when last food was eaten
Total cholesterol	5.2 mmol/l	
HDL-cholesterol	0.9 mmol/l	Unfavourable lipid profile with low HDL and high LDL
LDL-cholesterol	4.1 mmol/l	
Cholesterol:HDL ratio	5.78	
Urinary albumin:creatinine ratio	67	High

2. A chest X-ray in a patient with hypertension can potentially show evidence of an underlying cause such as coarctation of the aorta, in the form of rib notching. However, more commonly it identifies established cardiac consequences such as cardiomegaly or signs of cardiac failure. The absence of cardiomegaly on a chest X-ray does not rule out the possibility of left ventricular hypertrophy (LVH). The ECG has findings in keeping with LVH. The ECG is, however, only really a screening test for LVH, and echocardiography is necessary to establish its presence with certainty. LVH is confirmed on the echocardiogram. This signifies evidence of target organ damage from hypertension and suggests that measures should be taken to lower the pressure as soon as possible. The ultrasound study was normal, but might have shown findings such as a renal tumour, echobright kidneys (common in 'medical' kidney disease) or abnormal Doppler tracings (associated with renal artery stenosis).

   The biochemistry results show mild hypokalaemia and a sodium concentration towards the upper end of the normal range. The hypokalaemia is particularly surprising as the patient is taking an ACE inhibitor, which would be expected to cause hyperkalaemia if anything. The finding of hypokalaemia in a patient with hypertension should raise suspicions of an underlying diagnosis of primary hyperaldosteronism.

The glucose level is on the high side, but we are not given any information explaining whether this is a fasting level. However, it is not in the 'normal' range, and further steps should be taken to clarify the patient's glycaemic status. The lipid profile is suboptimal for a patient at risk of cardiovascular disease.

The urinary albumin:creatinine ratio is a measure of protein excretion from the kidneys. The level seen in this patient is in the 'microalbuminuric' range. The level requires repeating to ensure that it is truly abnormal. Assuming that it is a true value, however, this would be further evidence of target organ damage - this time to the kidney.

3. The patient has impaired glucose tolerance because, although the fasting glucose level is normal, the level after glucose loading is between 7.8 and 11.0 mmol/l.

Plasma renin activity	0.3 ng/ml per h	Low
Aldosterone	24 ng/l	High
Aldosterone:renin ratio	80	High

4. The test was performed in a patient suspected of having primary hyperaldosteronism. In this condition, aldosterone levels will be high and, because of negative feedback, renin levels will be low. The suggested cut-off value for an abnormal ratio, as detailed on page 65, is 30. In this case, the hormone patterns are in keeping with primary hyperaldosteronism and the ratio is greatly increased.

   The patient should be investigated further by arranging a further test such as a saline suppression test. Imaging of his adrenal glands to search for a tumour (it could be a carcinoma or more likely an adenoma) should then be undertaken. Adrenal hyperplasia can also cause this hormone abnormality. A CT scan would be the first imaging modality used in most instances. MRI is largely reserved for adrenal lesion characterisation. Nuclear imaging can also be used, and adrenal vein hormone sampling may also be required.

CASE SUMMARY

Hypertension
Left ventricular hypertrophy
Impaired glucose tolerance
Primary hyperaldosteronism

Index